Case Studies in Hepatology

Case Studies in Hepatology

Editor: Idris Roberts

AMERICAN
MEDICAL PUBLISHERS
www.americanmedicalpublishers.com

AMERICAN
MEDICAL PUBLISHERS
www.americanmedicalpublishers.com

Cataloging-in-Publication Data

Case studies in hepatology / edited by Idris Roberts.
p. cm.
Includes bibliographical references and index.
ISBN 979-8-88740-603-9
1. Hepatology. 2. Gastroenterology. I. Roberts, Idris.
RC802 .H47 2023
616.33--dc23

American Medical Publishers,
41 Flatbush Avenue,
1st Floor, New York,
NY 11217, USA

ISBN 979-8-88740-603-9 (Hardback)

Contents

Preface

This book aims to highlight the current researches and provides a platform to further the scope of innovations in this area. This book is a product of the combined efforts of many researchers and scientists, after going through thorough studies and analysis from different parts of the world. The objective of this book is to provide the readers with the latest information of the field.

Hepatology is the branch of medicine that focuses on the study, diagnosis and treatment of diseases and disorders related to the liver, gallbladder, biliary tree and pancreas. The liver plays a crucial role in various metabolic processes and is responsible for producing bile, which helps in the breakdown and absorption of nutrients from food. Hepatology encompasses a wide range of liver-related medical conditions, such as viral hepatitis, alcoholic liver disease, fatty liver disease, cirrhosis, liver cancer, autoimmune liver diseases, genetic liver diseases, and liver transplantation. Treatment options in hepatology depend on the specific liver condition and its severity. Lifestyle modifications, including dietary changes and abstaining from the consumption of alcohol are often suggested for patients with liver diseases such as fatty liver disease or alcoholic liver disease. Antiviral medications are used for the management of chronic viral hepatitis, while immunosuppressive drugs may be used to treat autoimmune liver diseases. This book unfolds the innovative aspects of hepatology which will be crucial for the progress of this field in the future. It will serve as a reference to a broad spectrum of readers.

I would like to express my sincere thanks to the authors for their dedicated efforts in the completion of this book. I acknowledge the efforts of the publisher for providing constant support. Lastly, I would like to thank my family for their support in all academic endeavors.

Editor

1

Treatment-Resistant Hepatitis C Viral Infection: A Case Report and Literature Review

Victoria Green[1] **and Marina Roytman**[2]

[1]*Department of Internal Medicine, University of California, San Francisco, Fresno, CA, USA*
[2]*Department of Gastroenterology and Hepatology, University of California, San Francisco, Fresno, CA, USA*

Correspondence should be addressed to Victoria Green; victoria.green@ucsf.edu

Academic Editor: Haruki Komatsu

Hepatitis C virus (HCV) is an ongoing global public health threat affecting millions worldwide. Increasing recognition of its impact and recent advances towards HCV prevention and cure have provided incentive for the World Health Organization to call for global elimination by 2030. The goal of therapy is to achieve a sustained virologic response (SVR-12), defined as undetectable HCV-RNA within 12 weeks after treatment completion. In 2011, approval was given for the first direct-acting antiviral agents (DAAs). More recently, in 2013, more effective DAAs, with pan-genomic properties, have been introduced, and these regimens boast increasing rates of SVR. The ultimate goal is that the history of HCV ends with the pan-genotypic efficacy of multiple, easy-to-use and tolerate, combination regimens. These regimens have already demonstrated the ability to cure previously challenging patient groups. However, limitations exist in the current portfolio of agents, with suboptimal outcomes for patients with HCV genotype 3. In addition to this, access to DAAs remains an obstacle for many patients. We present this case of a 61-year-old male with HCV genotype 3 who has had several treatment failures with standard HCV therapy who was eventually approved for compassionate use of a 16-week course of glecaprevir (GLE)/pibrentasvir (PIB), sofosbuvir (SOF), and ribavirin (RBV) which ultimately led to SVR-12.

1. Introduction

Hepatitis C virus (HCV) is an ongoing global public health threat affecting millions worldwide [1]. Chronic HCV infection is one of the leading causes of liver-related death and one of the primary reasons for liver transplantation [2]. HCV transmission is most commonly associated with direct exposure to blood, via blood transfusions, unsafe health-care-related injections, and intravenous drug use [3]. Increasing recognition of its impact and recent advances towards HCV prevention and cure have provided incentive for the World Health Organization (WHO) to call for global elimination as a public health threat by 2030 [4]. This virus exhibits high genetic diversity, and within the six known genotypes, genotype 3 represents 22–30% of all infection and is distinctive as it is associated with higher rates of steatosis, accelerated fibrosis, and increased oncogenesis [5].

The goal of therapy is to achieve sustained virologic response (SVR), defined as undetectable HCV-RNA within 12 weeks after treatment completion, at which point the patient is considered cured. In 2011, approval was given for the first direct-acting antiviral agents (DAAs), boceprevir, and telaprevir, for treatment of genotype 1, in combination with interferon and ribavirin. More recently, in 2013, more effective DAAs, with pan-genomic properties, have been introduced, and these regimens boast increasing rates of SVR [2]. However, currently approved novel DAAs have not demonstrated the uniform potency seen in genotype 1 disease for genotype 3 [6]. Due to the distinctive characteristics of genotype 3, especially in patients with comorbid conditions, treatment often requires longer duration with decreased response rates. [7].

The ultimate goal is that the history of HCV ends with the pan-genotypic efficacy of multiple, easy-to-use and tolerate, combination regimens. These regimens have already demonstrated the ability to cure previously challenging patient groups, including human immunodeficiency virus-HCV coinfection, decompensated cirrhosis, and post-liver transplantation. However, limitations exist in the current portfolio of agents, with suboptimal outcomes for genotype 3 [8]. In addition to this, access to DAAs remains an obstacle for many patients. We present this case of treatment-resistant HCV GT3 for its contribution to the literature.

2. Case Summary

A 61-year-old man with a past medical history of chronic HCV leading to compensated cirrhosis and a subsequent diagnosis of non-Hodgkin's lymphoma (NHL) presented to the liver clinic for further evaluation and management. He likely contracted HCV in Vietnam from unregulated tattooing. He denies prior intravenous drug use or blood transfusion. The patient consumed 7–14 drinks a week up until a month prior to the presentation when he was advised to stop. He has a significant 30-pack-year smoking history and he continues to smoke half-pack of cigarettes daily. His family history is negative for liver disease or liver malignancies.

During the initial clinic visit, his vital signs were stable and he weighed 74.8 kg with a calculated body mass index of 23.68 kg/m^2. His physical examination was positive for massive hepatosplenomegaly, however negative for scleral icterus, jaundice, ascites, peripheral edema, or asterixis. Laboratory studies of significant included creatinine 0.8 mg/dl, sodium 136 mmol/L, total bilirubin 1.5 mg/dl, international normalized ratio (INR) 1.2, platelets 115 $10^3/\mu$L, aspartate transaminase 107 U/L, alanine transaminase 73 U/L, and alkaline phosphatase 53 U/L. At this time, a model for end-stage liver disease (MELD) of 10 and Child-Pugh A were documented (see Table 1 for evolution of lab results).

Imaging included an abdominal ultrasound and magnetic resonance imaging/magnetic resonance cholangiopancreatography with and without contrast, both performed in 2018 and a computed tomography of the abdomen with and without contrast in 2019, all of which were consistent with cirrhosis and did not reveal any evidence of obstruction or malignancy. Small amount of ascites was noted on the 2019 imaging. The patient reports that, before entering this healthcare system, he was previously treated for HCV twice. In both treatment attempts, the viral load was undetectable during treatment and re-emerged after the discontinuation of antiviral therapy prior to 12-week posttreatment mark. The HCV genotype was retested each time and had remained GT3 which makes reinfection less likely and this is also compounded by his lack of risk factors for re-infection at the time. In 2019, his HCV-RNA was initially 338,000/IU and he was treated with a combination of sofosbuvir (SOF) and velpatasvir (VEL) for a duration of 12 weeks without achieving SVR-12. Subsequently, a combination of sofosbuvir/velpatasvir/voxilaprevir (SOF/VEL/VOX) and ribavirin (RBV) for a duration of 12 weeks was attempted and again did not lead to SVR-12. The patient reports meticulous compliance with both rounds of treatment. In both treatment attempts, the viral load was undetectable during treatment and re-emerged after the discontinuation of antiviral therapy prior to 12 weeks posttreatment. He underwent NS5A resistance testing which documented S62A and Y93H mutations predictive of resistance to VEL and daclatasvir (DCV). A 16-week combination therapy of glecaprevir/pibrentasvir (GLE/PIB) with SOF and RBV led to SVR-12 (see discussion below for the rationale).

With respect to complications of advanced liver disease, he has never experienced jaundice, clinically significant ascites or spontaneous bacterial peritonitis, variceal hemorrhage, or hepatic encephalopathy. Screening upper endoscopy did not reveal varices. He was diagnosed with NHL in 2019, which was attributing to ongoing HCV viremia. He had completed rituximab, cyclophosphamide, doxorubicin, vincristine (oncovin), and prednisolone (R-CHOP) therapy prior to achieving SVR-12 and is currently free of cancer as per his latest positron emission tomography scan.

3. Discussion

Achieving SVR improves overall survival and reduces the risk of liver failure, fibrosis progression, liver transplantation, and the incidence of hepatocellular carcinoma (HCC) [9]. Genotype 3 HCV infection is the second most prevalent HCV infection. However, cure rates are lower in some patients with genotype 3 such as those with cirrhosis or prior treatment experience. This therapeutic challenge may be in part explained by its unique characteristics such as its association with insulin resistance and alterations in lipid metabolism [10]. This patient was initially treated with SOF and VEL, a combination which in the ASTRAL-3 study led to SVR12 in 88% of participants with baseline velpatasvir-specific resistance associated substitutions (RASs) compared with 97% in those without NS5a RASs [11]. The patient did not achieve SVR12 leading to concern about the presence of NS5A RASs. As a result of the lower SVR12 in treatment-experienced individuals with cirrhosis in the ASTRAL-3 study, the addition of RBV was recommended for those with both treatment experience and cirrhosis [12].

DAA regimens containing NS5A inhibitors are highly effective treatments for HCV infection, but they are not 100% successful. Of the major HCV antiviral drug classes, there is only compelling evidence for the impact of NS5A inhibitor RASs on treatment outcome. In the POLARIS-1 phase 3 study, SOF/VEL/VOX for 12 weeks was highly effective in obtaining SVR in patients previously treated with a DAA regimen containing an NS5A inhibitor [13]. This multiclass combination given for 12 weeks without RBV led to a cure in 96% of the HCV infected who had a prior NS5A treatment failure [13]. This combination of SOF/VEL/VOX plus RBV was the second regimen offered to our patient, but again, it did not result in SVR-12.

According to Wyles et al., when NS5A inhibitor-based treatment fails, NS5A RASs frequently emerge and the presence of cirrhosis and prior HCV treatment increases the clinical impact of NS5A RASs [14]. Following failed NS5A-based treatment, up to 90% of individuals have NS5A RASs and they persist in most individuals for several years [15, 16].

TABLE 1: The evolution of pertinent lab results: pretreatment, during treatment, and posttreatment.

Labs	Dates													
	Pretreatment							During treatment				Posttreatment		
	Apr-19	Aug-19	Dec-19	Jan-20	Jul-20	Sep-20	Jan-21	Feb-21	Mar-21	Apr-21	May-21	Jun-21	Aug-21	Sep-21
AST, U/L	107	47	72	87	108	94	93	109	81	49	44	70	49	51
ALT, U/L	73	27	44	51	64	55	48	66	50	36	31	43	28	30
ALP, U/L	53	53	57	78	81	80	112	99	83	77	83	84	96	108
Total bilirubin, mg/dL	1.5	1	1.0	1.1	1.9	1.5	1.2	1.2	2.3	2.6	2.8	1	1.3	1.3
PT/INR	1.2	1.2	NT	NT	NT	1.2	1.1	1.2	1.2	1.1	1.1	1.2	1.2	1.1
Platelets, $10^3/\mu L$	115	197	67	54	78	100	106	108	103	107	117	105	92	107
Albumin, g/dL	3.6	4.2	3.5	3.3	3.4	3.6	3.3	3.6	3.6	3.5	3.6	3.8	3.6	3.5
Creatinine, mg/dL	0.8	1.4	0.7	0.6	0.9	0.8	0.8	1.0	0.9	0.8	0.8	0.9	1.2	0.9
eGFR, mL/min/1.73 m^2	>90	62	52	>90	85	92	95	85	85	85	93	83	61	80
Sodium, mmol/L	136	137	136	135	135	134	134	135	136	135	138	135	136	136
HCV-RNA quant (IU)	338,000	NT	6,510,00	NT	1,550,000	NT	NT	NT	ND	ND	ND	ND	ND	ND

NT, not tested; ND, not detected.

Fortunately, the impact of NS5A RAS is relative and can often be overcome by increasing the length of therapy or by adding RBV [17]. NS5A resistance testing is recommended at the time of failure of NS5A inhibitor-based treatment. The NS5A RAS of most clinical importance in HCV genotype 3 is Y93H, which confers a high level of resistance to DVR and VEL [18, 19]. In the case of virologic failure following treatment exposure to an NS5A inhibitor, the Y93H RAS emerges in the majority of individuals [14]. Our patient underwent NS5A resistance mutation testing which documented S62A and Y93H. VEL has an improved resistance profile compared with early generation NS5A inhibitors, although the Y93H variant in HCV genotype 3 infection still confers a high level of resistance to VEL [20]. Notably, data on the impact of baseline NS5A RASs on the outcome of NS5A inhibitor-containing therapy are limited.

This patient's treatment course was complicated by the development of diffuse large B-cell lymphoma (DLBCL), the most common type of NHL. The association between HCV and NHL is well documented and supported by epidemiological studies [21]. The exact pathogenetic mechanism is still unknown, but several mechanisms of HCV-related lymphomagenesis have been postulated [22]. The optimal management of HCV-related NHL is unclear; however, antiviral treatment may be satisfactory for low grade or asymptomatic cases, while immunotherapy is warranted in high grade cases [23]. The R-CHOP regimen is the gold standard for DLBCL as it has been shown to improve the clinical outcomes and prognosis [24]. Clinically significant flares of HCV during immunosuppressive therapy remain exceedingly uncommon, our patient did not experience it. He tolerated treatment well and was found to be free of cancer according to his latest positron emission tomography scan report.

Options for retreatment after failure of an NS5A inhibitor-based regimen are challenging. Newer generation NS5A inhibitors such as PIB retain activity against all NS5A RASs and therefore may retain activity despite resistance to current NS5A inhibitors [25]. Tailoring retreatment based on results of NS5A and NS3 resistance testing is recommended. As such, NS3 resistance testing may be an explorable avenue for this patient. The combination of GLE/PIB is the first pan-genotypic NS3/4A protease inhibitor-NS5A inhibitor combination to be approved that offers a potent ribavirin-free option [26]. A 2020 study by Toyoda et al. showed that the 12-week GLE/PIB regimen showed high virologic efficacy in patients with cirrhosis, experience of DAA, or HCV genotype 3 [27]. The MAGELLAN-3 trial showed that the addition of SOF and RBV led to SVR in 95% of patients [7, 14]. We felt that a combination of GLE/PIB with SOF plus RBV would offer our patient the best chance of cure based on his prior treatment experience and resistance analysis.

This combination therapy (GLE/PIB/SOF/RBV) was repeatedly denied by the patient's insurance due to the experimental nature of it and due to the patient having reached a lifetime limit of HCV treatment. Our concern for liver disease progression as manifested by the development of radiologically detectable ascites as well as concern to recurrence of NHL in the setting of ongoing viremia led to a last-ditch effort to obtain this combination through an appeal for compassionate use directly from pharmaceutical companies. The Food and Drug Administration (FDA) allows companies to provide their drugs to patients under certain circumstances such as having a serious disease, or whose life is immediately threatened by their disease or there is no comparable or satisfactory alternative therapy to diagnose, monitor, or treat the disease, and this is referred to as "compassionate use." Gaining access to these drugs through a compassionate use request can be a long and challenging process. Most patients will respond to treatment with SOF/VEL according to the ASTRAL-3 study [4]. In the POLARIS-1 phase 3 study, 96% of patients who fail SOF/VEL will achieve SVR with SOF/VEL/VOX [5]. This patient failed to respond to both regimens potentially due to presence of Y93H, the most clinically important resistance associated substitution [6]. In addition to this, the development of NHL also contributed to his complicated course.

In November 2020, compassionate use with third round of treatment for HCV with a 16-week course of GLE/PIB 100–40 mg daily, SOF 400 mg daily, and weight-based RBV at 600 mg twice daily was approved. The patient commenced therapy in January 2021 and continued to undergo close monitoring of liver enzymes, liver function tests, renal function tests, complete blood count, and HCV RNA every 2 weeks. The patient tolerated his 16-week treatment well with the only side effect endorsed being insomnia. August 2021 marked 12 weeks after the completion of treatment at which point his HCV RNA remained undetectable and he was considered cured. Reemergence of the virus after SVR-12 is extremely uncommon. According to Lin et al., PPV and NPV of SVR-12 predicting SVR-24 were 99.9% and 100%, respectively [28]. Retesting of HCV-RNA is generally driven by an unexplained rise in liver enzymes or high-risk behaviors. Neither of these situations is the case for the patient described in this case report. However given the rarity of this case, HCV-RNA will be retested at the SVR-24 time point.

The road to SVR for our patient was a difficult one, with several treatment failures and insurance obstacles. We remain hopeful for newer advancements that may benefit patients in this and similar predicaments.

The emergence of DAAs has made treatment effective and safe; however, treatment is costly and often inaccessible. Combining drugs from different classes produced by different pharmaceutical companies creates added barriers. In particular, individuals with HCV genotype 3 infection in whom NS5A inhibitor-based treatment has failed remain a population for whom we should increase our efforts to understand the virology and pathogenesis of, aiming at enhanced and more potent genotype-targeted treatments.

References

[1] N. J. Burstow, Z. Mohamed, A. Gomaa I et al., "Hepatitis C treatment: where are we now?" *International Journal of General Medicine*, vol. 10, pp. 39–52, 2017.

[2] R. González-Grande, M. Jiménez-Pérez, C. González Arjona, and J. Mostazo Torres, "New approaches in the treatment of hepatitis C," *World Journal of Gastroenterology*, vol. 22, no. 4, pp. 1421–1432, 2016.

[3] F. Roudot-Thoraval, "Epidemiology of hepatitis C virus infection," *Clinics and Research in Hepatology and Gastroenterology*, vol. 45, no. 3, Article ID 101596, 2021.

[4] H. Razavi, S. Robbins, S. Zeuzem et al., "Hepatitis C virus prevalence and level of intervention required to achieve the WHO targets for elimination in the European Union by 2030: a modelling study," *The Lancet Gastroenterology & Hepatology*, vol. 2, no. 5, pp. 325–336, 2017.

[5] A. Chan, K. Patel, and S. Naggie, "Genotype 3 infection: the last stand of hepatitis C virus," *Drugs*, vol. 77, no. 2, pp. 131–144, 2017.

[6] S. Kattakuzhy, R. Levy, E. Rosenthal, L. Tang, E. Wilson, and S. Kottilil, "Hepatitis C genotype 3 disease," *Hepatology International*, vol. 10, no. 6, pp. 861–870, 2016.

[7] H. Maddur and S. L. Flamm, "Hepatitis C genotype 3 infection," *Clinics in Liver Disease*, vol. 21, no. 4, pp. 645–657, 2017.

[8] A. J. Muir and S. Naggie, "Hepatitis C virus treatment: is it possible to cure all hepatitis C virus patients?" *Clinical Gastroenterology and Hepatology*, vol. 13, no. 12, pp. 2166–2172, 2015.

[9] S. K. Na and B.-C. Song, "Development and surveillance of hepatocellular carcinoma in patients with sustained virologic response after antiviral therapy for chronic hepatitis C," *Clinical and Molecular Hepatology*, vol. 25, no. 3, pp. 234–244, 2019.

[10] S. K. Bose and R. Ray, "Hepatitis C virus infection and insulin resistance," *World Journal of Diabetes*, vol. 5, no. 1, pp. 52–58, 2014.

[11] A. Bonaventura and F. Montecucco, "Sofosbuvir/velpatasvir: a promising combination," *World Journal of Hepatology*, vol. 8, no. 19, pp. 785–789, 2016.

[12] AASLD/IDSA, "HCV guidance: recommendations for testing, managing, and treating hepatitis C," 2017, http://hcvguidelines.org/.

[13] M. Bourlière, S. C. Gordon, S. L. Flamm et al., "Sofosbuvir, velpatasvir, and voxilaprevir for previously treated HCV infection," *New England Journal of Medicine*, vol. 376, no. 22, pp. 2134–2146, 2017.

[14] D. L. Wyles, O. Weiland, B. Yao et al., "Retreatment of hepatitis C infection in patients who failed glecaprevir/pibrentasvir," *Journal of Hepatology*, vol. 70, 2018.

[15] F. Lahser, A. Galloway, P. Hwang et al., "Interim analysis of a 3-year follow-up study of NS5A and NS3 resistance-associated variants (RAVs) after treatment with grazoprevir-containing regimens in patients with chronic hepatitis C virus (HCV) infection," *Hepatology*, vol. 64, no. suppl 1, 32A pages, 2016.

[16] P. Krishnan, R. Tripathi, G. Schnell et al., "0057: long-term follow-up of treatment-emergent resistance-associated variants in NS3, 0S5A and NS5B with paritaprevir/r-, ombitasvir- and dasabuvir-based regimens," *Journal of Hepatology*, vol. 62, no. suppl 2, S220 pages, 2015.

[17] C. Sarrazin, H. Dvory-Sobol, E. S. Svarovskaia et al., "Prevalence of resistance-associated substitutions in HCV NS5A, NS5B, or NS3 and outcomes of treatment with ledipasvir and sofosbuvir," *Gastroenterology*, vol. 151, no. 3, pp. 501–512, 2016.

[18] C. Hézode, S. Chevaliez, G. Scoazec et al., "Retreatment with sofosbuvir and simeprevir of patients with hepatitis C virus genotype 1 or 4 who previously failed a daclatasvir-containing regimen," *Hepatology*, vol. 63, no. 6, pp. 1809–1816, 2016.

[19] C. Wang, L. Jia, D. R. O'Boyle et al., "Comparison of daclatasvir resistance barriers on NS5A from hepatitis C virus genotypes 1 to 6: implications for cross-genotype activity," *Antimicrobial Agents and Chemotherapy*, vol. 58, no. 9, pp. 5155–5163, 2014.

[20] C. Hezode, N. Reau, E. S. Svarovskaia et al., "Resistance analysis in 1284 patients with genotype 1 to 6 HCV infection treated with sofosbuvir/velpatasvir in the phase 3 ASTRAL-1, ASTRAL-2, ASTRAL-3 and ASTRAL-4 studies," in *Proceedings of the International Liver Congress*, Barcelona, Spain, April 2016.
[21] D. S. Viswanatha and A. Dogan, "Hepatitis C virus and lymphoma," *Journal of Clinical Pathology*, vol. 60, no. 12, pp. 1378–1383, 2007.
[22] H. Khaled, F. Abu-Taleb, and R. Haggag, "Hepatitis C virus and non-Hodgkin's lymphomas: a minireview," *Journal of Advanced Research*, vol. 8, no. 2, pp. 131–137, 2017.
[23] S. Paydas, "Hepatitis C virus and lymphoma," *Critical Reviews In Oncology-Hematology*, vol. 93, no. 3, pp. 246–256, 2015.
[24] T. M. Habermann, E. A. Weller, V. A. Morrison et al., "Rituximab-CHOP versus CHOP alone or with maintenance rituximab in older patients with diffuse large B-cell lymphoma," *Journal of Clinical Oncology*, vol. 24, no. 19, pp. 3121–3127, 2006.
[25] T. Ng, P. Krishnan, and W. Kati, "ABT-530 an HCV NS5A inhibitor with potent pangenotypic activity and high barrier to resistance," in *Proceedings of the 21st Conference on Retroviruses and Opportunistic Infections (CROI)*, Boston, Massachusetts, March 2014.
[26] T. G. Cotter and D. M. Jensen, "Glecaprevir/pibrentasvir for the treatment of chronic hepatitis C: design, development, and place in therapy," *Drug Design, Development and Therapy*, vol. 13, pp. 2565–2577, 2019.
[27] H. Toyoda, M. Atsukawa, T. Watanabe et al., "Real-world experience of 12-week direct-acting antiviral regimen of glecaprevir and pibrentasvir in patients with chronic hepatitis C virus infection," *Journal of Gastroenterology and Hepatology*, vol. 35, no. 5, pp. 855–861, 2020.
[28] C.-P. Lin, P.-C. Liang, C.-I. Huang et al., "Concordance of SVR12, SVR24 and SVR durability in Taiwanese chronic hepatitis C patients with direct-acting antivirals," *PLoS One*, vol. 16, no. 2, Article ID e0245479, 2021.

2

Possible Paternal Hepatitis B Virus Infection with Different Clinical Courses between Siblings: A Report of Two Cases

Yoshiaki Sasaki and Hiroki Kajino

Department of Pediatrics, Abashiri-Kosei General Hospital, Abashiri, Hokkaido, Japan

Correspondence should be addressed to Yoshiaki Sasaki; cct33370@syd.odn.ne.jp

Academic Editor: Fumio Imazeki

The incidence of hepatitis B virus (HBV) infection is expected to decrease in the future owing to the preventive measures adopted against mother-to-child transmission of HBV and implementation of universal HBV vaccination for children. However, no countermeasure has been established against horizontal infection in nonvaccinated children. We report the case of two siblings who had different clinical courses of possible paternal HBV infection. The younger sibling developed acute hepatitis, whereas the older sibling was an asymptomatic HBV carrier. To eradicate HBV, HBV vaccination of all children and HBV infection screening of fathers and other family members should be encouraged.

1. Introduction

The incidence of hepatitis B virus (HBV) infection is expected to reduce in the future with the implementation of prevention projects against mother-to-child transmission of HBV and universal HBV vaccination [1]. In addition, the development of antiviral drugs for HBV has contributed to the reduction in the infection rate [1]. However, to date, no countermeasure has been established against horizontal infection, such as paternal infection of HBV in nonvaccinated children. Here, we report a case of possible paternal HBV infection that resulted in different clinical courses of HBV infection between siblings.

2. Case Presentation

2.1. Case 1. A 1-year and 4-month-old girl, with an unremarkable birth and medical history presented with vomiting of 3 days and diarrhea of 2 days before being admitted to our hospital with a diagnosis of acute rotavirus gastroenteritis. Her laboratory findings on admission showed severe liver dysfunction, with an alanine aminotransferase (ALT) level of 583 U/L and aspartate aminotransferase (AST) level of 406 U/L. Simultaneously, the tests for hepatitis B surface antigen (HBsAg) and immunoglobulin *M* antibody to hepatitis B core antigen were positive. Therefore, she was diagnosed with acute hepatitis B. She had not been vaccinated against HBV. With conservative treatment, such as rest and hydration, her symptoms improved without a fulminant course. She was discharged on the 10th day of admission. Three months afterwards, her test results revealed seroconversion of HBeAg/HBeAb. Eventually, at 8 years of age, she was declared HBsAg-negative, and virological remission was achieved (Table 1).

2.2. Case 2. The second patient, a 2-year-7-month-old girl, was the older sibling of the first patient. She was born with a low birth weight of 2,272 g and had no remarkable medical history. She was not vaccinated against HBV. Although she had no symptoms when the first patient was diagnosed with acute hepatitis B, her laboratory findings revealed mild liver dysfunction, with an ALT level of 87 U/L and an AST level of 79 U/L. She was HBsAg-positive, hepatitis B envelope antigen (HBeAg)-positive, and hepatitis B envelope antibody-negative. Her HBV DNA (PCR) was high (>8.2 log IU/L), and the HBV genotype was type B. Simultaneously, she was diagnosed as being an HBV carrier. Subsequently, she was

Table 1: Laboratory results of the first patient.

	HBsAg	Anti-HBs	IgM anti-HBc	HBeAg	Anti-HBe	HBV DNA (log IU/L)	ALT (IU/L)	AST (IU/L)
Age	–	–	–	–	–	–	–	–
1 year and 4 months	Positive	Negative	Positive	Positive	Negative	>8.2	583	406
1 year and 7 months	–	–	Negative	Negative	Positive	N.D.	11	29
8 years and 0 month	Negative	Positive	–	–	–	N.D.	13	25

HBsAg, hepatitis B surface antigen; Anti-HBs, antihepatitis B surface antibody; IgM anti-HBc, immunoglobulin M antibody to hepatitis B core antigen; HBeAg, hepatitis B envelope antigen; Anti-HBe, antihepatitis B envelope antibody; HBV DNA, hepatitis B virus-deoxyribonucleic acid; ALT, alanine aminotransferase; AST, aspartate aminotransferase; –, no result available; N.D, not detected.

Table 2: Laboratory results of the second patient.

	HBsAg	Anti-HBs	IgM anti-HBc	HBeAg	Anti-HBe	HBV DNA (log IU/L)	ALT (IU/L)	AST (IU/L)
Age	–	–	–	–	–	–	–	–
2 years and 7 months	Positive	Negative	Negative	Positive	Negative	>8.2	87	79
3 years and 10 months	–	–	Negative	Negative	Positive	N.D.	44	55
15 years and 10 months	Positive	Negative	Negative	Negative	Positive	3.27	10	17

HBsAg, hepatitis B surface antigen; Anti-HBs, antihepatitis B surface antibody; IgM anti-HBc, immunoglobulin M antibody to hepatitis B core antigen; HBeAg, hepatitis B envelope antigen; Anti-HBe, antihepatitis B envelope antibody; HBV DNA, hepatitis B virus-deoxyribonucleic acid; ALT, alanine aminotransferase; AST, aspartate aminotransferase; –, no result available; N.D, not detected.

followed up for inactive chronic hepatitis, and seroconversion of HBeAg/HBeAb was detected at the age of 3 years and 8 months (Table 2). To date, she is being followed up at an outpatient clinic as an inactive carrier of HBV. When the first patient developed acute hepatitis, her father was HBeAg-positive, whereas her mother was HBsAg-negative and antihepatitis B surface antibody-positive. Therefore, the HBV infection was considered to have been transmitted to the siblings from their father who was an asymptomatic HBV carrier; however, the actual source of the infection was unknown.

3. Discussion

In this report, we observed different clinical courses of horizontal HBV infection in siblings, transmitted from their father possibly. HBV is detected not only in blood but also in urine, saliva, nasopharynx, and tears, which may be sources of infection [2]. Therefore, the risk of HBV horizontal infection in daily life exists. In the literature, the prevalence of HBsAg carriage among children of 1 year or older has been reported to be higher than that among those aged <1 year [3]. This pattern of age distribution suggests that horizontal infection is an important route of HBV infection during early childhood [3]. Vaccine failure leading to mother-to-child infection is the major cause of chronic HBV infection in Japanese children, with paternal infection being the second most common mode of transmission [4]. Although the incidence of paternal infection has been reported to be lower than that of mother-to-child infection, 19.2% of HBeAg-positive fathers have been reported to transmit HBV infection to their children [5]. In our report, the HBV genotype of the siblings' father was not examined, but we diagnosed that the route of HBV transmission of the siblings was paternal, as no other HBV-infected person, except their father, was detected as a possible contact. Infants are susceptible to chronic persistent HBV infection owing to poor cytotoxic T cell (CTL) response [6]. Therefore, the CTL response of the second patient might have been weaker than that of her sibling. In addition, genetic variants in the HLA-DP locus, including HLA-DPA1 and HLA-DPB1, are associated with the chronicity of hepatitis B in literature [7]. Therefore, the second patient may have genetic variants in the HLA-DP gene.

To prevent mother-to-child HBV infection, HBV screening and preventive measures for pregnant women have been developed. However, HBV screening of fathers and other family members is necessary to prevent horizontal infection [8]. The World Health Organization recommends universal vaccination to eradicate HBV [1]. Despite routine immunization of infants with the HBV vaccine being initiated in 2016 in Japan, many children remain unvaccinated. Therefore, we must remember that many children do not benefit from the HBV vaccine program at this time, especially those who are not within their routine vaccination age.

In conclusion, we reported cases of possible paternal HBV infection that resulted in varying clinical presentations of HBV infection in the offspring. Our findings suggest that we should encourage HBV vaccination of all children and screening of HBV infection for all family members, including fathers. These measures are expected to minimize horizontal infection of HBV.

References

[1] World Health Organization, *Guidelines for the Prevention, Care and Treatment of Persons with Chronic Hepatitis B Infection*, World Health Organization, Geneva, Switzerland, 2015, https://www.who.int/hepatitis/publications/hepatitis-b-guidelines/en/.

[2] K. Kidd-Ljunggren, A. Holmberg, J. Bläckberg, and B. Lindqvist, "High levels of hepatitis B virus DNA in body fluids from chronic carriers," *Journal of Hospital Infection*, vol. 64, no. 4, pp. 352–357, 2006.

[3] G. B. Yao, "Importance of perinatal versus horizontal transmission of hepatitis B virus infection in China," *Gut*, vol. 38, no. Suppl 2, pp. S39–S42, 1996.

[4] H. Komatsu, A. Inui, T. Sogo, E. Hiejima, N. Kudo, and T. Fujisawa, "Source of transmission in children with chronic hepatitis B infection after the implementation of a strategy for prevention in those at high risk," *Hepatology Research*, vol. 39, no. 6, pp. 569–576, 2009.

[5] H.-W. L. Hann, R. S. Hann, and W. C. Maddrey, "Hepatitis B virus infection in 6,130 unvaccinated Korean-Americans surveyed between 1988 and 1990," *American Journal of Gastroenterology*, vol. 102, no. 4, pp. 767–772, 2007.

[6] B. Rehermann, K. M. Chang, J. McHutchinson et al., "Differential cytotoxic T-lymphocyte responsiveness to the hepatitis B and C viruses in chronically infected patients," *Journal of Virology*, vol. 70, no. 10, pp. 7092–7102, 1996.

[7] Y. Kamatani, S. Wattanapokayakit, H. Ochi et al., "A genome-wide association study identifies variants in the HLA-DP locus associated with chronic hepatitis B in Asians," *Nature Genetics*, vol. 41, no. 5, pp. 591–595, 2009.

[8] M. Bhat, P. Ghali, M. Deschenes, and P. Wong, "Prevention and management of chronic hepatitis B," *International Journal of Preventive Medicine*, vol. 5, pp. S200–7, 2014.

3

Cytomegalovirus Cholangiopathy in an Immunocompetent Patient: A Case Report and Literature Review

Ervin Alibegovic,[1,2] Admir Kurtcehajic,[2,3] Boris Ilic,[3] Ahmed Hujdurovic,[3] Edinka Smajic,[4] Amar Habibovic,[1] and Darja Perkunic[5]

[1] *Department of Gastroenterology and Hepatology, University Clinical Center Tuzla, Tuzla 75000, Bosnia and Herzegovina*
[2] *Medical Faculty, University of Tuzla, Tuzla 75000, Bosnia and Herzegovina*
[3] *Department of Internal Medicine, Medical Center "Plava Poliklinika", Plava Medical Group, Tuzla 75000, Bosnia and Herzegovina*
[4] *Department of Radiology, Medical Center "Plava Poliklinika", Plava Medical Group, Tuzla 75000, Bosnia and Herzegovina*
[5] *Department of Biochemistry, Medical Center "Plava Poliklinika", Plava Medical Group, Tuzla 75000, Bosnia and Herzegovina*

Correspondence should be addressed to Admir Kurtcehajic; admircg7@gmail.com

Academic Editor: Emilia Hadziyannis

A 37-year-old man presented with jaundice, upper right quadrant pain, and intermittent fever with chills. Laboratory assessment showed biliary stasis, with total bilirubin of 203 μmol/L (2–20), conjugated bilirubin of 105 μmol/L, and alkaline phosphatase of 556 U/L (30–120). Markers for hepatitis A–E viruses were negative. Serology assessment for rubeola, herpes simplex virus, Epstein-Barr virus, and *Toxoplasma gondii* showed negative IgM antibodies. HIV serology status was negative. For cytomegalovirus, both types of antibodies (IgM and IgG) were positive, with an IgM level >300 U/mL. pp65 antigen was also detected as well as CMV DNA. Diagnostic imaging of the abdomen except the dilated common bile duct showed a normal appearance of the gallbladder, liver, pancreas, spleen, and both kidneys. To our knowledge, cytomegalovirus cholangiopathy in the absence of any other underlying disease has not been reported. Therefore, the presence of cholangiopathy in our patient is interesting from an imaging, laboratory, and clinical point of view.

1. Introduction

Cytomegalovirus (CMV), also known as human herpesvirus type 5, has a seroprevalence of 30–100%, depending on the age, ethnicity, social, and immune status of the patient. CMV in immunocompetent patients typically manifests as an undifferentiated viral syndrome or a mononucleosis-like illness, which is usually self-limiting. However, in immunocompromised patients, CMV can cause severe complications such as encephalitis, pneumonitis, hepatitis, uveitis, retinitis, colitis, and graft rejection. In immunocompetent patients, the gastrointestinal tract is the primary site of involvement of a CMV infection. Specifically, or in more detail, medical literature has reported colitis and hepatitis in association with CMV infections [1–6].

Acute cholangitis is a morbid condition. It occurs when biliary stenosis, due to various benign causes or the presence of a tumour, results in cholestasis and biliary infection [7, 8]. To our knowledge, CMV cholangiopathy in the absence of any other underlying disease has not been reported. Here, we present the imaging, clinical, and laboratory features of CMV-related acute cholangitis in an immunocompetent patient.

2. Case Presentation

A 37-year-old man presented to our hospital with jaundice, upper right quadrant pain, and intermittent fever with chills. The symptoms had arisen 5–7 days before admission. He had no history of severe illness or surgery; his medical history was negative on the medications, alcohol, and tobacco.

On examination, the patient's temperature was 37.8°C, his blood pressure was 130/80 mmHg, his pulse rate was 100 beats per minute, and his respiratory rate was 16 breaths per minute. He was alert and oriented. Nonspecific inflammatory parameters were elevated, patient's white blood cells were 12.7 ($4–10 \times 10^9$/L), C-reactive protein was 77 (<0.5 mg/dL), and the erythrocyte sedimentation rate was 53 in the first hour. A complete blood count showed the following: red blood cells: 5.1 (4.2–5.4 million/mcL), hemoglobin: 12.5 (12–15 g/dL), hematocrit: 41 (36–47%), and platelets: 380 (150–400 × 109/L).

Laboratory assessment showed biliary stasis, where total bilirubin was 203 μmol/L (2–20), unconjugated bilirubin was 98 μmol/L, and conjugated bilirubin was 105 μmol/L. The results of other liver function tests were as follows: γ-glutamyl transferase: 702 U/L (2–30), alkaline phosphatase: 556 U/L (30–120), lactate dehydrogenase: 717 U/L (100–200), aspartate aminotransferase: 258 U/L (10–30), alanine aminotransferase: 207 U/L (10–40), serum amylase: 63 U/L (27–131), international normalized ratio: 1.01 (0.9–1.1), total protein: 6.9 g/dL [6–8], serum albumin: 4.1 g/dL (3.5–5.0), triglycerides: 119 mg/dL (‹160), and cholesterol: 167 mg/dL (‹200). Values for other biochemical tests were within the normal ranges. Markers for hepatitis A–E viruses were negative.

Real-time sonography of the abdomen indicated a dilated common bile duct (CBD; Figure 1(a)), but the gallbladder, liver, pancreas, spleen, and both kidneys appeared normal. Radiology assessment through magnetic resonance imaging (MRI) of the abdomen excluded malignant pathology and lymphadenopathy. Magnetic resonance cholangiopancreatography (MRCP) confirmed whole-length dilatation of the biliary tree and excluded choledocholithiasis (Figure 2). An endoscopy of the upper gastrointestinal tract and duodenal papilla was normal. Colour Doppler echocardiography and a chest X-ray were also normal.

The patient underwent conservative treatment, parenteral infusions, including ciprofloxacin 1 g/day, metamizole 500 mg/day, pantoprazole 40 mg/day, and liver supplements such as silymarin with vitamin B complex. Serology assessment (ELISA assay) for rubeola, the herpes simplex virus, and Epstein-Barr virus showed negative IgM and positive IgG antibodies. A serology assessment for *Toxoplasma gondii* showed negative IgM and IgG antibodies. The patient's HIV serology status was negative. For CMV, both types of antibodies (IgM and IgG) were positive, with an IgM level of 780 U/ml and an IgG level of 350 U/ml.

After 12 days, the patient was asymptomatic. His skin colour returned to normal, and he started eating.

Bilirubin levels normalized, as well as the other liver enzymes. Three weeks after beginning of the symptoms, a follow-up blood sample was again positive for CMV antibodies (IgM 400 and IgG 500). pp65 antigen was also positive, and real-time polymerase chain reaction (PCR) confirmed the presence of CMV DNA. Control sonography of the abdominal organs showed that the CBD had a normal appearance (Figure 1(b)). On day 15, the patient was discharged, with a diagnosis of CMV cholangiopathy. Six months later, a control exam with real-time sonography showed that the biliary tract had a normal appearance, and liver enzymes were also within the normal ranges.

3. Discussion

According to the Tokyo guidelines 2018, the diagnostic criteria for acute cholangitis includes systemic inflammation (fever and/or shaking chills) and cholestasis (jaundice, abnormal liver function tests) on diagnostic imaging [7], as imaging findings and laboratory markers are distinct criteria.

On admission, our patient had jaundice, upper right quadrant pain, and intermittent fever, a condition known as Charcot's triad. Biochemical observations indicated hyperbilirubinaemia and increased levels of enzymes associated with biliary stasis.

From the laboratory point of view, interesting feature was more elevated aspartate aminotransferase than alanine aminotransferase, and both bilirubin (indirect/direct) were almost equal; it has not been seen frequently in nonalcoholic and noncirrhotic patients.

Imaging plays a pivotal part in the diagnosis of cholangitis by identifying predisposing factors and revealing complications. Sonography is highly sensitive and specifically used for imaging of the gallbladder and assessing bile duct dilatation [7, 8]. Our diagnostic imaging was based on real-time sonography, MRI, and MRCP, which excluded the presence of stones in the biliary tract, benign strictures, and a possible malignancy as a cause of obstruction. According to the diagnostic criteria in the 2018 Tokyo guidelines, our patient had acute cholangitis, with clear clinical, biochemical, and imaging signs.

The cause of this type of biliary stasis was unclear. Endoscopic retrograde cholangiopancreatography (ERCP) was initially planned as part of the diagnostic and therapeutic protocol, but after a week, the patient felt clinically better, and all bilirubin levels subsequently decreased.

Based on the recommended diagnostic approach, all known causes of acute cholangitis, such as cholelithiasis, benign biliary stricture, malignant occlusion, pancreatitis, duodenal diverticulum, and iatrogenic factors [7, 8], were ruled out. Serological studies indicative of acute CMV infection include the identification of CMV pp65 antigen in blood sample as a marker of active viral replication, positive IgM antibodies, or a significant increase in the titre of IgG antibodies in paired samples obtained during the infection. Active CMV infection is defined by detection of pp65 antigen-positive and/or CMV DNA in the blood [1, 3, 5, 6].

A follow-up blood sample beside the increased level of IgG antibodies and positive pp65 antigen showed the presence of CMV DNA via real-time PCR. After reviewing the patient's medical history and serology status, the only factor that seemed to have a link with this type of cholangiopathy was a CMV infection—pp65 antigenemia and positive IgM and IgG antibodies; CMV DNA was also detected via real-time PCR. Oku and colleagues [9] reported CMV cholangitis in an immunocompetent patient with diabetes mellitus and essential hypertension. Diagnostic

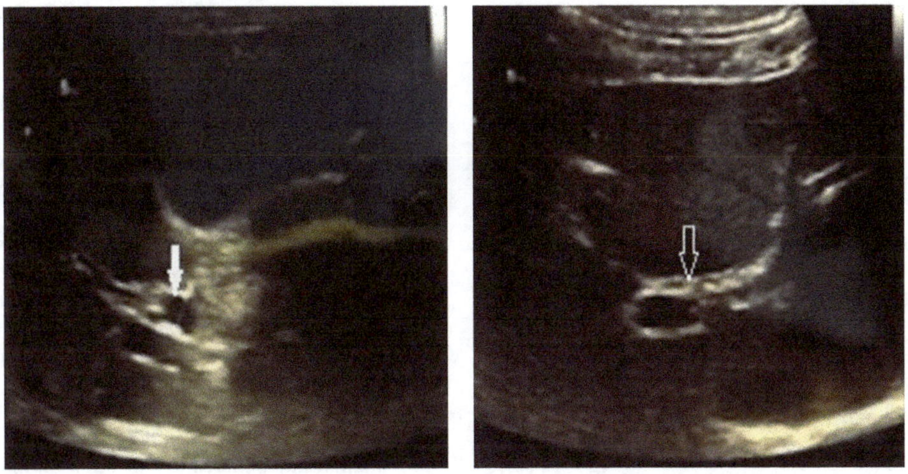

(a) (b)

FIGURE 1: Abdominal ultrasound showing (a) dilated common bile duct (white arrow) (b) on the 12th hospital day normal appearance of common bile duct (arrow).

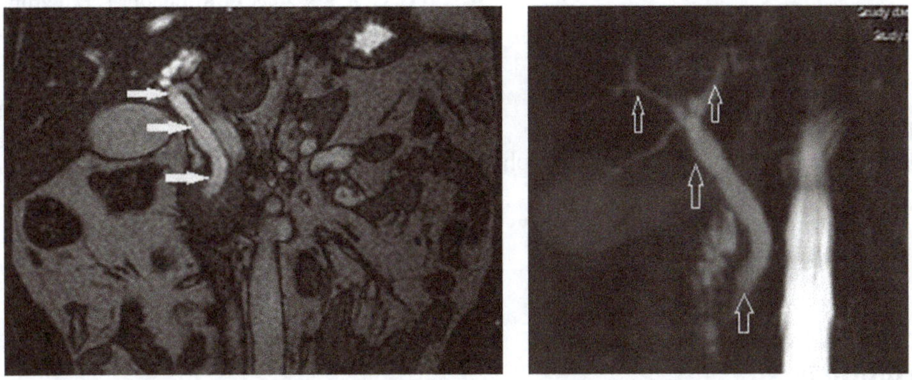

(a) (b)

FIGURE 2: MRI image showing (a) dilation of hepatic and common bile duct (white arrows). MRCP image showing (b) full-length dilation of biliary tree (arrows).

imaging (based on computed tomography and ERCP) showed cholelithiasis and a focal narrowing of the distal CBD, followed by pancreatitis. CMV was also detected. The real cause of this type of adverse event remains unclear; it could be the result of cholelithiasis and stricture of CBD or the result of CMV infection. Imaging assessment in our case showed an absence of any strictures of the CBD and no presence of the stone in the complete biliary tract, which could be a predisposing factor for cholangitis.

Jensen and colleagues [4] reported acute CMV hepatitis in a patient with a previous cholecystectomy caused by gallstones. MRCP was performed to address the question of the pathology of the biliary duct system, but this did not show any pathological results. There was no cholangiopathy, and this case did not provide any imaging support.

Regarding the gastrointestinal tract, Pasticci and colleagues [10] reported acute appendicitis due to CMV in an apparently immunocompetent patient. The biliary tract was also involved in this patient; six years previously, the patient had been diagnosed with primary sclerosing cholangitis and ulcerative colitis, with suspected retroperitoneal fibrosis, bile sludge, and splenomegaly. Prasad and colleagues [11] found CMV hemobilia in a patient who had undergone long-term steroid therapy; on admission, the patient presented with hematemesis, fever, and retroperitoneal fluid collection.

Tleyjeh and colleagues [12] reported a case of CMV cholangitis that occurred in a patient undergoing chronic corticosteroid therapy who presented with recurrent hemobilia and biliary obstruction and was successfully treated with ganciclovir and a cholecystostomy.

Unlike these last three cases, aside from CMV cholangiopathy, our patient did not have any other underlying disease and/or the immunosuppressive therapy.

A review article by Rafailidis and colleagues [1] about CMV infection in immunocompetent patients noted possible CMV gastrointestinal complications such as colitis, gastroenteritis, duodenitis, ileitis, proctitis, and hepatitis. However, CMV cholangitis was not present. Therefore, the presence of cholangiopathy in our patient is interesting from an imaging, biochemical, and clinical point of view.

Although it is currently thought that CMV infection in immunocompetent patients does not require treatment, the risks and benefits of specific antiviral treatment for severely ill patients have not been adequately addressed [1]. Our patient had a good response to conservative treatment, which included infusions, antibiotics, liver supplements, and a proton pump inhibitor.

4. Conclusion

In conclusion, all patients with onset cholestasis should undergo diagnostic assessment based on a thorough laboratory analysis, different imaging modalities, an upper gastrointestinal endoscopy, and conventional assessment of serology status, checking for hepatitis viruses A–E and HIV. In the absence of clear jaundice aetiology, CMV antibodies, pp65 antigen, and CMV DNA should be considered as part of the diagnostic protocol.

Abbreviations

CBD: Common bile duct
CMV: Cytomegalovirus
ERCP: Endoscopic retrograde cholangiopancreatography
HIV: Human immunodeficiency virus
MRCP: Magnetic resonance cholangiopancreatography
MRI: Magnetic resonance imaging.

Authors' Contributions

EA and AK drafted the article and provided the intellectual input; DP and A. Habibovic analyzed and interpreted data; ES performed diagnostic imaging and chose images; AK, BI, and A. Hujdurovic wrote and approved the manuscript.

References

[1] P. I. Rafailidis, E. G. Mourtzoukou, I. C. Varbobitis, and M. E. Falagas, "Severe cytomegalovirus infection in apparently immunocompetent patients: a systematic review," *Virology Journal*, vol. 5, no. 1, p. 47, 2008.

[2] T. G. Wreghitt, E. L. Teare, O. Sule, R. Devi, and P. Rice, "Cytomegalovirus infection in Immunocompetent patients," *Clinical Infectious Diseases*, vol. 37, no. 12, pp. 1603–1606, 2003.

[3] D. Lancini, H. M. Faddy, R. Flower, and C. Hogan, "Cytomegalovirus disease in Immunocompetent adults," *Medical Journal of Australia*, vol. 201, no. 10, pp. 578–580, 2014.

[4] K. O. Jensen, E. Angst, F. H. Hetzer, and C. Gingert, "Acute cytomegalovirus hepatitis in an immunocompetent host as a reason for upper right abdominal pain," *Case Reports in Gastroenterology*, vol. 10, no. 1, pp. 36–43, 2016.

[5] G. Breda, B. Almeida, S. Carstensen et al., "Human cytomegalovirus detection by real-time PCR and pp65-antigen test in hematopoietic stem cell transplant recipients: a challenge in low and middle-income countries," *Pathogens and Global Health*, vol. 107, no. 6, pp. 312–319, 2013.

[6] L. von Müller, A. Klemm, M. Weiss et al., "Active cytomegalovirus infection in patients with septic shock," *Emerging Infectious Diseases*, vol. 12, no. 10, pp. 1517–1522, 2006.

[7] M. Yokoe, J. Hata, T. Takada et al., "Tokyo Guidelines 2018: diagnostic criteria and severity grading of acute cholecystitis (with videos)," *Journal of Hepato-Biliary-Pancreatic Sciences*, vol. 25, no. 1, pp. 41–54, 2018.

[8] M. Gupta and A. Sachdev, "Acute cholangitis- an overview of diagnosis and medical Management," *Journal of Medical College Chandigarh*, vol. 6, no. 2, pp. 1–8, 2016.

[9] T. Oku, M. Maeda, E. Waga et al., "Cytomegalovirus cholangitis and pancreatitis in an immunocompetent patient," *Journal of Gastroenterology*, vol. 40, no. 10, pp. 987–992, 2005.

[10] M. B. Pasticci, S. Corsi, F. Spigarelli et al., "Acute appendicitis due to cytomegalovirus in an apparently immunocompetent patient: a case report," *Journal of Medical Case Reports*, vol. 8, no. 1, p. 92, 2014.

[11] G. A. Prasad, S. C. Abraham, T. H. Baron, and M. D. Topazian, "Hemobilia caused by cytomegalovirus cholangiopathy," *American Journal of Gastroenterology*, vol. 100, no. 11, pp. 2592–2595, 2005.

[12] I. M. Tleyjeh, G. Georgescu, A. Virk et al., "Cytomegalovirus cholangitis presenting with recurrent hemobilia," *European Journal of Clinical Microbiology & Infectious Diseases*, vol. 24, no. 9, pp. 634–636, 2005.

4

Endometrioma of the Liver: A Case Report and Review of the Literature

Prachi Rana, [1] **Shida Haghighat,** [1] **and Hyosun Han** [2]

[1] *Department of Internal Medicine, Los Angeles County Hospital/University of Southern California, USA*
[2] *Department of Gastroenterology and Liver Diseases, Los Angeles County Hospital/University of Southern California, USA*

Correspondence should be addressed to Prachi Rana; prachi.rana@med.usc.edu

Academic Editor: Melanie Deutsch

Hepatic endometriosis is a rare form of endometriosis first described by Finkel in 1986. A thorough review of the literature revealed 28 cases of hepatic endometriosis. This unusual condition offers several diagnostic challenges due to its variable appearance on imaging and need for histologic analysis to establish a definitive diagnosis. We present a 42-year-old female initially treated for presumed hydatid cyst that was later found to be endometriosis in the liver. The case highlights the importance of considering endometriosis in the differential for a patient presenting with a solitary liver mass regardless of age and previous history of endometriosis.

1. Introduction

Endometriosis is characterized by the presence of endometrial tissue outside of the uterine cavity. It is a benign condition most commonly noted in the uterus, fallopian tubes, ovaries, and local pelvic peritoneum. Atypical endometriosis, when the condition is found in extrapelvic regions, is rare [1]. While uncommon, atypical endometriosis has been described in remote sites including the GI tract, diaphragm, skin, lung, pleura, kidney, and pancreas. The only organ in the abdomen that is refractory to endometriosis is the spleen [2].

Hepatic endometriosis is one of the most rare forms of extrapelvic endometriosis, first described in 1986 [3]. Only 28 cases have been reported in the English literature. We herein present the 29th case of hepatic endometriosis, a 42-year-old female initially treated for presumed hydatid cyst that was later found to be endometriosis in the liver. This rare condition offers several diagnostic challenges. We offer an exhaustive review of the literature focusing on advances in the clinical manifestation, patient characteristics, pathogenesis, and diagnostic workup of the condition.

2. Case Presentation

A 42-year-old multiparous woman presented with episodic, severe right upper quadrant pain associated with nausea and vomiting. Her past surgical history included a hysterectomy and left oophorectomy for unclear reasons. Several months prior she presented to another hospital for similar symptoms and was diagnosed with a hepatic mass. Physical examination demonstrated right upper quadrant tenderness without any palpable masses. Liver function and viral serologies for hepatitis B and C were normal. Tumor markers demonstrated normal CA 19-9 and AFP, with mildly elevated CA-125 40 U/mL (normal <38U/mL).

Computed tomography with intravenous contrast showed a 3.2cm x 4cm x 1.8cm multiseptated cystic lesion in the left hepatic lobe and an ill-defined heterogeneous hyperdensity within the peripheral right hepatic lobe measuring 3cm x 1.3cm (Figure 1). Ultrasound-guided fine needle aspiration and core biopsy of the left hepatic lesion were inconclusive.

Further workup revealed a positive Echinococcal IgG antibody and she was started on Albendazole for a presumed hydatid cyst. After completion of therapy, she was scheduled for complete left lateral hepatic resection. However, she presented again several weeks later with progressive right upper quadrant pain. At this time repeat computed tomography redemonstrated the left hepatic mass which was unchanged in size but did not show the right hepatic lesion. Imaging also revealed a new pericardial effusion that was

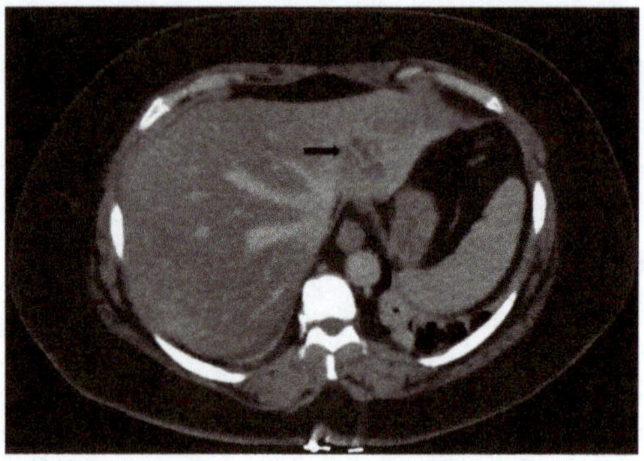

FIGURE 1: Computed tomography showing 3.2 x 4.0 x 1.8 cm multiseptated cystic lesion in the left hepatic lobe.

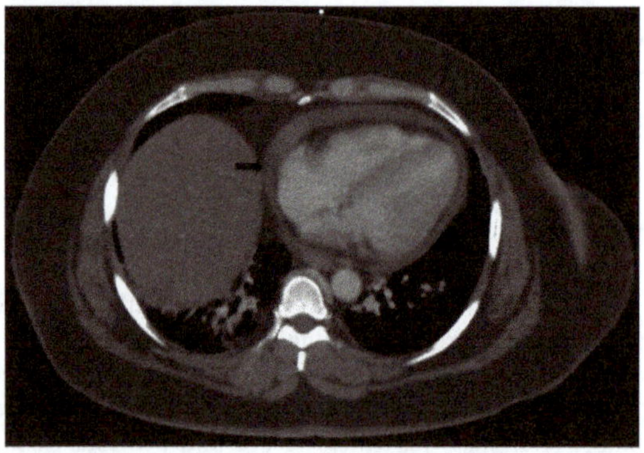

FIGURE 2: Computed tomography showing small pericardial effusion.

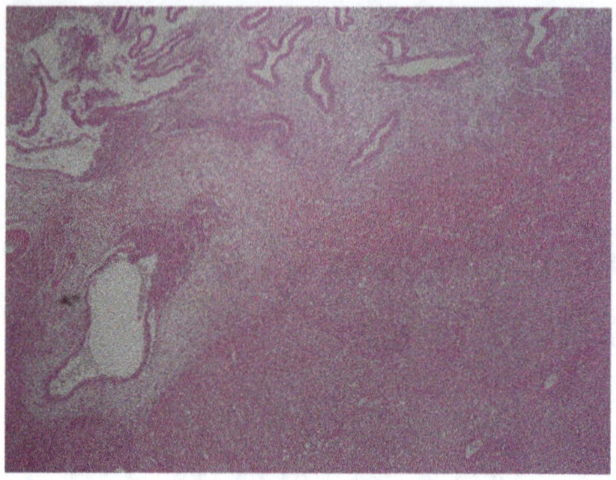

FIGURE 3: Low-power view of the interface between an endometriotic nodule and liver parenchyma. Notice the large endometrial type glands surrounded by endometrial type stroma in the superior portion of the image. These are separated from the liver parenchyma (lower right portion) by a band of fibrosis. *The liver parenchyma displays macrovesicular steatosis.* Hematoxylin & Eosin, 40x.

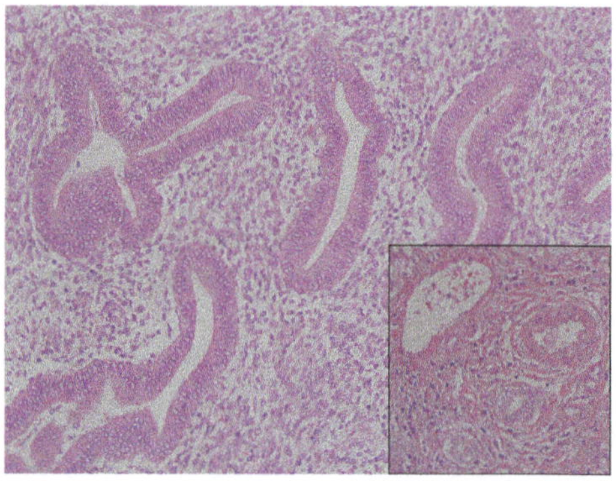

FIGURE 4: High-power view of an endometriotic nodule. Endometrioid type glands of varying shape and size show characteristic columnar lining, within a cellular endometrial type stroma. *The inset shows a portal tract for comparison (from top to bottom: vein, artery, bile ducts); notice the small round shape of the bile ducts and lack of cellular stroma.* Hematoxylin & Eosin, 200x.

not present on previous imaging (Figure 2). Her liver tests were the following: AST 485 U/L (normal 10-40 U/L), ALT 308 U/L (normal 5-40 U/L), ALP 50 U/L (normal 35-104 U/L), and total bilirubin 0.5 mg/dL (normal <1.0 mg/dL). Given the concern for pericardial involvement, she urgently underwent a laparoscopic left partial hepatectomy (segment II and partial segment III). The postoperative course was uneventful. Final pathology was consistent with hepatic endometriosis (Figures 3 and 4). After 2 months of follow-up, the patient was asymptomatic and liver tests normalized. She was started on medroxyprogesterone acetate and remains well to date.

3. Discussion

Endometriosis is a common gynecologic disease characterized by the presence of endometrial glands and stroma outside of the uterus. It affects 5-15% of women of reproductive age. Pelvic endometriosis involves the ovaries, fallopian tubes, uterine ligaments, Pouch of Douglas, and surrounding peritoneum [4]. A more rare form of endometriosis, extrapelvic, includes involvement of gastrointestinal tract, urinary system, thoracic cavity, kidneys, and pancreas. The exact prevalence of extrapelvic endometriosis is unknown but is thought to present in an older population with a median age of 34-40 years [4].

There is no clear consensus or unifying theory of the exact pathophysiology of extrapelvic endometriosis. Several theories have been proposed; however no theory alone accounts for the development of extrapelvic endometriosis, suggesting a multifactorial nature to the disease.

The classic theory of retrograde menstruation proposes that reflux of endometrial fragments through the fallopian tubes during menstruation results in implantation of the peritoneal cavity. Though retrograde menstruation is a common phenomenon seen in up to 90% of healthy women, not all of these women develop extrapelvic endometriosis [5].

The coelomic metaplasia theory suggests that endometriosis develops from metaplasia of the peritoneal epithelium possibly due to environmental or genetic factors [5, 6]. The induction theory suggests that defects in embryogenesis give rise to endometrial like tissue. The Müllerian ducts give rise to the female genitourinary tract.

In males, this structure dissolves under the influence of anti-Müllerian hormone. However remnants of this structure may persist and differentiate later in life into endometriotic like tissue due to the presence of excesses in endogenous or exogenous estrogen as is seen in men with chronic liver disease and prostate cancer [5, 7].

While these theories account for endometriosis within the peritoneal and pelvic cavity and provide some insight into its pathogenesis in men, they do not account for the cases of disseminated endometriosis seen in cases of lymph nodes, thoracic cavity, and liver involvement, as seen in our patient. Whether these original cells originate in the uterus or the peritoneal cavity, the theory that endometriotic tissue disseminates through lymphatic spread offers a plausible explanation for the manifestation of hepatic endometriosis [5].

A thorough review of the literature revealed 28 cases of hepatic endometriosis. Our report adds one case to this rare clinical finding; herein we present the twenty-ninth case of hepatic endometriosis. Tables 1 and 2 summarize the previously reported cases and ours, comparing the presentation, imaging, treatment, and pathologic features. In this review, the patient age ranged from 21 to 62 years, with a mean of 41.5 years. Of the 19 cases that reported parity, ten were nulligravid and nine were either uni- or multiparous, thus demonstrating that pregnancy and childbirth have no bearing on hepatic endometriosis. Six of 29 (21%) patients were postmenopausal, thus showing this condition is not limited to women of reproductive age and that the diagnosis should be considered in postmenopausal women. Twelve of 29 (41%) had a prior history of endometriosis; thus the diagnosis should not be limited only to patients with a known history of endometriosis. A significant portion of these patients had prior abdominopelvic surgery—at least half (51%) had prior pelvic surgery, and 41% had a hysterectomy, suggesting that endometrial tissue seeding during surgery later resulted in the development of hepatic endometriosis. The majority (90%) of patients described in the literature had epigastric or right upper quadrant pain; only two patients complained of characteristic cyclic pain related to menses. Only three patients were asymptomatic and their condition was diagnosed incidentally. In one peculiar case, however, the patient presented with flu-like symptoms and right shoulder pain, misdiagnosed as pneumonia initially [8].

Abdominal US, CT, and MRI are the imaging modalities most frequently used. Typical US findings include well-defined cystic masses with solid components and septations. The majority of CT reports show low density, heterogenous cystic lesions that are either nonenhancing or poorly enhancing. Calcifications have been reported along with irregular soft tissue components but can be variable. Finally, MRI usually demonstrates signal intensity on T1- and T2-weighted images, similar to that of normal endometrium. However, because endometrial implants can exhibit various degrees of hemorrhage due to hormonal stimulation, implants may demonstrate a spectrum of appearances depending on the age of the hemorrhage but can be variable [9].

Of the 19 cases that reported lab values, 79% had normal liver tests. Three cases exhibited mild transaminitis, and a fourth case, ours, had markedly elevated transaminases with AST 485 U/L and ALT 305 U/L.

Excluding two, all patients underwent surgery for treatment. The most common surgery was hepatectomy via laparotomy (59%). Other surgical techniques included ultrasonic cyst manipulation. In the two nonsurgical cases, those patients were treated with danazol alone [9, 10]. Tumor size ranged from 1 to 30cm, with mean tumor size 9.8 cm.

The final diagnosis can only be made by histopathologic analysis. The differential diagnosis includes both benign and malignant conditions, as echinococcal cyst, abscess, hematoma, cystadenoma, and malignant cystic neoplasm, such as cystadenocarcinoma or metastatic disease. Method of diagnosis was largely by histologic analysis after surgery in 90% of cases. Only four patients underwent CT-guided percutaneous biopsy prior to surgery, with only three yielding a diagnosis of endometriosis and one case, ours, yielding inconclusive results. Histopathologic examination of the tumors was consistent with endometriosis as evidenced largely by fibrous capsules with internal epithelial lining containing endometrial glands and stroma. Furthermore, although malignant transformation of endometriosis is a rare event, occurring commonly in the ovary, there were two cases of malignancy reported, one adenosarcoma and one low-grade endometrial stroma sarcoma [11, 12]. Of the eight cases that reported on immunostaining, all eight cases were positive for estrogen and progesterone receptor, consistent with endometriosis. Five cases reported on further immunohistochemistry markers that included CD10 (in endometrial tissue) and/or CK7 (in glandular tissue) [13–17].

Hepatic endometriosis is a rare form of endometriosis. This unusual condition offers several diagnostic challenges but should be considered in the differential in any female presenting with a solitary hepatic mass, regardless of age and previous history of endometriosis.

Disclosure

Institutional Mailing Address: LAC + USC Medical Center, 1200 N. State St., CT A7D - GME, Los Angeles, CA 90033.

Table 1: Patient characteristics, presentation, and treatment of case reports of hepatic endometriosis.

Author, Year	Age	Parity	Pre/Post-Menopausal	Prior Pelvic Surgery	Hysterectomy	History of Endometriosis	Symptoms	Method of Diagnosis	Treatment
Asran, 2010	61	Unknown	Post	Salpingo-oophorectomy	Yes	Yes	Post prandial epigastric pain	CT guided percutaneous liver biopsy	N/A
Bouras, 2013	35	Nulliparous	Pre	No	No	No	Recurrent, intermittent epigastric pain	Surgery	L lateral hepatic sectionectomy by laparotomy
Chung, 1998	40	Multiparous	Pre	L ovarian cystectomy	No	Yes	Asymptomatic	Surgery	Cyst enucleation
De Riggi, 2016	27	Nulliparous	Pre	No	No	No	Painless abdominal mass	Surgery	L hepatectomy by laparotomy
Finkel, 1986	21	Uniparous	Pre	L fallopian tube cyst removal	No	No	Episodic sharp, epigastric pain associated with nausea and vomiting not related to menses	Surgery	Cyst enucleation + Danazol
Fluegen, 2013	32	Nulliparous	Pre	No	No	No	RUQ pain	Surgery	Ultrasonic pericystectomy
Goldsmith, 2009	48	Nulliparous	N/A	Salpingo-oophorectomy	Yes	Yes	Relapsing/remitting chronic RUQ pain	Surgery	Nonanatomic resection, laparotomy, ultrasonic cyst aspiration
Groves, 2003	52	N/A	N/A	Oophorectomy	Yes	No	RUQ pain	Surgery	R hepatectomy
Hertel, 2012	44	N/A	N/A	Oophorectomy	Partial	no	Sudden onset upper abdominal pain	Surgery	Partial hepatectomy
Huang, 2002	56	N/A	Post	Salpingo-oophorectomy	Yes	Yes	Intermittent epigastric pain not associated with menses	Surgery	L hepatic lobectomy by laparotomy
Inal, 2000	25	N/A	Pre	No	No	Yes	Pelvic pain, mass and rectal hemorrhage	Percutaneous CT guided biopsy	Danazol
Jelovsek, 2004	52	Uniparous	Post	Salpingo-oophorectomy	Yes	Yes	Flu like symptoms, pleuritic chest pain	Surgery	Leuprolide, then resection via laparotomy
Keramidaris, 2018	40	Multiparous	Pre	No	No	No	Asymptomatic, incidental	Surgery	Cystectomy by laparotomy
Khan, 2002	31	N/A	N/A	Hysterectomy, salpingo-oophorectomy	Yes	Yes	Malaise, abdominal distention	Surgery	R hepatectomy + goserelin
Khan, 2002	61	N/A	Post	No	No	Yes	RUQ pain	Surgery	R hepatectomy
Liu, 2015	36	Uniparous	Pre	No	No	No	RUQ pain prior to menstruation	Surgery	Pericystectomy
N'Senda, 2002	54	Uniparous	Post	Hysterectomy, oophorectomy	Yes	No	RUQ pain for 1 year	Surgery	Right hepatectomy by thoracolaparotomy
Nezhat, 2005 (1)	36	Nulliparous	N/A	No	No	No	Cyclic epigastric pain for 1 year	Surgery	Cyst removal by CO2 laser laparoscopically
Nezhat, 2005 (2)	30	Nulliparous	N/A	No	No	Yes	Chronic pelvic pain, dysmenorrhea, and painful bowel movements	Surgery	Laparoscopic removal of liver mass
Reid, 2003	46	Nulliparous	N/A	Oophorectomy	Yes	yes	RUQ pain	Surgery	R hepatectomy + goserelin
Rivkine, 2013	51	Multiparous	N/A	Hysterectomy	Yes	no	Epigastric pain, vomiting	Surgery	L lobectomy by laparotomy
Roesch-Dietlan, 2011	25	Nulliparous	Pre	No	No	No	Relapsing/remitting RUQ pain	Surgery	Incidentally found during laparoscopic cholecystectomy, treated with danazol
Rovati, 1990	37	Nulliparous	Pre	No	No	Yes	Chronic, acyclic epigastric pain	Surgery	Segmentectomy by laparotomy + Danazol

Table 1: Continued.

Author, Year	Age	Parity	Pre/Post-Menopausal	Prior Pelvic Surgery	Hysterectomy	History of Endometriosis	Symptoms	Method of Diagnosis	Treatment
Schuld, 2011	39	Uniparous	Pre	No	No	No	RUQ pain, cough	Surgery	Segmentectomy, transdiaphragmatic pulmonary wedge resection
Sherif, 2016	44	N/A	Pre	Hysterectomy	Yes	Yes	RUQ pain and vomiting	CT guided core biopsy	Segmentectomy
Tuech, 2003	42	Nulliparous	N/A	No	No	No	Chronic, acyclic epigastric pain	Surgery	Deroofing & cystectomy
Verbeke, 1996 (1)	34	N/A	Pre	No	No	No	Acute abdomen	Surgery	R hemihepatectomy
Verbeke, 1996 (2)	62	N/A	Post	Yes	No	No	RUQ pain	Surgery	Cholecystectomy, L hepatectomy
Rana, 2019	42	Multiparous	Pre	Hysterectomy, L oophorectomy	Yes	No	Severe RUQ pain, N/V	Surgery	L partial hepatectomy

TABLE 2: Imaging features of case reports of hepatic endometriosis.

Author, Year	US	CT	MRI
Asran, 2010	N/A	Multiple, irregularly shaped, heterogeneous, low density lesions scattered throughout the liver	N/A
Bouras, 2013	N/A	10cm cystic lesion with a fatty component and calcifications	10cm cystic lesion with a fatty component and calcifications
Chung, 1998	6.4 cm x 3 cm x 2.5 cm septated cyst	Low density hepatic cyst, with undulating wall but no obvious septations	N/A
De Riggi, 2016	N/A	30cm hepatic cyts in the L love reaching segments IV, V, VIII	
Finkel, 1986	12.5 x12x9.5 cm cystic mass in L lobe with possible septations	12cm smooth-walled cystic lesion without septations	N/A
Fluegen, 2013	N/A	N/A	9.5cm x 12cm lobulated cyst in segments IV, V, VIII
Goldsmith, 2009	9 x 11cm cystic mass in segment IV. The wall appeared thick with complex septae.	N/A	11 x13 cm cystic mass in segments IV and VIII with incomplete septations
Groves, 2003	Bilateral lesions, largest in R posterior lobe 12 x 9cm	N/A	N/A
Hertel, 2012	N/A	N/A	9.5x9.1x11.2cm cystic mass with a thickened wall in R hepatic lobe
Huang, 2002	N/A	9x6cm well circumscribed cystic mass with irregular soft tissue components	N/A
Inal, 2000	Round, well defined and heterogeneous including anechoic cystic and echogenic solid components with septations and solid components	Round, well circumscribed heterogeneous mass with septations. Fine punctate/nodular calcifications at the periphery of the lesion	A lobulated but well-demarcated subcapsular mass in the posterior segment of R lobe of the liver
Jelovsek, 2004	N/A	11 x7cm mass	N/A
Keramidaris, 2018	Large cystic lesion between L and R lobe of the liver	none	Multiseptated cystic lesion 10.3x7.8x7.7 cm in the L lobe, segments IV, II, III
Khan, 2002	Large mass in R lobe and small in L lobe	large non-enhancing lobulated mass in R lobe and mass in L lobe; portal vein thrombosis	N/A
Khan, 2002	N/A	Large mass occupying the entire R lobe	N/A
Liu, 2015	6 cm lesion in L lobe (segment III)	6.5 x6cm loculated cystic lesion in segment III, wall with thick complex septae	N/A
N'Senda, 2002	N/A	Huge heterogeneous hypodense mass partially enhanced after contrast injection; cystic changes w/ fluid levels	Heterogeneous mass on both T1-, T2- and T1-weighted image after gadolinium injection; cystic changes w/ fluid levels
Nezhat, 2005 (1)	3-cm hepatic cyst in the far caudal aspect of the right lobe of the liver	3-cm hepatic cyst in the far caudal aspect of the right lobe of the liver	N/A
Nezhat, 2005 (2)	Normal findings	N/A	Normal findings
Reid, 2003	10cm mass with echogenic margins and internal debris	Low density lesion	N/A
Rivkine, 2013	80 x 75 mm intraparenchymal hepatic necrotic tumor	Hypovascularized, cystic mass in the L liver lobe with hemorrhagic contents, no septations	Cystic mass in segments II and III

Table 2: Continued.

Author, Year	US	CT	MRI
Roesch-Dietlan, 2011	No masses, multiple small gallstones	N/A	N/A
Rovati, 1990	10cm cystic mass with septations	Multilocular 10cm cyst with fine calcifications in the wall	N/A
Schuld, 2011	N/A	N/A	6.8 x2.3 cm in diameter in the right basal lung and peripheral bile ducts
Sherif, 2016	3cm complex cyst in R lobes	3cm well defined hypodense subcapsular lesion in R lobe with heterogeneous peripheral enhancement in the venous and delayed phases	Subcapsular partially cystic focal lesion with possible hemorrhagic content and heterogeneous peripheral enhancement
Tuech, 2003	N/A	24cm smooth walled cystic lesion without septations in the R lobe	N/A
Verbeke, 1996 (1)	N/A	Cystic tumor in R lobe of liver, with reactive enlargement of L hepatic lobe	Cystic tumor in R lobe of liver, with reactive enlargement of L hepatic lobe
Verbeke, 1996 (2)	Cyst (12 x 10 x 7.5 cm) in the left liver lobe, located near the gallbladder and the liver hilus, which partially compressed the proximal ductus choledochus.	Cyst (12 x 10 x 7.5 cm) in the left liver lobe, located near the gallbladder and the liver hilus, which partially compressed the proximal ductus choledochus.	N/A
Rana 2019	N/A	3.2cm x 4cm x 1.8cm multi-septated cystic lesion in the left hepatic lobe	N/A

Authors' Contributions

Prachi Rana and Shida Haghighat equally contributed to the collection of the data and writing of the manuscript. Hyosun Han reviewed and edited the manuscript.

Acknowledgments

We thank Dr. Yangling Ma and Dr. Esteban Gnass for the review and interpretation of the pathologic reports.

References

[1] S. K. Sonavane, K. P. Kantawala, and C. O. Menias, "Beyond the boundaries-endometriosis: typical and atypical locations," *Current Problems in Diagnostic Radiology*, vol. 40, no. 6, pp. 219–232, 2011.

[2] S. M. Markham, "Extrapelvic endometriosis," *Modern Approaches to Endometriosis*, pp. 151–182, 1991.

[3] L. Finkel, A. Marchevsky, and B. Cohen, "Endometrial cyst of the liver," *American Journal of Gastroenterology*, vol. 81, no. 7, pp. 576–578, 1986.

[4] D. Charatsi, O. Koukoura, I. G. Ntavela et al., "Gastrointestinal and urinary tract endometriosis: a review on the commonest locations of extrapelvic endometriosis," *Advances in Medicine*, vol. 2018, 11 pages, 2018.

[5] R. O. Burney and L. C. Giudice, "Pathogenesis and pathophysiology of endometriosis," *Fertility and Sterility*, vol. 98, no. 3, pp. 511–519, 2012.

[6] P. G. Signorile and A. Baldi, "Endometriosis: new concepts in the pathogenesis," *The International Journal of Biochemistry & Cell Biology*, vol. 42, no. 6, pp. 778–780, 2010.

[7] C. Rei, T. Williams, and M. Feloney, "Endometriosis in a man as a rare source of abdominal pain: a case report and review of the literature," *Case Reports in Obstetrics and Gynecology*, vol. 2018, Article ID 2083121, 6 pages, 2018.

[8] J. E. Jelovsek, C. Winans, J. Brainard, and T. Falcone, "Endometriosis of the liver containing mullerian adenosarcoma: Case report," *American Journal of Obstetrics & Gynecology*, vol. 191, no. 5, pp. 1725–1727, 2004.

[9] M. Inal, K. Biçakçi, S. Soyupak et al., "Hepatic endometrioma: A case report and review of the literature," *European Radiology*, vol. 10, no. 3, pp. 431–434, 2000.

[10] F. Roesch-Dietlen, A. Jiménez-García, A. Pérez-Morales, P. Grube-Pagola, K. L. Ramírez-Cervantes, and J. M. Remes-Troche, "Hepatic endometriosis," *Annals of Hepatology*, vol. 10, no. 3, pp. 347-348, 2011.

[11] A. W. Khan, M. Craig, M. Jarmulowicz, and B. R. Davidson, "Liver tumours due to endometriosis and endometrial stromal sarcoma," *HPB*, vol. 4, no. 1, pp. 43–45, 2002.

[12] P. Nsenda, D. Wendum, P. Balladur, H. Dahan, J.-M. Tubiana, and L. Arrivé, "Adenosarcoma arising in hepatic endometriosis," *European Radiology*, vol. 10, no. 8, pp. 1287–1289, 2000.

[13] M. Asran, A. Rashid, and J. Szklaruk, "Hepatic endometriosis mimicking metastatic disease: A case report and review of the literature," *Journal of Radiology Case Reports*, vol. 4, no. 11, pp. 26–31, 2010.

[14] G. Fluegen, F. Jankowiak, L. Zacarias Foehrding, F. Kroepil, W. T. Knoefel, and S. A. Topp, "Intrahepatic endometriosis as differential diagnosis: Case report and literature review," *World Journal of Gastroenterology*, vol. 19, no. 29, pp. 4818–4822, 2013.

[15] D. Keramidaris, S. Gourgiotis, A. Koutela et al., "Rare case of hepatic endometriosis as an incidental finding: Difficult diagnosis of a diagnostic dilemma," *Annals of Hepatology*, vol. 17, no. 5, pp. 884–887, 2018.

[16] K. Liu, W. Zhang, S. Liu, B. Dong, and Y. Liu, "Hepatic endometriosis: A rare case and review of the literature," *European Journal of Medical Research*, vol. 20, no. 1, 2015.

[17] E. Rivkine, D. Jakubowicz, L. Marciano et al., "Hepatic endometrioma: A case report and review of the literature: Report of a case," *Surgery Today*, vol. 43, no. 10, pp. 1188–1193, 2013.

5

Turmeric Induced Liver Injury: A Report of Two Cases

Raphael P. Luber,[1,2,3] Clarissa Rentsch,[1,3,4] Steve Lontos,[2] Jeffrey D. Pope,[5,6] Ar Kar Aung,[7,8] Hans G. Schneider,[5,7] William Kemp,[1,3] Stuart K. Roberts,[1,3] and Ammar Majeed,[1,3]

[1]*Department of Gastroenterology, The Alfred Hospital, 55 Commercial Road, Melbourne, Victoria, Australia*
[2]*Department of Gastroenterology and Liver Transplantation, The Austin Hospital, 145 Studley Road, Heidelberg, Melbourne, Victoria, Australia*
[3]*Central Clinical School, Monash University, The Alfred Hospital, 99 Commercial Road, Melbourne, Victoria, Australia*
[4]*Department of Pharmacy, The Alfred Hospital, 55 Commercial Road, Melbourne, Victoria, Australia*
[5]*Clinical Biochemistry Unit, The Alfred Hospital, 55 Commercial Road, Melbourne, Victoria, Australia*
[6]*Department of Forensic Medicine, Monash University, Melbourne, Australia*
[7]*Department of Epidemiology and Preventive Medicine, Monash University, Melbourne, Australia*
[8]*Department of General Medicine, The Alfred Hospital, 55 Commercial Road, Melbourne, Victoria, Australia*

Correspondence should be addressed to Raphael P. Luber; raphaelluber@gmail.com

Academic Editor: Sorabh Kapoor

Turmeric is a commonly used oral herbal supplement with purported anti-inflammatory and antineoplastic properties. It is promoted as safe, with limited reports of severe adverse effects directly related to oral turmeric thus far in the literature. Herein we report two cases of turmeric supplement induced severe hepatitis. These cases highlight the need for physicians to be aware of patients taking this common supplement and the potential risks that exist.

1. Introduction

Idiosyncratic drug induced liver injury (DILI) is estimated to occur in 1 in 10,000 to 1 in 100,000 people who take a medication [1]. It is the most frequent adverse event leading to abandonment of new drugs and is implicated in 13% of acute liver failure cases in the United States [2]. Herbal and dietary supplements (HDS) account for at least 9% of cases overall [1], with this rate thought to be an underestimate due to their popularity and underreporting.

Turmeric, with its major active ingredient curcumin, is one of the most commonly used HDS [3]. In recent years it has gained attention for its anti-inflammatory, anti-cancer, and other properties across a variety of disorders [4]. Regarding safety, dosing studies and randomized controlled trials have thus far concluded that curcumin treatment is safe, with minimal reported severe adverse effects [4–7].

We report two cases of likely turmeric supplement induced severe liver injury, including one in which a positive rechallenge occurred.

2. Case 1

A 52-year-old Caucasian female presented to her general practitioner with a one-week history of nausea, pruritus, and painless jaundice with associated pale stools and dark urine. This occurred approximately one month following commencement of a turmeric supplement among other medications. She rarely consumed alcohol, was a nonsmoker, and had no history of tattoos, illicit drug use, or recent travel. She had no prior history of liver disease and had normal liver function tests three months before. Her medical history was notable only for oligoarticular osteoarthritis.

On presentation she was found to have a bilirubin of 162 μmol/L with a hepatocellular profile on liver function

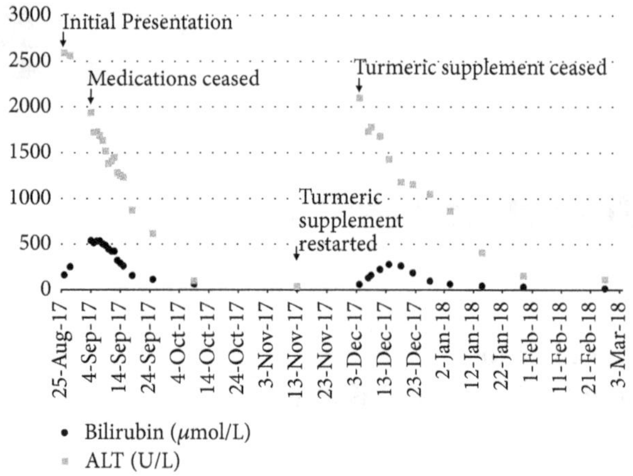

FIGURE 1: Bilirubin and ALT trend in relation to turmeric supplement use in Case 1.

tests (ALT 2591U/L, AST 1770U/L, ALP 263U/L, and GGT 370U/L) and preserved hepatic synthetic function (INR 1.0, albumin 32 g/L) (Figure 1). She was jaundiced, with no hepatomegaly or clinical features of chronic liver disease on examination. With progressive jaundice over the subsequent days she was referred to the emergency department, at which point her bilirubin peaked at 536 μmol/L.

Approximately one month prior to presentation she had commenced one tablet per day of Ancient Wisdom Modern Medicine® High Potency Turmeric (375mg curcuminoids and 4 mg black pepper per tablet), along with a flaxseed oil supplement and occasional diclofenac use for arthritic pain. Her long-term medications of cholecalciferol 50mcg daily and ascorbic acid 500 mg daily along with a levonorgestrel 52 mg intrauterine device had been unchanged for at least a year. There was no recent history of paracetamol use.

Upon admission, all oral medications and supplements were ceased. Apart from a detectable hepatitis B core antibody (surface antigen negative, surface antibody positive, and HBV viral load, not detectable), the remainder of this screen was unremarkable with negative hepatitis A, C, and E serology, negative CMV, EBV, VZV, and HSV IgM and PCR, negative liver-kidney, mitochondrial, smooth muscle, antinuclear, anti-tissue transglutaminase and anti-deamidated gliadin antibodies. Plasma eosinophil count, serum copper, and ceruloplasmin were all within normal limits, and paracetamol level was undetectable. Abdominal ultrasonography showed patent portal and hepatic veins with no biliary duct dilatation.

Due to lack of significant improvement by day four of admission (bilirubin 534μmol/L, ALT 1686U/L, ALP 252U/L, and GGT 400U/L) a liver biopsy was performed. Histology showed nonspecific inflammatory changes with generally preserved hepatic architecture and no fibrosis. A florid inflammatory cell infiltrate comprising lymphocytes, histiocytes, neutrophils, scattered eosinophils, and minimal plasma cells were noted in the portal tracts with associated interface hepatitis and reactive changes in bile duct epithelium. A drug reaction was the favored differential.

She was discharged day 12 of admission (bilirubin 260μmol/L, ALT 1232U/L) with the presumptive diagnosis of diclofenac induced liver injury. By two months after admission her LFTs had normalized (bilirubin 21μmol/L, ALT 33U/L) and she was discharged from the clinic.

At this point she recommenced the turmeric supplement (1125mg curcuminoids per day) as sole therapy for her arthritis. Three weeks later her nausea recurred and repeat liver function tests showed an acute hepatitis (ALT 2093U/L, AST 1030U/L, and bilirubin 60μmol/L). Repeat viral serology was unremarkable. She was advised to cease the turmeric supplement, and two months later her liver function tests had again normalized. The calculated Roussel UCLAF causality assessment method (RUCAM) score pertaining to the causal implication of the turmeric supplement was 9 or "highly probable", augmented by the rechallenge [8].

The turmeric supplements were sent for analysis. A sample of the supplement was pulverized, dissolved in methanol to a concentration of 1 mg/mL, and filtered through a 0.45 μm polyvinylidene fluoride filter. The filtrate was diluted and analyzed by a validated liquid chromatography quadruple time-of-flight (LC-QTOF) mass spectrometry method. Results were compared to a toxicology library containing approximately 1400 compounds, including medications, illicit drugs, and over-the-counter medicines. A detailed method is published elsewhere [9]. A further sample was analyzed by inductively coupled plasma (ICP) mass spectrometry for the presence of trace and toxic elements. The turmeric supplement tested negative for drugs, adulterants, or toxic heavy metals.

3. Case 2

A 55-year-old man of Italian background presented to his general practitioner for a routine checkup and was found to have an asymptomatic transaminitis on blood panel (ALT of 1149U/L, bilirubin 23μmol/L, ALP 145U/L, and GGT 302U/L). He occasionally drank alcohol, was a nonsmoker, and had no recent travel history or risk factors for viral hepatitis. Examination was unremarkable. His background history included idiopathic thrombocytopenic purpura, hypertension, gout, and osteoarthritis, with regular medications including long-term Telmisartan, Atenolol, and Lercanidipine. He had no known liver history with normal liver function tests one year prior. His only new medication was commencement of a turmeric supplement five months prior.

He was referred to a hepatologist and underwent a screen for causes of acute hepatitis. Apart from a positive ANA titre of 1:160, screening was unremarkable. Hepatic synthetic function was preserved with a normal INR and albumin of 45 g/L. Abdominal ultrasonography showed diffuse steatosis, but no ductal or vascular pathology. A drug reaction was suspected, and the turmeric supplement was ceased.

Close follow-up occurred over the subsequent four months. Near normalization of liver function tests occurred by one month (ALT 96U/L, bilirubin 10μmol/L) with further improvement by four months after cessation (ALT 46U/L, bilirubin 11 μmol/L). The turmeric supplement was the presumed cause of the hepatitis and as such the patient was not rechallenged. The RUCAM score was 6, or "probable"

[8]. The turmeric supplement was not known, and therefore further analysis could not be performed on the supplement.

4. Discussion

Turmeric rhizome has been used for thousands of years as a spice, a dye and for its purported medicinal properties. An increasing body of *in vivo* data and emerging clinical evidence exists for the anti-inflammatory, antioxidant, immunomodulatory, wound healing, antiproliferative, and antimicrobial activities of its major active curcuminoid constituent, curcumin, across a number of conditions [4, 10].

Products containing turmeric are generally listed by the curcuminoid content, commonly making up only 3-5% of turmeric rhizome and giving turmeric its yellow appearance [10]. Curcumin exhibits poor bioavailability, undergoing extensive first pass metabolism with doses of at least 4 g per day required for detectability in plasma [5, 6]. Formulation modifications to improve bioavailability include the use of liposomal encapsulation, nanoparticles, emulsions, and sustained released preparations [10–12]. When delivered with the alkaloid piperine, derived from *piper nigrum* (black pepper) and other piper species, plasma levels of curcumin have been shown to be augmented in humans and rats due to increased intestinal absorption and inhibition of hepatic glucuronidation by piperine [13].

Paradoxically to the presented cases, curcumin has been studied for its benefits in a number of hepatic pathologies. In humans, a combination formula of 1 g each of curcumin and *Tinospora cordifolia* has been shown to reduce hepatotoxicity in patients with active tuberculosis undergoing antituberculous treatment [14]. In another human pilot study, patients with nonalcoholic fatty liver disease randomized to 70 mg curcumin daily for 8 weeks displayed a significant reduction in sonographic liver fat content compared to placebo [15].

Regarding adverse effects, a number of severe adverse effects have been reported when given orally [16–18], topically [19], vaginally [20], and intravenously [21]. Mild liver function test derangement has been reported in approximately 5% of cases in randomized controlled trials [22], with one report of drug induced autoimmune hepatitis reported recently [22]. The potential for drug interactions has been recognized, with dose-dependent inhibition of cytochrome p450 subtypes CYP3A4 and CYP1A2 in the liver [23] and intestines [24] identified. Accordingly, the addition of curcumin to medications metabolized by CYP3A4 can lead to an increase in plasma levels, with curcumin associated with acute calcineurin inhibitor nephrotoxicity due to CYP3A4 inhibition [25].

However, while clinical studies may assess pure curcumin compounds, the products available to patients in pharmacies and nutritional food stores contain varying concentrations of curcumin plus numerous additives, potentially accounting for differing real-life risk profiles [26]. In case 1, the supplement used contained 4 mg of piperine in addition to 375 mg of curcumin. A dose of 20 mg of piperine in a similar ratio to curcumin has been shown to increase curcumin bioavailability 20-fold compared to curcumin alone due to inhibition of first pass metabolism in the intestines and liver [13]. Given the known pharmacological mechanisms of piperine and lack of any reported direct adverse effects in the literature, the hepatotoxicity in case 1 is felt more likely to be due to augmented effects of curcumin than the piperine itself. Furthermore, no other known toxic substances or toxic levels of heavy metals were found in the supplement on LC-QTOF and ICP mass spectrometry, respectively, essentially excluding a contaminant albeit for rare, unknown compounds. The curcumin supplement used in case 2 is not known, and hence comment on additives cannot be made.

The presented cases are "highly probable" and "probable," respectively, for turmeric induced hepatotoxicity based on RUCAM scores. In both cases the timing of turmeric supplement use with respect to onset and offset of liver injury was compatible, and both underwent extensive serological screening excluding other causes of deranged liver function. The rechallenge in case 1, along with the histology consistent with drug toxicity and lack of any other known toxins on further analysis of the supplement, provides an even stronger case for the turmeric inducing hepatotoxicity and negates any relationship between other medications and the liver injury.

With high community interest in HDS therapies and emerging evidenced based support for turmeric across specialties, there will likely be increasing use by patients. In this context, the reported cases of turmeric induced hepatotoxicity highlight the need for the physician to be aware of patients taking this therapy and the potential risks that exist.

Acknowledgments

The authors acknowledge Linda Graudins, convenor of The Alfred Hospital Adverse Drug Reaction Review Committee.

References

[1] N. Chalasani, R. J. Fontana, and H. L. Bonkovsky, "Causes, clinical features, and outcomes from a prospective study of drug-induced liver injury in the United States," *Gastroenterology*, vol. 135, no. 6, pp. 1924–1934.e4, 2008.

[2] G. Ostapowicz, R. J. Fontana, F. V. Schioødt et al., "Results of a prospective study of acute liver failure at 17 tertiary care centers in the United States," *Annals of Internal Medicine*, vol. 137, no. 12, pp. 947–954, 2002.

[3] T. Smith, K. Kawa, V. Eckl et al., "Herbal supplement sales in US increase 7.7% in 2016," *HerbalGram*, vol. 115, pp. 56–65, 2016.

[4] S. C. Gupta, S. Patchva, and B. B. Aggarwal, "Therapeutic roles of curcumin: lessons learned from clinical trials," *The AAPS Journal*, vol. 15, no. 1, pp. 195–218, 2013.

[5] C. D. Lao, M. T. Ruffin IV, D. Normolle et al., "Dose escalation of a curcuminoid formulation," *BMC Complementary and Alternative Medicine*, vol. 6, article 10, 2006.

[6] B. T. Kurien, D. Danda, and R. H. Scofield, "Therapeutic potential of curcumin and curcumin analogues in rheumatology," *International Journal of Rheumatic Diseases*, vol. 18, no. 6, pp. 591–593, 2015.

[7] A. S. Cheifetz, R. Gianotti, R. Luber, and P. R. Gibson, "Complementary and alternative medicines used by patients with inflammatory bowel diseases," *Gastroenterology*, vol. 152, no. 2, pp. 415–429.e15, 2017.

[8] G. Danan and C. Benichou, "Causality assessment of adverse reactions to drugs—I: a novel method based on the conclusions of international consensus meetings: application to drug-induced liver injuries," *Journal of Clinical Epidemiology*, vol. 46, no. 11, pp. 1323–1330, 1993.

[9] J. D. Pope, K. Weng Choy, O. H. Drummer, and H. G. Schneider, "Novel benzodiazepines (clonazolam and flubromazolam) identified in candy-like pills," *The Journal of Applied Laboratory Medicine*, vol. 3, no. 1, pp. 48–55, 2018.

[10] L. Braun and M. Cohen, *Herbs and Natural Supplements, Volume 2: An Evidence-Based Guide*, vol. 2, Elsevier Health Sciences, 2015.

[11] N. Pescosolido, R. Giannotti, A. M. Plateroti, A. Pascarella, and M. Nebbioso, "Curcumin: therapeutical potential in ophthalmology," *Planta Medica*, vol. 80, no. 4, pp. 249–254, 2014.

[12] D.-W. Zhang, M. Fu, S.-H. Gao, and J.-L. Liu, "Curcumin and diabetes: a systematic review," *Evidence-Based Complementary and Alternative Medicine*, vol. 2013, Article ID 636053, 16 pages, 2013.

[13] G. Shoba, D. Joy, T. Joseph, M. Majeed, R. Rajendran, and P. S. S. R. Srinivas, "Influence of piperine on the pharmacokinetics of curcumin in animals and human volunteers," *Planta Medica*, vol. 64, no. 4, pp. 353–356, 1998.

[14] M. R. Adhvaryu, N. M. Reddy, and B. C. Vakharia, "Prevention of hepatotoxicity due to anti tuberculosis treatment: a novel integrative approach," *World Journal of Gastroenterology*, vol. 14, no. 30, pp. 4753–4762, 2008.

[15] S. Rahmani, S. Asgary, G. Askari et al., "Treatment of non-alcoholic fatty liver disease with curcumin: a randomized placebo-controlled trial," *Phytotherapy Research*, vol. 30, no. 9, pp. 1540–1548, 2016.

[16] L. Horev, Y. Ramot, and L. Klapholz, "Yellow feet in a patient with breast and thyroid carcinoma, due to oral intake of turmeric," *Drug Safety - Case Reports*, vol. 2, no. 1, p. 4, 2015.

[17] S.-W. Lee, S.-S. Nah, J.-S. Byon et al., "Transient complete atrioventricular block associated with curcumin intake," *International Journal of Cardiology*, vol. 150, no. 2, pp. e50–e52, 2011.

[18] E. J. Kim, D. J. Lewis, B. S. Dabaja, and M. Duvic, "Curcumin for the treatment of tumor-stage mycosis fungoides," *Dermatologic Therapy*, vol. 30, no. 4, p. e12511, 2017.

[19] J. Huber, R. Deshazo, D. Powell, K. Duffy, and C. Hull, "Erythema multiforme-like allergic contact dermatitis to turmeric essential oil," *Dermatitis*, vol. 27, no. 6, pp. 385-386, 2016.

[20] L. Gattoc, P. M. Frew, S. N. Thomas et al., "Phase I dose-escalation trial of intravaginal curcumin in women for cervical dysplasia," *Open Access Journal of Clinical Trials*, vol. 9, pp. 1–10, 2017.

[21] D. R. Lasoff, F. L. Cantrell, and B. T. Ly, "Death associated with intravenous turmeric (Curcumin) preparation," *Clinical Toxicology*, vol. 56, no. 5, pp. 384-385, 2018.

[22] A. L. Lukefahr, S. McEvoy, C. Alfafara, and J. L. Funk, "Drug-induced autoimmune hepatitis associated with turmeric dietary supplement use," *BMJ Case Reports*, vol. 2018, 2018.

[23] T. Sugiyama, J.-I. Nagata, A. Yamagishi et al., "Selective protection of curcumin against carbon tetrachloride-induced inactivation of hepatic cytochrome P450 isozymes in rats," *Life Sciences*, vol. 78, no. 19, pp. 2188–2193, 2006.

[24] W. Zhang, T. M. C. Tan, and L.-Y. Lim, "Impact of curcumin-induced changes in P-glycoprotein and CYP3A expression on the pharmacokinetics of peroral celiprolol and midazolam in rats," *Drug Metabolism and Disposition*, vol. 35, no. 1, pp. 110–115, 2007.

[25] A. Nayeri, S. Wu, E. Adams et al., "Acute calcineurin inhibitor nephrotoxicity secondary to turmeric intake: a case report," *Transplantation Proceedings*, vol. 49, no. 1, pp. 198–200, 2017.

[26] P. R. Holt, "Curcumin for inflammatory bowel disease: a caution," *Clinical Gastroenterology and Hepatology*, vol. 14, no. 1, p. 168, 2016.

6

Acute Hepatitis Secondary to the Use of *Ilex paraguariensis* (Mate Tea): A Case Report and Review of Literature

Eduardo A. Rodriguez, Raquel Teixeira Yokoda, David E. Payton, Rish Pai, and Thomas J. Byrne

Mayo Clinic Arizona, 5777 E Mayo Blvd, Phoenix, AZ 85054, USA

Correspondence should be addressed to Eduardo A. Rodriguez; erodrigu18@yahoo.com

Academic Editor: Mauro Vigano

Drug induced liver injury is a very frequent cause of hepatotoxicity and within that group, herbal and dietary supplements are a well described subcategory. The following clinical vignette describes the case of a young man with acute hepatitis secondary to the use of *Ilex paraguariensis*, also known as yerba mate, which is a herbal product commonly drunk in South America. This is the first written case of mate tea induced hepatotoxicity.

1. Introduction

Drug induced liver injury (DILI) can occur following the use of both prescription and/or over the counter medications. Even though it is not as frequent as other more common causes of liver injury such as viral hepatitis, it remains to be an important differential diagnosis category that the smart clinician should always consider. Within this category herbal and dietary supplements (HDS) are a frequent cause of hepatotoxicity [1]. The following clinical vignette describes the case of acute hepatitis secondary to the use of *Ilex paraguariensis*, also known as yerba mate.

2. Case Presentation

A 21-year-old American gentleman without significant past medical history was transferred from northern Argentina for further investigation of elevated liver enzymes. He had spent the last four months over there as part of his church mission and during the latter two weeks of vacation had initially noted mildly icteric sclera, followed by generalized malaise, jaundice, pruritus, and dark urine. He denied fever, chills, diaphoresis, alcohol intake, over the counter medications, illicit drug use including IV drugs, and recent sexual encounters. He also denied other abdominal complaints such as pain, bloating, nausea, vomiting, and diarrhea. Initial workup abroad included negative viral hepatitis serologies, negative autoimmune markers as well as negative magnetic resonance cholangiopancreatography. Due to the lack of improvement, the family of the patient decided to return him to the U.S. for further evaluation.

On presentation his vital signs were stable. His physical exam was normal except for jaundice. He did not have any neurological deficit. The laboratory findings were as follows: total bilirubin, 32.9 mg/dL: direct bilirubin > 18.0 mg/dL, alanine aminotransferase (ALT), 2685 U/L; aspartate aminotransferase (AST), 1842 U/L, alkaline phosphatase (ALP) 129 U/L. RUCAM score was 65.4. He had negative viral hepatitis markers including hepatitis A, B, C, E, cytomegalovirus, herpes simplex, adenovirus, and varicella zoster virus.

Autoimmune panel including anti smooth muscle antibody (ASMA), anti nuclear antibody (ANA), anti mitochondrial antibody (AMA) and LKM1 antibody were all negative/unremarkable. Further serologies for *Entamoeba histolitica* and *Schistosoma mansoni* were also obtained given the geographical location of his mission, and these were negative. Urine toxicology screen was negative for alcohol, amphetamines, barbiturates, benzodiazepenes, cocaine, opiates, and tetrahydrocannabinol. Acetaminophen level in blood was undetectable (Table 1).

TABLE 1: Laboratory data on admission.

Complete blood count		
White blood cell count	5900	/μL
Hemoglobin	14.2	g/dL
Platelets	350	$10^3/\mu L$
Coagulation		
PT	13.6	sec
INR	1.2	
Complete metabolic panel		
Albumin	4.7	g/dL
Total bilirubin	32.9	mg/dL
Direct bilirubin	>18	mg/dL
AST	1842	U/L
ALT	2685	U/L
ALP	129	U/L
Lipase	20	U/L
BUN	7.5	mg/dL
Creatinine	0.69	mg/dL
eGFR	>90	mL/min
Immunology		
ANA	0.4	Dil
AMA	<0.1	Index
anti-LKM1 Ab	<5.0	Index
ASMA	Negative	Index
Alpha-antitrypsin	177	mg/dL
Infectious markers		
HCVAb	Negative	
HCV-RNA	Undetectable	
HBsAg	Negative	
HBcgM Ab	Negative	
HAV-IgM	Negative	
HEV-IgM	Negative	
HTLV-1 Ab	Negative	
EBV-IgG	Negative	
EBV-IgM	Negative	
CMV-IgG	Negative	
CMV-IgM	Negative	
VZV-IgG	Negative	
VZV-IgM	Negative	
HSV-IgG	Negative	
HSV-IgM	Negative	
Adenovirus PCR	Negative	
Toxicology and drug testing		
Acetominophen, S	<5.0	mcg/mL
Ethanol, U	Undetectable	
Amphetamines, U	Undetectable	
Barbiturates, U	Undetectable	
Benzodiazepines, U	Undetectable	
Cocaine, U	Undetectable	
Methadone metabolite, U	Undetectable	
Opiates, U	Undetectable	
Tetrahydrocannabinnol, U	Undetectable	

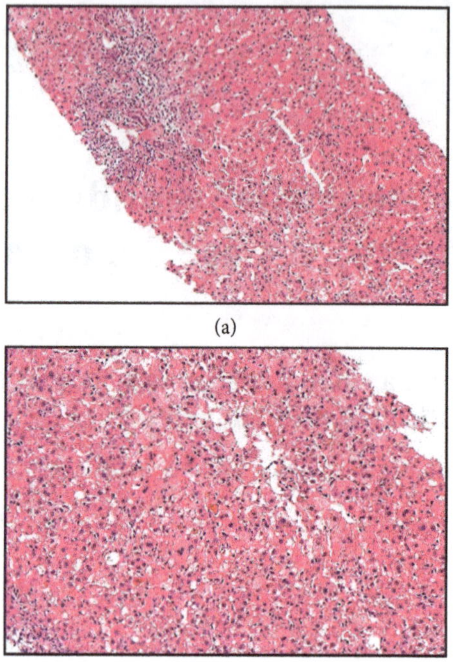

(a)

(b)

FIGURE 1: Acute cholestatic hepatitis. (a) Portal inflammation with bile ductular reaction and periportal hepatocyte injury (H&E 100X). (b) Lobular disarray characterized by lobular inflammation, acidophil bodies, and cholestasis (H&E 200X).

Upon further questioning he reported daily yerba mate tea during the four months he spent in Argentina, sometimes twice a day and symptoms began during the last two weeks he stayed there. He continued drinking the tea until the last day of his vacations, before coming back to the United States. He also added the fact that all of his co-workers had drunk the same tea on a daily basis however no one else developed similar complaints.

In order to further investigate the etiology of his acute hepatitis an ultrasound-guided liver biopsy was obtained. Histological evaluation revealed an acute cholestatic hepatitis pattern, without typical features for autoimmune hepatitis. It demonstrated expanded portal tracts with a mixed inflammatory cell infiltrate composed of lymphocytes as well as occasional eosinophils and neutrophils. A mild bile ductular reaction was also present at the periphery of these portal areas, likely in response to the hepatocellular injury and likely explaining the elevated RUCAM score. Significant lobular disarray with numerous foci of lobular inflammation and acidophil bodies was appreciated. Iron stain demonstrated scattered Kupffer cell iron. PAS with diastase stain was negative for intracytoplasmic globules. Plasma cells were not prominent. The trichrome and reticulin stains confirmed the absence of fibrosis. Overall, the morphologic changes noted were thought to be found most commonly in the setting of medication or toxin-induced injury (including herbal medication) (Figure 1).

Even though liver markers initially rose, after two days hepatic panel numbers started to downtrend, and the patient was discharged from the hospital. In the outpatient setting

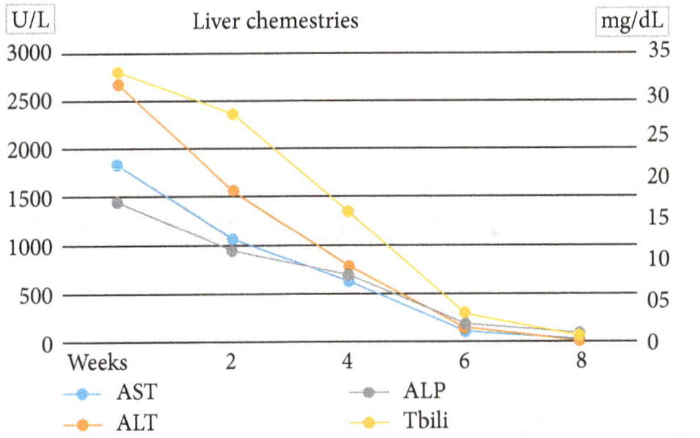

FIGURE 2: Trend of liver enzymes during admission and in the outpatient setting.

patient was monitored closely with liver panel labs. After two months of close follow up, all numbers came back to normal levels, and patient was discharged from clinic (Figure 2). Except for the temporary jaundice and malaise, he remained asymptomatic throughout.

3. Discussion

HDS liver injury shares the same underlying biochemical process with DILI in which the foreign chemical needs to be metabolized in order to be eliminated. It is during that process that potential hepatotoxic metabolites can be produced and cause injury in susceptible patients [2]. Most cases of herbal hepatotoxicity reflect an idiosyncratic pattern, which means reactions can occur unpredictably in the population. The other group includes those products that cause intrinsic injury, which means predictable reactions in humans or in animal models when enough dose of the offending agent is administered. Acetaminophen is the prototypic cause of intrinsic injury [1]. In order to consider DILI, other more common etiologies should be rule ruled out first. In this case, we performed a thorough evaluation including viral hepatitis panel as well as autoimmune markers due to the significantly elevated transaminases initially noted, and given the young age of the patient.

After an extensive evaluation which included a liver biopsy that ultimately suggested medication/toxin (including possible HDS) effect, we consider that the main cause of the acute hepatitis in this case was *Ilex paraguariensis,* also known as yerba mate, which the patient drank while in Argentina. The present case describes the first reported case of HDS injury secondary to the use of yerba mate, a common herbal product that is drunk as a tea in the southern portion of South America, namely Argentina, Brazil, Paraguay, and Uruguay [3]. In these countries the leaves and stems of the plant are processed in the production of several types of beverages including mate or chimarrao (warm), as well as various types of teas and carbonated drinks. Some of the attributed biological properties include an antioxidant and hypocholesterolemic capacity as well as possible cancer prevention properties [4]. It is also possible that some of these drinks might have the presence of adulterants that may be incorporated into the final product, either intentionally or unintentionally.

Pathogenesis is difficult to characterize in HDS injury as this is mainly a human and not animal process and thus experimental data on animals are limited. However, some of the available experimental studies have described an intrinsic pattern of HDS with the possible involvement of unsaturated pyrrolizidine alkaloids (PAs). These can damage the endothelial cells of the liver and reduce the sinusoidal blood flow, causing clinical features of hepatic sinusoidal obstruction syndrome [2]. In our case, the hepatotoxic pattern was cholestatic which correlates with a possible hepatic sinusoidal obstruction syndrome-like presentation.

Liver injury from HDS is a growing and challenging problem. Further clinical and basic science research as well as better monitoring and regulatory efforts is needed in order to insure consumer safety [5].

References

[1] N. P. Chalasani, P. H. Hayashi, H. L. Bonkovsky, V. J. Navarro, W. M. Lee, and R. J. Fontana, "ACG clinical guideline: the diagnosis and management of idiosyncratic drug-induced liver Injury," *American Journal of Gastroenterology*, vol. 109, no. 7, pp. 950–966, 2014.

[2] C. Frenzel and R. Teschke, "Herbal hepatotoxicity: clinical characteristics and listing compilation," *International Journal of Molecular Sciences*, vol. 17, no. 5, p. 588, 2016.

[3] C. I. Heck and E. G. de Mejia, "Yerba mate tea (*Ilex paraguariensis*): a comprehensive review on chemistry, health implications, and technological considerations," *Journal of Food Science*, vol. 72, no. 9, pp. R138–R151, 2007.

[4] A. T. Valduga, I. L. Goncalves, E. Magri, and J. R. Delalibera Finzer, "Chemistry, pharmacology and new trends in traditional functional and medicinal beverages," *Food Research International*, vol. 120, pp. 478–503, 2019.

[5] V. J. Navarro, I. Khan, E. Bjornsson, L. B. Seeff, J. Serrano, and J. H. Hoofnagle, "Liver injury from herbal and dietary supplements," *Hepatology*, vol. 65, no. 1, pp. 363–373, 2017.

7

Benefit of *N*-Acetylcysteine in Postoperative Hepatic Dysfunction: Case Report and Review of Literature

Deanna K. Bauerlein,[1] Hashem N. Akbar,[2] Erik C. von Rosenvinge,[3] Nora D. Loughry,[4] and Preeti R. John[3]

[1]*Veterans Affairs New Jersey Healthcare System, USA*
[2]*Tufts University Medical Center, USA*
[3]*Veterans Affairs Maryland Healthcare System, University of Maryland School of Medicine, USA*
[4]*Emory University School of Medicine, USA*

Correspondence should be addressed to Preeti R. John; preeti.john@va.gov

Academic Editor: Melanie Deutsch

N-Acetylcysteine (NAC) is reported to have multiple clinical applications in addition to being the specific antidote for acetaminophen toxicity. NAC stimulates glutathione biosynthesis, promotes detoxification, and acts directly as a scavenger of free radicals. It is a powerful antioxidant and a potential treatment option for diseases characterized by the generation of free oxygen radicals. We present a case of postoperative hepatic dysfunction of multifactorial etiology in a patient with therapeutic acetaminophen levels, where hepatic function improved considerably following administration of intravenous NAC. This case suggests that NAC should be considered for treatment of acute liver dysfunction in the postoperative setting, even in the absence of elevated acetaminophen levels.

1. Introduction

N-Acetylcysteine (NAC) is the antidote for acetaminophen (APAP) toxicity and has been used as a beneficial drug treatment for liver disorders. Its use and benefits have been reported in multiple other conditions and is attributed to the fact that it increases levels of glutathione, the body's major antioxidant [1].

We present a patient who developed hepatic dysfunction of multifactorial etiology in the postoperative period, whose hepatic function improved soon after administration of intravenous (IV) NAC. The patient had hepatitis C virus (HCV), alcohol use disorder (AUD) with liver function tests suggestive of alcoholic hepatitis, and borderline malnutrition. He received oral APAP for postoperative analgesia. It is believed that these factors combined to cause the development of acute hepatic dysfunction postoperatively. Following NAC administration, hepatic function improved rapidly.

2. Case Description

A 58-year-old male underwent elective left lower lobe resection via video-assisted thoracoscopic surgery (VATS) for a 9 mm lung nodule suspicious for malignancy. The patient's past medical history included hypertension, gastroesophageal reflux disease, depression, anxiety, chronic hepatitis C, and AUD. Liver biopsy and Fibroscan had not been performed to assess for cirrhosis, preoperatively. His last admission was six months prior to surgery for alcohol withdrawal syndrome. The patient reported drinking 10 beers a day with his last drink on the day before surgery. He denied tobacco, but reported using marijuana. He had no known allergies or adverse drug reactions.

His baseline liver function tests (LFTs) before surgery were: AST 111 U/L, ALT 50 U/L, total bilirubin (TBili) 0.5 mg/dl, INR 1.11 (Table 1). AST/ALT ratio suggested alcoholic hepatitis. Nutritional status was marginal, with albumin 3.1 g/dL. Platelet count was 120,000 k/cmm. Outpatient medications included aripiprazole, sertraline, and a multivitamin.

There were no hypotensive episodes or other complications during VATS. Blood loss was less than 50 ml. He received general anesthesia with sevofluorane. There were no other concomitant medications given intraoperatively or postoperatively that could have contributed to deteriorating hepatic function.

The following analgesics were given to optimize pain control postoperatively: APAP 1 g orally every six hours for three

Table 1: Pertinent laboratory values.

Labs (reference range)	Prior to surgery	POD 1	POD 2	POD 3	POD 4	POD 5	POD 6	POD 7
AST (0–37 U/L)	111			3169	5417	3318	1432	863
ALT (17–63 U/L)	50			758	1372	1209	766	607
Total bilirubin (0–1.3 mg/dl)	0.5			2.8	3.5	3.6	3.5	3.3
INR (0.83–1.18)	1.11				2.83	2.23	1.24	1.24
Alk phos (38–126 U/L)				110	119	104	137	215
Albumin (3.5–4.8 g/dl)				3.4	2.6	2.5	2.4	2.7
BUN (6–20 mg/dl)	4	3	6	9	10	8	5	2
Cr (0.9–1.3 mg/dl)	1.36	0.86	1.03	1.08	1.28	0.94	0.79	0.78
Glucose (70–105 mg/dl)	79	105	82	80	58	112	95	99
NH_3 (9–35 mcMol/l)						52		
Lactate (0.5–2 mmol/L)					6.1	3.1		

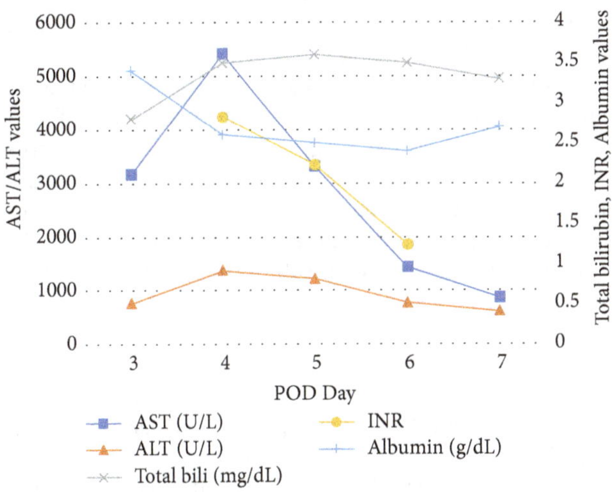

Figure 1: Selected laboratory trends.

days, oxycodone 5–10 mg orally every four hours as needed, and hydromorphone 0.5 mg IV every four hours as needed for breakthrough pain.

On postoperative day 2 (POD 2), the patient remained hemodynamically stable. On POD 3, he developed nausea and discomfort in the right upper quadrant. LFTs were checked and noted to be elevated: AST 3169 U/L, ALT 758 U/L, TBili 2.8 mg/dL (Table 1, Figure 1). He had received a total of 9 g of APAP over a period of 3 days, with no more than 4 g over a 24-hour period. APAP was discontinued at this time due to LFT elevation and concern for iatrogenic hepatotoxicity.

On POD 4, LFTs peaked: AST 5417 U/L, ALT 1372 U/L, TBili 3.5 mg/dL; albumin 2.6 g/dL, INR 2.83, lactate 6.1 mmol/L; and glucose 58 mg/dl. Renal function and arterial blood gas remained within normal limits. Urine toxicology screen was negative. The patient reported right-sided abdominal pain and nausea, and had two episodes of emesis. He was noted to have scleral icterus and grade I encephalopathy. He had a syncopal episode secondary to hypoglycemia, which promptly responded to intravenous dextrose administration. A CT scan of the abdomen and pelvis was done, revealing fatty liver without portal vein thrombosis or other biliary tract abnormalities. Ischemic hepatitis (shock liver) was thought unlikely as the patient was never hypotensive.

The hepatology service was consulted and a diagnosis of acetaminophen-induced hepatotoxicity was suspected based on the clinical picture, laboratory values, and negative imaging. However, APAP level was within normal limits at 12.9 mg/L (normal therapeutic range 5–20 mg/L) [2]. Despite a nontoxic APAP level, NAC was recommended. On POD 4, he was treated with 3 weight-based doses of IV NAC: 9 g (150 mg/kg) over one hour, then 3 g (50 mg/kg) over four hours, followed by 6 g (100 mg/kg) over sixteen hours. A one-time dose of oral vitamin K 10 mg was also administered.

On POD 5, APAP level decreased to 0.5 mg/L and LFTs were noted to be declining. He was discharged on POD 7, at which time he was clinically stable and asymptomatic. LFTs continued to improve and the patient's renal function remained at baseline and within normal limits. One month after discharge, LFTs further decreased to: AST 427 U/L, ALT 82 U/L, TBili 2 mg/dL.

Throughout the patient's hospital stay, renal function remained at baseline (0.8–1.4 mg/dl).

3. Discussion

This case report describes the beneficial effect of IV NAC when used in the postoperative period, in a patient who developed hepatic dysfunction following oral APAP use for analgesia. Our patient had preexisting risk factors for acetaminophen-induced hepatotoxicity including HCV, AUD with possible alcoholic hepatitis, and malnutrition. Expert opinion recommends limitation of APAP dosage to 2 g/day in patients with chronic or acute alcohol abuse [2]. However, this patient received APAP 4 g/day in adherence with current FDA recommendations for APAP use in adults. When measured, his APAP level was within normal limits at 12.9 mg/L. Therapeutic APAP blood concentration is ≤20 mg/L and toxic blood concentrations are typically in the range of 25–150 mg/L [3]. Although it is unlikely that APAP toxicity was the sole cause of his acute liver dysfunction, it likely contributed to it.

Treatment with NAC was recommended by hepatologists based on documented benefits of NAC use in liver dysfunction caused by various etiologies. Regardless of the etiology of acute liver dysfunction in this patient who underwent surgery, the use of IV NAC in the postoperative period was associated with rapidly improving liver function. The discontinuation of APAP also likely contributed to improving liver function.

There are only two case reports in the published literature that we are aware of, describing beneficial effects of IV NAC when used in the postoperative period in patients who developed hepatic dysfunction associated with APAP use. Both describe patients who developed hepatic dysfunction associated with intravenous (IV) APAP use. In this case report, we describe hepatic dysfunction associated with oral APAP use in the postoperative period.

The first case report describes a 36-year-old woman who underwent laparoscopic appendectomy and received a total of 16 g of IV APAP for pain control over 5 days in the peri-operative period. APAP level was 34 mg/L [4]. The patient had transaminase elevations that resolved with IV NAC administration. Malnutrition was the only known hepatotoxic risk factor in this patient [4].

The second report describes a 92-year-old female who received a total of 13 g of IV APAP (1 g every six hours) for pain control after laparoscopic reduction of internal hernias, which resulted in elevated LFTs. APAP level was within normal range. She had no history of hepatic disease or alcohol abuse. Her advanced age, postoperative status and likely catabolic state were thought to have caused susceptibility to acetaminophen-induced hepatotoxicity. LFTs improved with the administration of IV NAC [5].

NAC is a potential treatment option for both acute and chronic diseases characterized by the generation of free oxygen radicals [1]. There are several reports in the literature about benefits of NAC treatment for APAP toxicity [3, 6] and treatment of this condition constitutes its only FDA approved use in liver dysfunction.

NAC has antioxidant properties, which has been attributed to its role as a precursor of glutathione [7]. Oxidative stress is one of the pathogenetic mechanisms causing liver damage. It contributes to initiation and progression of steatosis, fibrosis, and hepatic dysfunction in a variety of liver disorders [8].

NAC stimulates glutathione biosynthesis by providing cysteine, which is involved in a rate-limiting step in glutathione synthesis. Glutathione is essential for the body's antioxidant defenses [9].

In addition to oxidative stress, nitrosative stress mechanisms are involved in the pathogenesis of chronic liver diseases. In the presence of reactive oxygen species, nitric oxide forms peroxynitrites which have deleterious effects [10]. Nitric oxide contributes to liver ischemia-reperfusion injury. Inhibition of inducible nitric oxide synthase (iNOS) shows beneficial effects and NAC modulates expression of iNOS in human hepatocytes stimulated by proinflammatory cytokines [10]. This may be the basis of beneficial effects of NAC in chronic liver diseases [10].

NAC has been used successfully for chronic liver disorders such as chronic hepatitis C [11, 12].

The American Association for the Study of Liver Diseases (AASLD) recommends NAC for all cases of acute liver failure, even if APAP is not the cause [13]. They suggest NAC administration if increasing aminotransferases are suggestive of liver injury, even if serum APAP level or amount of APAP ingested does not indicate APAP toxicity. This recommendation is based on the fact that NAC has the potential to improve liver function in nonacetaminophen-induced liver dysfunction [13].

A prospective, double-blind randomized controlled trial (RCT) concluded that IV NAC increased the transplant-free survival rate in patients who had nonacetaminophen-induced acute liver failure with coma grade I-II compared to placebo [14].

Another prospective, double-blind RCT showed that IV NAC improved hepatic function as shown by decreasing ALT and bilirubin values (but not AST, INR, or creatinine) and decreasing transplant rates in patients with nonacetaminophen-induced acute liver failure with coma grade I-II compared to placebo [15].

A third prospective, RCT demonstrated that IV NAC decreases mortality and hospital length of stay compared to placebo in patients with nonacetaminophen-induced acute liver failure with coma grade I–IV [16].

Furthermore, NAC may play a role in preventing postoperative complications. One study on the prevention of acute renal failure after cardiac surgery showed marked reduction in renal failure in a subgroup of patients placed on cardiopulmonary bypass, who received NAC [17]. Another small study of twenty-two patients concluded that NAC may be useful in preventing pulmonary complications in patients undergoing esophagectomy for cancer [18].

Multiple other benefits of NAC supplementation in various disorders have been supported by varying levels of scientific evidence. These include treatment of pulmonary conditions (chronic obstructive pulmonary disease, chronic bronchitis, asthma, idiopathic pulmonary fibrosis, influenza virus, renal conditions (contrast induced nephropathy prevention), and treatment of infertility in patients with polycystic ovarian syndrome [1]. There have also been reports about the benefit of NAC in some psychiatric disorders such as schizophrenia and bipolar disorder [9].

With regard to drug safety, NAC is relatively safe. In its oral form, mild gastrointestinal symptoms are the most common side effects [9]. When given intravenously at high doses (>3 g/day), anaphylactoid reactions can occur.

4. Conclusion

Intravenous NAC was beneficial in this patient who developed acute hepatic dysfunction in the postoperative period. Given its favorable risk/benefit ratio in both acute and chronic hepatic dysfunction as reflected in multiple published reports, the use of intravenous NAC should be considered in postoperative patients with worsening hepatic dysfunction of multifactorial etiology.

References

[1] P. J. Millea, "*N*-Acetylcysteine: multiple clinical applications," *American Family Physician*, vol. 80, no. 3, pp. 265–269, 2009.

[2] N. Chandok and K. D. S. Watt, "Pain management in the cirrhotic patient," *Mayo Clinic Proceedings*, vol. 85, no. 5, pp. 451–458, 2010.

[3] K. J. Heard, "Acetylcysteine for acetaminophen poisoning," *The New England Journal of Medicine*, vol. 359, no. 3, pp. 285–292, 2008.

[4] P. J. Lee, M. Shen, S. Wang et al., "Possible hepatoxicty associated with intravenous acetaminophen in a 36-year-old female patient," *P&T*, vol. 40, no. 2, pp. 125–132, 2015.

[5] S. A. Seifert, D. Kovnat, V. E. Anderson, J. L. Green, R. C. Dart, and K. J. Heard, "Acute hepatoxicity associated with therapeutic doses of intravenous acetaminophen," *Clinical Toxicology*, vol. 54, no. 3, pp. 282–285, 2016.

[6] J. L. Green, K. J. Heard, K. M. Reynolds, and D. Albert, "Oral and intravenous acetylcysteine for treatment of acetaminophen toxicity: a systematic review and meta-analysis," *The Western Journal of Emergency Medicine*, vol. 14, no. 3, pp. 218–226, 2013.

[7] V. Mokhtari, P. Afsharian, M. Shahhoseini, S. M. Kalantar, and A. Moini, "A review on various uses of *N*-acetylcysteine," *Cell Journal*, vol. 19, no. 1, pp. 11–17, 2017.

[8] J. Medina and R. Moreno-Otero, "Pathophysiological basis for antioxidant therapy in chronic liver disease," *Drugs*, vol. 65, no. 17, pp. 2445–2461, 2005.

[9] S. Dodd, O. Dean, D. L. Copolov, G. S. Malhi, and M. Berk, "*N*-acetylcysteine for antioxidant therapy: pharmacology and clinical utility," *Expert Opinion on Biological Therapy*, vol. 8, no. 12, pp. 1955–1962, 2008.

[10] R. Moreno-Otero, "Hepatoprotective effects of antioxidants in chronic hepatitis C," *World Journal of Gastroenterology*, vol. 16, no. 15, pp. 1937–1938, 2010.

[11] T. Nabi, S. Nabi, N. Rafiq, and A. Shah, "Role of *N*-acetylcysteine treatment in nonacetaminophen-induced acute liver failure: a prospective study," *Saudi Journal of Gastroenterology*, vol. 23, no. 3, pp. 169–175, 2017.

[12] A. Melhem, M. Stern, O. Shibolet et al., "Treatment of CHC virus infection via antioxidants: results of a phase I clinical trial," *Journal of Clinical Gastroenterology*, vol. 39, no. 8, pp. 737–742, 2005.

[13] W. M. Lee, A. M. Larson, and R. T. Stravitz, "AASLD position paper: the management of acute liver failure: update 2011," pp. 1–88, 2011, https://www.aasld.org/sites/default/files/2019-06/AcuteLiverFailureUpdate201journalformat1.pdf, February 12, 2019.

[14] W. M. Lee, L. S. Hynan, L. Rossaro et al., "Intravenous *N*-acetylcysteine improves transplant-free survival in early stage nonacetaminophen acute liver failure," *Gastroenterology*, vol. 137, no. 3, pp. 856–864, 2009.

[15] S. Singh, L. S. Hynan, and W. M. Lee, "Improvements in hepatic biomarkers are associated with clinical benefit of intravenous *N*-acetylcysteine in early stage nonacetaminophen acute liver failure," *Digestive Diseases and Sciences*, vol. 58, no. 5, pp. 1397–1402, 2013.

[16] G. K. Glantzounis, H. J. Salacinski, W. Yang, B. R. Davidson, and A. M. Seifalian, "The contemporary role of antioxidant therapy in attenuating liver ischemia reperfusion injury: a review," *Liver Transplantation*, vol. 11, no. 9, pp. 1031–1047, 2005.

[17] E. Sisillo, R. Ceriani, F. Bortone et al., "NAC for prevention of acute renal failure in patients with chronic renal insufficiency undergoing cardiac surgery: a prospective, randomized clinical trial," *Critical Care Medicine*, vol. 36, no. 1, pp. 81–86, 2008.

[18] U. Zingg, C. Hofer, K. Seifert, B. U. Metzger, and A. Zollinger, "High dose NAC to prevent pulmonary complications in partial or total transthoracic esophagectomy: results of a prospective observational study," *Diseases of the Esophagus*, vol. 20, no. 5, pp. 399–405, 2007.

8

Autoimmune Hepatitis (AIH) in Acquired Immune Deficiency Syndrome (AIDS): A Case Report and Review of Literature

Jordan Roussel,[1] Sudha Pandit,[2] Paul Jordan,[2] Moheb Boktor,[2] Kurt Knowles,[3] Nester Dela Cruz,[3] and Hrishikesh Samant[2]

[1]*Department of Internal Medicine, Louisiana State University Health Sciences Center, Shreveport, LA, USA*
[2]*Department of Gastroenterology and Hepatology, Louisiana State University Health Sciences Center, Shreveport, LA, USA*
[3]*Department of Pathology, Louisiana State University Health Sciences Center, Shreveport, LA, USA*

Correspondence should be addressed to Hrishikesh Samant; samanthrishi@gmail.com

Academic Editor: Melanie Deutsch

The common causes of abnormal liver chemistries in human immunodeficiency virus (HIV) infected patients are multifactorial. Diagnosis of autoimmune hepatitis (AIH) in HIV infected patients is intriguing but data is scarce. Unmasking of AIH during immune reconstitution in HIV patients after starting antiretroviral therapy is reported but not with advanced acquired immunodeficiency syndrome (AIDS). Here we present a fascinating case of 32-year-old African-American man with advanced AIDS who presented with elevated transaminases. He was diagnosed with AIH before starting antiretroviral therapy and successfully treated with prednisolone and azathioprine with antiretroviral therapy despite very low CD4 count.

1. Introduction

Patients with human immunodeficiency virus (HIV) infection have a wide variety of causes for elevated liver chemistries. Some common etiologies are coinfections such as hepatitis B (HBV), Hepatitis C (HCV), opportunistic infection, and alcoholic and nonalcoholic fatty liver disease, and less common causes include cholecystitis, AIDS related cholangiopathy, and antiretroviral drug toxicity. Autoimmune hepatitis (AIH) is rarely reported as cause of liver function derangement in HIV patient. The relation between HIV and AIH is interesting. The pathophysiology of AIH begins with loss of self-tolerance of T-lymphocytes causing an overwhelming immune cascade leading to autoantibodies to liver cells [1]. On the other hand, HIV is a disease that causes decreased activity of the immune system by infecting and destroying T-lymphocytes and also sometimes developing various antibodies by polyclonal stimulation of B cells. The diagnosis of AIDS is made when a patient with an HIV infection becomes significantly immunocompromised with a severely reduced CD4 count. This very low CD4 cells and severely immunocompromised state is the basis of why developing AIH in a patient with AIDS may be extremely rare. AIH with advanced AIDS, to our knowledge, has never been reported. Furthermore, treating AIH with high dose immunosuppressive medication is usually risky in AIDS patient. We herein report the case of advanced AIDS patient who was diagnosed with AIH before starting antiretroviral therapy and successfully achieved remission of transaminitis on standard immunosuppressive therapy for AIH and antiretroviral therapy without any side effects.

2. Case Presentation

Our patient is a 32-year-old African-American male with past medical history of HIV/AIDS, hypertension, and focal segmental glomerulosclerosis (FSGS) related chronic kidney disease stage 3, who presented to our institution complaining of a two-week history of generalized abdominal pain, associated with jaundice, pruritus, nausea, and vomiting. The patient's HIV/AIDS status was significant for a very low CD4 count of 11 cells/mm3 with a viral load of 64000 IU/ml. Patient had history of nonadherence to antiretroviral therapy and was not taking his medications since his diagnosis of HIV. Review of systems was otherwise normal. Travel history or use of nonprescription medications was negative. Family history was

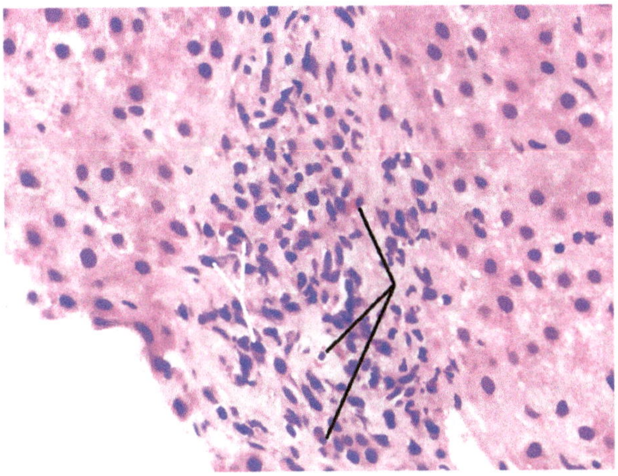

FIGURE 1: Liver biopsy. The portal triad demonstrates plasma cells (white arrows) and eosinophils (black arrows) consistent with autoimmune hepatitis. H&E stain, high power (400X).

noncontributory. Surgical history included a knee surgery. He had 20-pack year history of cigarette smoking but denied alcohol, illicit drug use, or hepatotoxic medications. Pertinent positives in the physical examination included icteric sclera, hepatomegaly 2 cm below costal margin, and jaundiced skin. Admission labs revealed abnormal liver chemistries: aspartate transferase (AST) 255 U/L, alanine transferase (ALT) 461 U/L, alkaline phosphatase 123 U/L, gamma glutamyl transferase 34 U/L, and total bilirubin 17.4 mg/dL. Viral hepatitis workup was negative which included IgM/Total hepatitis A, IgM hepatitis E, anti-HCV antibody, HCV RNA, HEV RNA, hepatitis B surface antigen, IgM/total hepatitis B core antibody, and HBV DNA viral load. Other infectious disease workups including cytomegalovirus (CMV), Herpes Simplex (HSV), Epstein Barr (EBV), syphilis, and varicella were all negative. Ultrasound liver revealed hepatomegaly. MRCP done for borderline elevated alkaline phosphatase and pruritis but was negative for any biliary pathology. Urine drug screen was negative. Amongst autoimmune markers, anti-nuclear antibody (ANA), and liver kidney microsomal (LKM)-1, anti-mitochondrial antibody (AMA) was negative, but anti-smooth muscle antibody (SMA) titers by ELISA came positive at 1:84 with elevated immunoglobulin G levels of 3540 g/L (twice upper limit of normal levels). Further evaluation with core liver biopsy revealed chronic lymphoplasmacytic inflammation with abundant plasma cells and minimal interface activity without bile duct damage, necrosis, or fibrosis suggestive of autoimmune hepatitis (Figure 1). Patient fulfilled the Revised Original Score for Autoimmune Hepatitis with score of 20 giving diagnosis as "Definite for AIH" [16, 17]. The patient was started on standard dose of highly active antiretroviral treatment (HAART) and prednisone 30 mg oral daily with close monitoring of liver enzymes. After starting prednisone, the patient improved symptomatically with improvement in liver functions and immunoglobulin levels. Patients CD4 count remained < 50 during the period of liver function improvement. Azathioprine was introduced gradually at 1-1.5 mg/kg on week 2 after confirming normal thiopurine methyltransferase (TPMT) phenotype and subsequently steroid was tapered off successfully. Patient's liver enzymes normalized completely after 9 months with continued azathioprine and HAART.

3. Discussion

Autoimmune hepatitis is a rare cause of transaminitis in HIV infected patients with the more common causes being a coinfection such as HBV and HCV due to the same route of transmission as HIV. Also, opportunistic infection, steatohepatitis, and medications toxicity may coexist causing abnormal liver enzymes in HIV population [18]. In recent study by Virot and collogues investigating the prevalence of autoimmune diseases in HIV patients, only one case of AIH was identified in a cohort of 5186 patients [19].

The HIV virus causes the destruction of the host's T-lymphocytes resulting in an immunocompromised state. Once the CD4 T-lymphocytes are less than 200 or the patient develops an AIDS-defining condition, the term acquired immunodeficiency syndrome (AIDS) can be used. Once the CD4 count drops below 50, it is called "advanced AIDS". Since AIH results from overactivation of T-lymphocytes, whereas AIDS is a result of depletion of T-lymphocytes, these contrasting processes may be the reason for the low prevalence of AIH in HIV patients. Although it is uncommon, autoimmune disorders like immune thrombocytopenic purpura, antiphospholipid syndrome, sarcoidosis, SLE, and Graves' disease have been described in HIV [20]. Pathogenesis of AIDS is known to initiate autoimmune phenomenon by polyclonal stimulation of B cells by HIV virus itself and development of hypergammaglobulinemia in proinflammatory milieu. In HIV, immune system is known to attack itself and form circulating autoimmune antibodies [21]. Vergani and collogues showed cross-reaction between anti-liver kidney microsome (LKM)-1 antibodies (involved in type 2 AIH) against CYP2D6 and HCV, HSV, and CMV [22]. Nowadays more cases of autoimmune diseases in HIV are reported with increasing use of HAART for treatment of HIV, suggesting unmasking of an underlying autoimmune dysfunction with immune reconstitution which predominantly involve CD8 cells [2, 4]. However, in the present case, at the time of diagnosis of AIH, patient was not taking HAART and had very low CD4 count without any evidence of coinfection.

We searched PubMed database for relevant English literature with the search terms of "Autoimmune hepatitis" and "human immunodeficiency virus", "Acquired Immunodeficiency syndrome" and identified 14 case reports/series of 35 patients with the concomitant diagnosis of AIH and HIV only without any coinfection (Table 1). In these previous reported cases/series, the range of CD4 count at the time of AIH diagnosis was between 174 and 1011 cells/mm3 with a viral load between undetectable and 27,000 IU/ml [2–15]. Our patient's CD4 count was just 11 cells/mm3 and viral load was 64,000 IU/ml at the time of AIH diagnosis. Also, cases described in the literature thus far only had HIV infection

Table 1: Review of reported cases/case series of HIV with AIH.

Author	Case	Age	Sex	CD4 at diagnosis (cells/mm3)	Viral Load diagnosis (IU/ml)	AIH score	ART	AIH Treatment	Outcome
Daas et al. [2]	1	42	F	232	Undetectable	Definite	Yes	Steroids	Remission
Tan-Tam et al [3]	1	59	M	>150	-	-	Yes	Transplant	Transplant
Puius et al. [4]	3	29	M	174	27,732	Probable	Yes	None	Remission
		45	F	297	Undetectable	Probable	Yes	Steroids +AZT	Remission
		65	F	922	Undetectable	Definite	Yes	Steroids	Remission
Wan et al. [5]	2	54	M	357	5,104	Probable	Yes	Steroids	Remission
		49	F	286	69,318	Definite	Yes	Steroids	Remission
Kaku et al. [6]	1	43	M	638	13,000	Probable	Yes	Steroids	Remission
O'Leary et al. [7]	1	44	F	526	Undetectable	Definite	Yes[1]	Steroids +AZT	Remission
German et al. [8]	1	38	M	216	Undetectable	Probable	Yes	None	Remission
Parekh et al. [9]	2	21	M	753	7,900	Probable	No	Steroids +AZT	Remission
		59	F	483	Undetectable	Definite	Yes	Steroids +AZT	Remission
Hagel et al [10]	1	52	M	641	Undetectable	Probable	Yes	Steroids	Remission
Kia et al. [11]	5	33 to 60	M	1011	Undetectable	-	Yes	Steroids +AZT	Remission
			F	456	Undetectable		Yes		
			F	783	Undetectable		Yes		
			F	688	Undetectable		Yes		
			F	653	Undetectable		Yes		
Ofori et al. [12]	2	40	M	832	Undetectable	Probable	Yes	Steroids	Remission
		44	F	823	Undetectable	Probable	Yes	Steroids	Remission
Murunga [13]	9	23 to 45	1 M 8 F	253-876	Undetectable	-	Yes	Steroids	Remission
Iordche [14]	4	-	-	488.4	Undetectable	-	Yes	Steroids +AZT	Remission
Zoboli [15]	2	38	M	762	8072	Definite	Yes	Steroids +AZT	Remission
		70	F	938	<50	Definite	Yes	Steroids	Remission
Our patient	1	32	M	11	64,000	Definite	No	Steroids +AZT	Remission

AZT: azathioprine, AIH: autoimmune hepatitis, and ART: antiretroviral therapy.

with AIH diagnosis, but our patient is unique in the sense that he had advanced AIDS when he was diagnosed with AIH.

Although there are more common causes of transaminitis in HIV/AIDS patients, an autoimmune hepatitis can still be a possibility. Physicians must be aware of this completely treatable but challenging "AIH in HIV/AIDS" diagnosis which frequently will need detailed biochemical, viral, autoimmune workup, and likely liver biopsy. Furthermore, there are no guidelines in the treatment of AIH in HIV patients. Standard immunosuppressive therapy, such as steroids and azathioprine, is usually thought to be high-risk in already immunocompromised HIV patients. There are only two reported cases, where patient's condition improved with HAART alone [3, 7]. Prior retrospective case reports showed that standard AIH therapy was successful in well controlled HIV on HAART (CD4 >250 and undetectable HIV viral load). In our case, despite very low CD4 count and high viral load, the patient showed complete remission of liver functions following the administration of prednisolone and azathioprine for AIH and starting HAART for AIDS.

4. Conclusion

Our case highlights that etiological workup for elevated liver chemistry in HIV/AIDS should include autoimmune hepatitis, irrespective of degree of immunosuppression and despite severe immunocompromised state, standard treatment for AIH can be used safely with HAART under close supervision.

Disclosure

This study was presented as poster in American College of Gastroenterology (ACG) Conference-Oct 2017.

Authors' Contributions

Jordan Roussel and Sudha Pandit wrote the article and literature review and have equal contribution. Kurt Knowles and Nester Dela Cruz provided the histopathology images. Paul Jordan reviewed the manuscript. Hrishikesh Samant reviewed and edited the manuscript. All authors read and approved the final manuscript.

References

[1] E. L. Krawitt, "Autoimmune hepatitis," *The New England Journal of Medicine*, vol. 354, no. 1, pp. 54–66, 2006.

[2] H. Daas, R. Khatib, H. Nasser, F. Kamran, M. Higgins, and L. Saravolatz, "Human immunodeficiency virus infection and autoimmune hepatitis during highly active anti-retroviral treatment: A case report and review of the literature," *Journal of Medical Case Reports*, vol. 5, p. 233, 2011.

[3] C. Tan-Tam, P. Liao, J. S. Montaner et al., "HIV and liver transplantation: the british columbia experience, 2004 to 2013," *Canadian Journal of Infectious Diseases & Medical Microbiology*, vol. 25, Article ID 373898, pp. 159–162, 2014.

[4] Y. A. Puius, L. M. Dove, D. G. Brust, D. P. Shah, and J. H. Lefkowitch, "Three cases of autoimmune hepatitis in HIV-infected patients," *Journal of Clinical Gastroenterology*, vol. 42, no. 4, pp. 425–429, 2008.

[5] D. W. Wan, K. Marks, R. K. Yantiss, and A. H. Talal, "Autoimmune hepatitis in the hiv-infected patient: A therapeutic dilemma," *AIDS Patient Care and STDs*, vol. 23, no. 6, pp. 407–413, 2009.

[6] Y. Kaku, S. Kodama, M. Higuchi et al., "Corticoid therapy for overlapping syndromes in an HIV-positive patient," *Internal Medicine*, vol. 54, no. 2, pp. 223–230, 2015.

[7] J. G. O'Leary, K. Zachary, J. Misdraji, and R. T. Chung, "De novo autoimmune hepatitis during immune reconstitution in an HIV-infected patient receiving highly active antiretroviral therapy," *Clinical Infectious Diseases*, vol. 46, no. 1, pp. e12–e14, 2008.

[8] V. German, A. Vassiloyanakopoulos, D. Sampaziotis, and G. Giannakos, "Autoimmune hepatitis in an HIV infected patient that responded to antiretroviral therapy," *Infectious Diseases*, vol. 37, no. 2, pp. 148–151, 2005.

[9] S. Parekh, Z. Spiritos, P. Reynolds, S. Parekh, A. Perricone, and B. Quigley, "HIV and autoimmune hepatitis: a case series and literature review," *Journal of Biomedical Sciencies*, vol. 6, no. 2, 2017.

[10] S. Hagel, T. Bruns, A. Herrmann, A. Tannapfel, and A. Stallmach, "Autoimmune hepatitis in an HIV-infected patient: An intriguing association," *International Journal of STD & AIDS*, vol. 23, no. 6, pp. 448–450, 2012.

[11] L. Kia, A. Beattie, and R. M. Green, "Autoimmune hepatitis in patients with human immunodeficiency virus (HIV): Case reports of a rare, but important diagnosis with therapeutic implications," *Medicine (United States)*, vol. 96, no. 7, article no. e6011, 2017.

[12] E. Ofori, D. Ramai, M. A. Ona, and M. Reddy, "Autoimmune hepatitis in the setting of human immunodeficiency virus infection: A case series," *World Journal of Hepatology*, vol. 9, no. 36, pp. 1367–1371, 2017.

[13] E. Murunga, M. Andersson, and C. V. Rensburg, "Autoimmune hepatitis: a manifestation of immune reconstitution inflammatory syndrome in HIV infected patients?" *Scandinavian Journal of Gastroenterology*, vol. 51, no. 7, pp. 814–818, 2016.

[14] L. Iordache, O. Launay, O. Bouchaud et al., "Autoimmune diseases in HIV-infected patients: 52 cases and literature review," *Autoimmunity Reviews*, vol. 13, no. 8, pp. 850–857, 2014.

[15] F. Zoboli, D. Ripamonti, S. V. Benatti, L. Comi, and M. Rizzi, "Autoimmune hepatitis and HIV infection: Two case reports and review of the literature," *AIDS*, vol. 31, no. 15, pp. 2172–2175, 2017.

[16] F. Alvarez, "International autoimmune hepatitis group report: review criteria for diagnosis of autoimmune hepatitis," *Journal of Hepatology*, vol. 31, no. 5, pp. 929–938, 1999.

[17] A. J. Czaja, "Performance parameters of the diagnostic scoring systems for autoimmune hepatitis," *Hepatology*, vol. 48, no. 5, pp. 1540–1548, 2008.

[18] N. Crum-Cianflone, G. Collins, S. Medina et al., "Prevalence and factors associated with liver test abnormalities among human immunodeficiency virus-infected persons," *Clinical Gastroenterology and Hepatology*, vol. 8, no. 2, pp. 183–191, 2010.

[19] E. Virot, A. Duclos, L. Adelaide et al., "Autoimmune diseases and HIV infection a cross-sectional study," *Medicine (Baltimore)*, vol. 96, article no. e5769, 2017.

[20] G. Zandman-Goddard and Y. Shoenfeld, "HIV and autoimmunity," *Autoimmunity Reviews*, vol. 1, no. 6, pp. 392–437, 2002.

[21] R. Root-Bernstein, "Antigenic complementarity between HIV and other AIDS-associated infections results in idiotype-antiidiotype antibody complexes that cross react with lymphocyte proteins," *Vaccine*, vol. 23, no. 17-18, pp. 2160–2163, 2005.

[22] D. Vergani and G. Mieli-Vergani, "Aetiopathogenesis of autoimmune hepatitis," *World Journal of Gastroenterology*, vol. 14, no. 21, pp. 3306–3312, 2008.

9

Acute Hepatitis A Causing Severe Hemolysis and Renal Failure in Undiagnosed Glucose-6-Phosphate Dehydrogenase Deficient Patient: A Case Report and Review of the Literature

Iman Abutineh,[1] Kyle Kreitman,[2] Jiten P. Kothadia,[2] Bilal Ali,[2] Richa Jain,[3] Ian Clark,[3] Benedict J. Maliakkal,[2] and Satheesh P. Nair[2]

[1]*Department of Internal Medicine, University of Tennessee Health Science Center, Memphis, TN, USA*
[2]*Methodist University Hospital, James D. Eason Transplant Institute, University of Tennessee Health Science Center, Memphis, TN, USA*
[3]*Department of Pathology, Memphis Pathology Group, University of Tennessee Health Science Center, Methodist University Hospital, Memphis, TN, USA*

Correspondence should be addressed to Kyle Kreitman; kkreitma@uthsc.edu

Academic Editor: Haruki Komatsu

Infection with hepatitis A virus is usually a self-limited illness that rarely results in fulminant liver failure. Severe hemolysis is an uncommon complication but has been reported in patients with glucose-6-phosphate dehydrogenase (G6PD) deficiency. Here, we report a case with undiagnosed G6PD deficiency who presented with hyperbilirubinemia, severe hemolysis, and acute renal failure precipitated by acute hepatitis A infection.

1. Introduction

Hepatitis A is one of the most frequent causes of foodborne infection, with an estimated 1.5 million cases each year [1]. Infection most commonly manifests with symptoms such as fever, malaise, anorexia, abdominal discomfort, diarrhea, dark-colored urine, and jaundice. Acute hepatitis A is usually a self-resolving illness without chronic sequelae. Acute liver failure develops in approximately one percent of cases [2].

A mild to moderate degree of hemolysis is a known complication of acute viral hepatitis. In a few cases, patients may present with severe hemolysis, which is more frequent in patients with coexisting glucose-6-phosphate dehydrogenase (G6PD) deficiency [2–9]. It has been postulated that viral infection itself can cause severe hemolysis in a patient with G6PD deficiency. In addition, the administration of certain drugs and particular foods may aggravate the condition [2]. It has also been noted that G6PD deficiency impedes the repair of the damaged hepatocytes and can lead to fulminant hepatitis and liver failure in patients with acute viral hepatitis [10, 11]. Here, we describe a patient with undiagnosed G6PD deficiency who presented with hyperbilirubinemia, severe hemolysis, and acute renal failure precipitated by acute hepatitis A infection.

2. Case Report

A 55-year-old African American male with a medical history of hypertension, hyperlipidemia, chronic hepatitis B, and well-controlled HIV on ART presented to the hospital with a one-week history of fatigue, fever, myalgias, shortness of breath, and dark-colored urine. He denied any history of alcohol, illicit drug use, or family history of liver disease.

On physical exam, he had scleral icterus and mild lower abdominal pain without guarding, rebound, or rigidity. He was alert and oriented without focal deficit or asterixis. He had no ascites. Vital signs were within normal limits. Lab work was significant for creatinine at 6.38 mg/dL (0.7–1.3), BUN 48 mg/dL (7–18), total bilirubin 51.8 mg/dL (0.2–1), direct bilirubin 40.4 mg/dL (≤0.2), lactate dehydrogenase 2678 unit/L (87–241), haptoglobin <7.7 mg/dL, alkaline phosphatase 195 unit/L, AST 216 unit/L (15–37), ALT 6,244 unit/L (16–61), lactic acid 5.5 mmol/L (0.4–2), WBC 16.6 thou/mcL (4.2–10.2), hemoglobin 7.5 g/dL (12.8–16.4), platelet 344×10^3/microL (150–400), and INR 1.6 (0.8–1). His model for end-stage liver disease (MELD) score was 40. Urine drug screen, acetaminophen, and alcohol level were negative. Serologic studies for *Treponema pallidum*, cytomegalovirus, Epstein-Barr virus, herpes simplex virus, and parvovirus were negative. Influenza and COVID-19 PCR were negative. The hepatitis panel was positive for hepatitis A IgM, hepatitis A total antibody, and hepatitis B core IgG antibody. Hepatitis C antibody, hepatitis E IgG/IgM, and HBV DNA were negative. His autoimmune markers including antinuclear antibody, antismooth muscle antibody, antimitochondrial antibody, and myeloperoxidase autoantibody were negative. Serum ceruloplasmin was also negative. Erythrocyte G6 PD level was normal due to acute hemolysis. A computed tomography (CT) scan of the abdomen and pelvis showed normal appearing liver with nondilated bile ducts and patent hepatic vasculature. A transthoracic echocardiogram (TTE) showed LVEF 60–65% with normal wall motion, no diastolic dysfunction, valvular disease, or thrombus.

The patient was treated empirically with antibiotics and intravenous fluids. Patient continued to be oliguric and hemodialysis was initiated. Peripheral smear showed fragmented erythrocytes, spherocytes, bite cells, and target cells indicative of hemolysis. Fibrinogen was normal, and Coomb's test was negative. Liver biopsy showed cholestatic hepatitis with areas of resolving necrosis (Figure 1). Renal biopsy showed acute tubular injury with bilirubin and hemoglobin casts (Figure 2). The patient was initially listed for transplant but clinically improved with supportive measures alone. Over the next few weeks, patient's liver functions test and hemolysis labs steadily improved (Figures 3 and 4). He was discharged to a rehab facility and has since followed up in our clinic. His most recent liver function tests, 3 months after hospitalization, are normal. Erythrocyte G6PD is 3.3 U/g Hb, confirming the diagnosis of G6PD deficiency. His renal function also improved, and he is no longer on dialysis.

3. Discussion

Hepatitis A is the most common cause of viral hepatitis worldwide, generally causing a mild self-limited illness akin to other foodborne illnesses. Chronic sequelae are rare, and mortality related to hepatitis A accounts for only 0.5% of deaths secondary to viral hepatitis [10]. However, recent data suggest a dramatic increase in the number of outbreaks occurring worldwide. The recent CDC morbidity and mortality report warn of a considerable increase in hepatitis A in the United States, with cases climbing by 294% in 2016–2018 compared to the country's nadir in 2013–2015 [12, 13]. Acute liver failure secondary to hepatitis A is rare, but with higher rates in older adults >40 years of age or those with chronic liver disease [10, 14]. Hemolytic anemia has been associated with viral hepatitis, but the degree is usually mild to moderate [3]. When the disease course is complicated by severe hemolysis, a diagnosis in addition to hepatitis should be sought out [3, 15]. A more common occurrence seemed to be the finding of underlying G6PD deficiency in patients who developed severe hemolysis [2–4, 6–9, 15].

To our knowledge, this is the first reported case of severe hemolysis and renal failure precipitated by acute HAV in an undiagnosed G6PD deficient and HIV-positive patient in the United States. G6PD deficiency is the most common human enzyme defect, affecting more than 400 million people worldwide. This X-linked hereditary defect impairs catalyzation of the first step in the pentose phosphate pathway, which is crucial for the production of NADPH, protecting cells from oxidative stress, and regenerating glutathione for reduction of reactive oxygen species [16, 17]. While usually a clinically silent disorder, certain stressors, including drugs (particularly primaquine or trimethoprim-sulfamethoxazole), ingestion of food (fava beans, bitter melon, blueberries, and falafel), or viral infection can trigger an acute hemolytic crisis [18–20]. The global prevalence of the disorder is 4.9%, with African and Mediterranean descent at the highest risk [21], an estimated 10% of black Americans and as high as 70% of Kurdish Jews may carry the mutation [16].

Despite a high prevalence of G6PD deficiency in the African American population, there are no current universal screening guidelines for the disease. However, evidence suggests that these patients have a more complicated course when infected by hepatitis A than a non-G6PD deficient patient [3, 5, 22]. In a retrospective study by Gotsman and Muskat of patients with acute hepatitis A admitted between 1980 and 1999, those with G6PD deficiency demonstrated a more severe clinical course with severe hemolysis and higher bilirubin level [5]. It has been hypothesized that G6PD deficient hepatocytes have reduced levels of glutathione, thereby causing an accumulation of free radicals and delayed hepatocyte repair with viral insult. There is ongoing discussion regarding the utility of blood transfusions or plasmapheresis in cases with severe hemolysis to prevent long-standing complications including renal failure [8].

On review of literature, there are 80 cases related to viral hepatitis, and G6PD deficiency causing severe hemolysis has been reported (Table 1) [2–9, 23–35]. The patient's median age was 19.5 years (IQR: 14.25–35). Among these patients, 32 had hepatitis A, 19 had hepatitis E, and 29 had unspecified viral hepatitis as a precipitating cause for severe hemolysis. 22.5% (18/80) of the patients had renal failure as a complication, and of that, 12 were treated with dialysis. One patient was treated with plasmapheresis. Of the 80 total patients, 72 (90%) made a full recovery, while 8 died of complications from renal/liver failure, seizures, sepsis, and cerebral hemorrhage. Our case was an immunocompromised patient with HIV treated with empiric antibiotics, blood transfusion, and hemodialysis with subsequent clinical improvement.

With a large population at risk and an alarming rise in acute HAV cases in the United States, it is of utmost importance for clinicians to be cognizant of typical and atypical features of the infection. Although most acute HAV cases

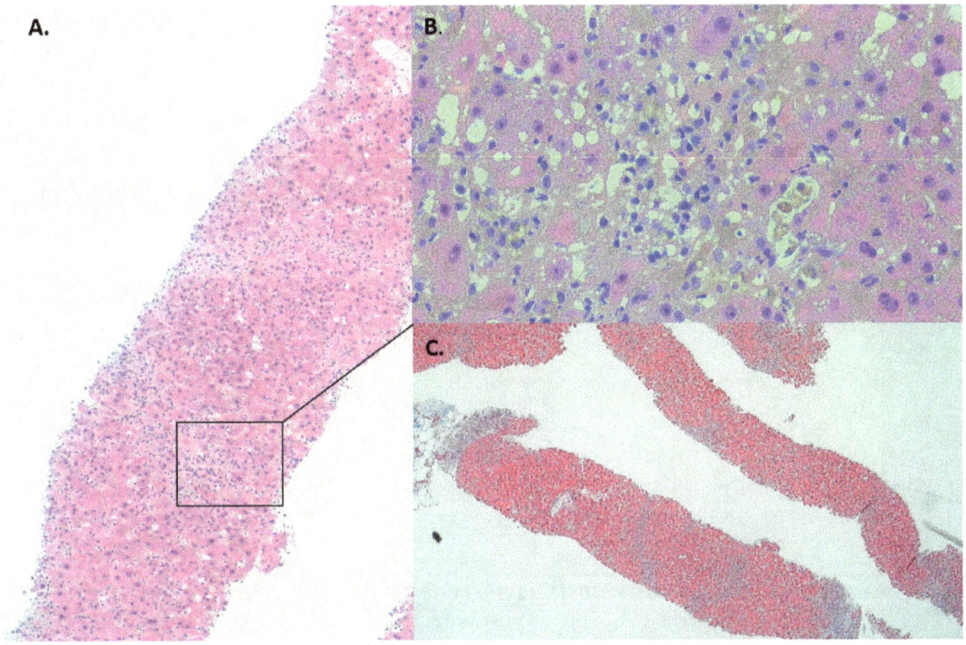

FIGURE 1: (a) Liver biopsy (H&E, x40) showing bridging necrosis and collapse of parenchyma with cholestasis and sparse inflammatory infiltrate rich in lymphocytes and plasma cells ((b) inset x200). (c) A trichrome stain (x20) showing lack of fibrosis supporting acute nature of the illness.

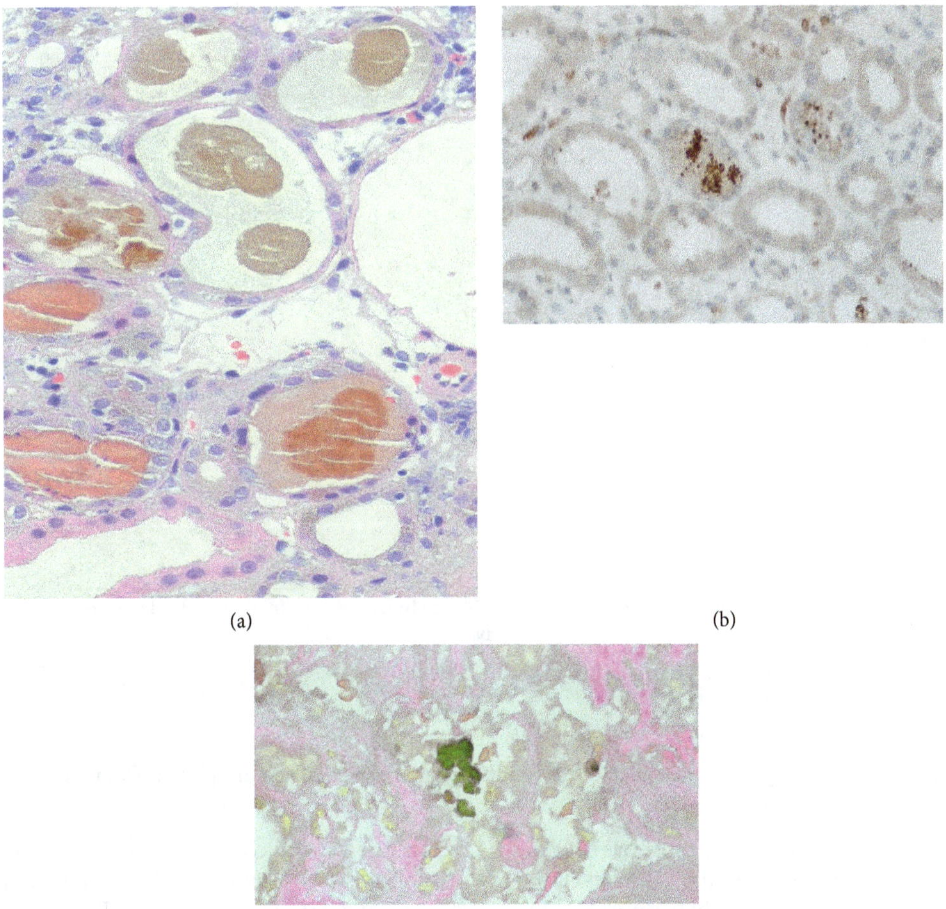

(a) (b)

(c)

FIGURE 2: (a) Renal biopsy showing tubular casts comprising of hemoglobin (hemoglobin immunostained (b)) and bile pigment (Fouchet stained (c)). Glomeruli and vasculature were within normal limits.

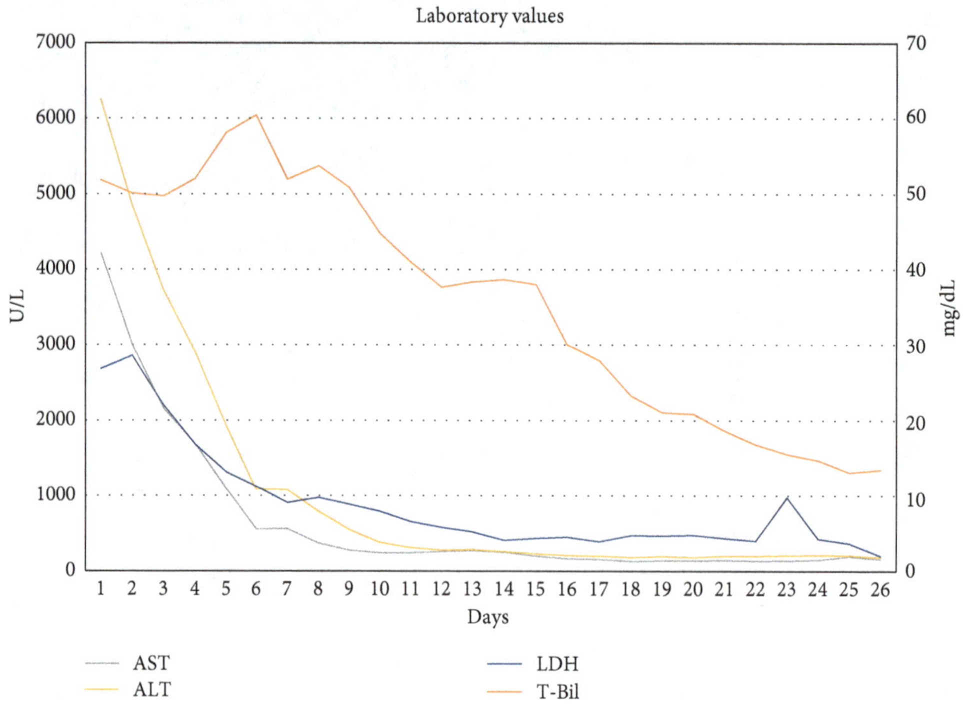

Figure 3: Changes in AST, ALT, LDH, and T-Bil during hospitalization are plotted from admission at days 1–25.

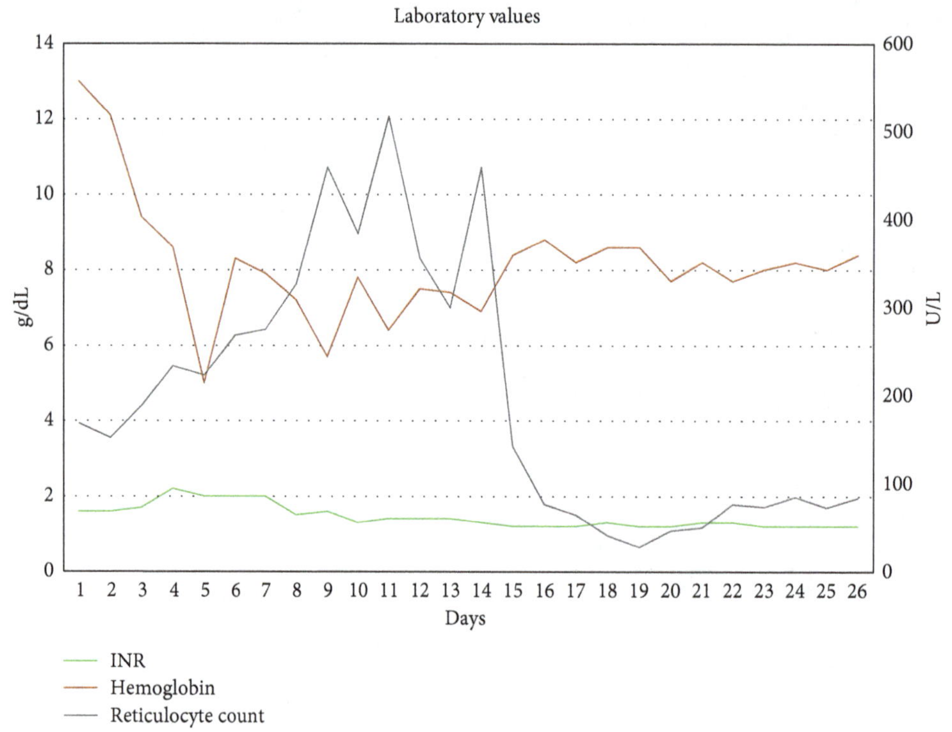

Figure 4: Changes in INR, hemoglobin, and reticulocyte counts during hospitalization are plotted from admission at days 1–25.

will resolve with supportive care alone, those with underlying G6PD deficiency are at an increased risk for developing severe intravascular hemolysis, marked hyperbilirubinemia, and increased risk of developing acute renal failure. Oxidant medications and nephrotoxins should be avoided. Treatment is generally supportive, but corticosteroids and plasma exchange can be considered in certain instances [15]. We recommend the hepatitis A vaccine in all patients with underlying G6PD deficiency. Ultimately, a high clinical suspicion and early recognition of patients at risk for severe manifestations of viral hepatitis can alter the course of the disease and aid in preventing chronic sequelae.

Table 1: Summary of reported cases with concomitant viral hepatitis and G6PD deficiency causing severe hemolysis.

Year	Author	Number of cases	Age (y)	Sex	Presenting symptoms	Geographic region	Cause of viral hepatitis	Presence of renal failure	Treatment	Need for transplant	Outcome
1966	Salen [23]	3	38, 28, 39	F, M, M	Fever, anorexia, and dark urine	USA	Did not specify	Yes (1 patient)	F: peritoneal dialysis, prednisone 40 mg qday; M-28: IVF; M-39: IVF and blood transfusion	No	Full recovery
1969	Clearfield et al. [4]	3	29, 31, 24	M, M, M	Myalgia, nausea, pruritis, dark urine, and jaundice	USA	Did not specify	No	Supportive care for all three patients	No	Full recovery
1975	Chan and Todd [3]	18	N/A	N/A	Fever and jaundice	Hong Kong	Did not specify	No	Supportive care for all 18 patients	No	15 had full recovery and 3 died from renal failure and hemolysis
1985	Agarwal et al. [24]	5	9, 19, 10, 10, 8	5 M	Fever, jaundice, and vomiting	India	Did not specify	Yes (2 patients)	4 patients required blood transfusions and 1 patient required peritoneal dialysis, blood transfusions, and antibiotics	No	4 had full recovery and 1 died of liver and renal failure
2001	Gotsman Muszkat [5]	18	Average 15.1	13 M, 5 F	Fever and jaundice	Israel	A	No	3 patients required blood transfusion, IVF fluids, and antibiotics. 15 patients required supportive care	No	Full recovery
2002	Abid and Khan [25]	5	26,16, 14, 22, 35	5 M	Fatigue, fever, jaundice, and vomiting	Pakistan	E	Yes (5 patients)	Supportive care for all 5 patients and 2 patients required hemodialysis	No	Full recovery
2003	Monga et al. [26]	1	35	M	Fever, abdominal pain, fatigue, jaundice, and dark urine	India	E	No	Supportive care	No	Full recovery
2008	Ozbay Hosnut et al. [8]	2	10, 5	M, F	Jaundice, emesis, and abdominal pain	Europe	A	Yes (1 patient)	Male: IVF, blood transfusion, and plasmapheresis; female: antibiotic therapy, vitamin K, lactulose, IVF, and blood transfusion	No	Full recovery
2009	Thapa et al. [27]	1	7	M	Jaundice	India	E	No	Supportive care	No	Full recovery
2011	Somani et al. [29]	1	17	M	Fever, abdominal pain, anorexia, jaundice, and dark urine	India	E	Yes	Supportive care	No	Full recovery
2011	Au et al. [28]	1	54	M	Jaundice, cyanosis, and confusion	Hong Kong	E	Yes	Hemodialysis	No	Died of cerebral hemorrhage
2012	Jain et al [6]	10	Average 16.1	8 M, 2 F	N/A	India	A, E	No	Supportive care	No	Full recovery

Table 1: Continued.

Year	Author	Number of cases	Age (y)	Sex	Presenting symptoms	Geographic region	Cause of viral hepatitis	Presence of renal failure	Treatment	Need for transplant	Outcome
2012	Wing-Yan and Chan [34]	2	53, 54	M	Right upper quadrant pain and flu-like symptoms	Hong Kong	E	Yes (1 patient)	Blood transfusion and hemodialysis	No	53-year-old died of seizures and sepsis. 54-year-old died of renal and liver failure
2014	Tomar et al. [31]	1	15	M	Fever, jaundice, dark urine, nausea, fatigue, and decreased PO intake	India	E	Yes	Blood transfusion and hemodialysis	No	Full recovery
2015	Dea [30]	1	20	M	Fever, jaundice, and dark urine	India	A	No	Supportive care	No	Full recovery
2016	Karki et al. [32]	1	48	M	Jaundice, dark urine, fever, and confusion	India	E	Yes	Blood transfusion, hemodialysis, and antibiotics	No	Full recovery
2017	Moiz and Ali [7]	1	10	F	Fever, abdominal pain, and lethargy	Pakistan	A	No	Supportive care	No	Full recovery
2017	Ahmad et al. [33]	1	28	M	Jaundice and abdominal pain	Pakistan	E	Yes	Blood transfusion and hemodialysis	No	Full recovery
2018	Sharma et al. [9]	1	39	M	Fever, jaundice, and dark urine	India	A	Yes	Blood transfusion and intermittent hemodialysis	No	Full recovery
2019	Bajpai et al. [2]	1	16	M	Fever, jaundice, and dark urine	India	A	Yes	IVF, ventilation, antibiotics, continuous renal replacement, and plasma and blood transfusion	No	Full recovery
2020	Kamani et al. [35]	2	19, 15	2 M	Jaundice, nausea, and vomiting	Pakistan	E	No	IVF and blood transfusion	No	19-year-old died from liver failure. 15-year-old made a full recovery
2020	Abutineh et al. (present case)	1	55	M	Fatigue, fever, malaise, jaundice, and abdominal pain	US	A	Yes	IVF, antibiotics, blood transfusion, and hemodialysis	No	Full recovery

4. Conclusions

While this may be the first reported case with an HIV-positive patient in the United States, the phenomenon is one that has been reported in foreign literature for decades. With a high prevalence of G6PD deficiency and an increased incidence of hepatitis A in the past few years, it is imperative for clinicians to be mindful of the potential complications to prevent chronic sequelae and adverse outcomes. In conclusion, intravascular hemolysis due to G6PD deficiency should be considered in patients with acute hepatitis A infection who present with marked hyperbilirubinemia and renal failure.

Abbreviations

ART: Antiretroviral therapy
ATN: Acute tubular necrosis
G6PD: Glucose-6-phosphate dehydrogenase
HBV: Hepatitis B virus
HIV: Human immunodeficiency virus.

Disclosure

This case report was presented at ACG 2020.

Authors' Contributions

Drafting the case report and acquisition of available literature were carried out by Iman Abutineh, MD and Kyle Kreitman, DO. Drafting the case report and critical revision of the manuscript for important intellectual content were carried out by Jiten P. Kothadia, MD. Histopathology images were provided and the manuscript was reviewed by Richa Jain, MD, Ian Clark MD. The manuscript was reviewed by Satheesh P. Nair, MD, Benedict J. Maliakkal, MD, and Bilal Ali, MD.

References

[1] A. H. Havelaar, "World Health Organization Global estimates and regional comparisons of the burden of foodborne disease in 2010," *PLoS Medicine*, vol. 12, no. 12, Article ID e1001923, 2015.

[2] M. Bajpai, B. Kakkar, and D. Patale, "Role of high-volume plasma exchange in a case of a G6PD deficient patient presenting with HAV related acute liver failure and concomitant acute renal failure," *Transfusion and Apheresis Science*, vol. 58, no. 6, Article ID 102677, 2019.

[3] T. K. Chan and D. Todd, "Haemolysis complicating viral hepatitis in patients with glucose-6-phosphate dehydrogenase deficiency," *Bmj*, vol. 1, no. 5950, pp. 131–133, 1975.

[4] H. R. Clearfield, J. I. Brody, and H. J. Tumen, "Acute viral hepatitis, glucose-6-phosphate dehydrogenase deficiency, and hemolytic anemia," *Archives of Internal Medicine*, vol. 123, no. 6, pp. 689–691, 1969.

[5] I. Gotsman and M. Muszkat, "Glucose-6-phosphate dehydrogenase deficiency is associated with increased initial clinical severity of acute viral hepatitis A," *Journal of Gastroenterology and Hepatology*, vol. 16, no. 11, pp. 1239–1243, 2001.

[6] A. K. Jain, S. Sircar, M. Jain, S. Adkar, C. Waghmare, and F. Chahwala, "Increased morbidity in acute viral hepatitis with glucose-6-phosphate dehydrogenase deficiency," *Indian Journal of Gastroenterology*, vol. 32, no. 2, pp. 133-134, 2013.

[7] B. Moiz and S. A. Ali, "Fulminant hemolysis in glucose-6-phosphate dehydrogenase deficiency," *Clinical Case Reports*, vol. 6, no. 1, pp. 224-225, 2018.

[8] F. Ozbay Hosnut, F. Ozcay, U. Selda Bayrakci, Z. Avci, and N. Özbek, "Etiology of hemolysis in two patients with hepatitis A infection: glucose-6-phosphate dehydrogenase deficiency or autoimmune hemolytic anemia," *European Journal of Pediatrics*, vol. 167, no. 12, pp. 1435–1439, 2008.

[9] D. Sharma, O Singh, D Juneja, A Goel, S. K Garg, and S Shekhar, "Hepatitis A virus-induced severe hemolysis complicated by severe glucose-6-phosphate dehydrogenase deficiency," *Indian Journal of Critical Care Medicine : Peer-Reviewed, Official Publication of Indian Society of Critical Care Medicine*, vol. 22, no. 9, pp. 670–673, 2018.

[10] E. C. Shin and S. H. Jeong, "Natural history, clinical manifestations, and pathogenesis of hepatitis A," *Cold Spring Harbor Perspectives in Medicine*, vol. 8, no. 9, 2018.

[11] A. Serious Hepatitis, "An analysis of patients hospitalized during an urban epidemic in the United States," *Annals of Internal Medicine*, vol. 128, no. 2, pp. 111–114, 1998.

[12] N. P. Nelson, "Prevention of hepatitis A virus infection in the United States," *Recommendations of the Advisory Committee on Immunization Practices*, vol. 2020, 2020.

[13] M. A. Foster, M. G. Hofmeister, B. A. Kupronis et al., "Increase in Hepatitis a virus infections-United States, 2013–2018," *MMWR. Morbidity and Mortality Weekly Report*, vol. 68, no. 18, pp. 413–415, 2019.

[14] S. M. Lemon, "Type a viral hepatitis: a summary and update on the molecular virology, epidemiology, pathogenesis and prevention," *Journal of Hepatology*, vol. 17, 2017.

[15] "Acute hemolytic anemia complicating viral hepatitis in patients with glucose-6-phosphate dehydrogenase deficiency," *Annals of Internal Medicine*, vol. 65, no. 6, pp. 1210–1220, 1966.

[16] E. Beutler, "G6PD deficiency," *Blood*, vol. 84, no. 11, pp. 3613–3636, 1994.

[17] M. Cappellini and G. Fiorelli, "Glucose-6-phosphate dehydrogenase deficiency," *The Lancet*, vol. 371, no. 9606, pp. 64–74, 2008.

[18] L. Luzzatto and P. Arese, "Favism and glucose-6-phosphate dehydrogenase deficiency," *New England Journal of Medicine*, vol. 378, no. 1, pp. 60–71, 2018.

[19] T. Babu, G. M. Panachiyil, J. Sebastian, and M. D. Ravi, "Probable blueberry-induced haemolysis in a G6PD deficient child: a case report," *Nutrition and Health*, vol. 25, no. 4, pp. 303–305, 2019.

[20] S. N. Stone, K. V. Reisig, H. L. Saffel, and C. M. Miles, "Management of athletes with G6PD deficiency: does missing an enzyme mean missing more games?" *Sports Health: A Multidisciplinary Approach*, vol. 12, no. 2, pp. 149–153, 2020.

[21] E. T. Nkhoma, C. Poole, V. Vannappagari, S. A. Hall, and E. Beutler, "The global prevalence of glucose-6-phosphate dehydrogenase deficiency: a systematic review and meta-analysis," *Blood Cells, Molecules, and Diseases*, vol. 42, no. 3, pp. 267–278, 2009.

[22] C. A. Kattamis and F. Tjortjatou, "The hemolytic process of viral hepatitis inchildren with normal or deficient glucose-6-

phosphate dehydrogenase activity," *The Journal of Pediatrics*, vol. 77, no. 3, pp. 422–430, 1970.

[23] G. Salen, "Acute hemolytic anemia complicating viral hepatitis in patients with glucose-6-phosphate dehydrogenase deficiency," *Annals of Internal Medicine*, vol. 65, no. 6, pp. 1210–1220, 1966.

[24] R. K. Agarwal, A. Moudgil, K. Kishore, R. N. Srivastava, and R. K. Tandon, "Acute viral hepatitis, intravascular haemolysis, severe hyperbilirubinaemia and renal failure in glucose-6-phosphate dehydrogenase deficient patients," *Postgraduate Medical Journal*, vol. 61, no. 721, pp. 971–975, 1985.

[25] S. Abid and A. H. Khan, "Severe hemolysis and renal failure in glucose-6-phosphate dehydrogenase deficient patients with hepatitis E," *The American Journal of Gastroenterology*, vol. 97, no. 6, pp. 1544–1547, 2002.

[26] A. Monga, R. P. Makkar, A. Arora, S. Mukhopadhyay, and A. K. Gupta, "Case report: acute hepatitis E infection with co-existent glucose-6-phosphate dehydrogenase deficiency," *Canadian Journal of Infectious Diseases*, vol. 14, no. 4, pp. 230-231, 2003.

[27] R. Thapa, S. Pramanik, B. Biswas, and D. Mallick, "Hepatitis E virus infection in a 7-year-old boy with glucose 6-phosphate dehydrogenase deficiency," *Journal of Pediatric Hematology/oncology*, vol. 31, no. 3, pp. 223-224, 2009.

[28] W. Y. Au, C.-W. Ngai, W.-M. Chan, R. Y. Y. Leung, and S.-C. Chan, "Hemolysis and methemoglobinemia due to hepatitis E virus infection in patient with G6PD deficiency," *Annals of Hematology*, vol. 90, no. 10, pp. 1237-1238, 2011.

[29] S. K. Somani, "Hepatitis e virus infection leads to severe hemolysis in glucose-6-phosphate dehydrogenase deficiency patients," 2011.

[30] B. Dea, "Severe hemolysis as the first manifestation of acute hepatitis A in an adult with G6PD deficiency and positive ANA," *American Journal of Medical Case Reports*, vol. 3, pp. 158-159, 2015.

[31] L. R. Tomar, A. Aggarwal, P. Jain, S. Rajpal, and M. P. Agarwal, "Acute viral hepatitis E presenting with haemolytic anaemia and acute renal failure in a patient with glucose-6-phosphate dehydrogenase deficiency," *Tropical Doctor*, vol. 45, no. 4, pp. 245-246, 2015.

[32] P. Karki, S Malik, B Mallick, V Sharma, and S. S Rana, "Massive Hemolysis causing renal failure in acute hepatitis E infection," *Journal of Clinical and Translational Hepatology*, vol. 4, no. 4, pp. 345–347, 2016.

[33] B. S. Ahmad, A Ahmad, S Jamil, S. A Abubakar Mohsin Ehsanullah, and A Munir, "Severe haemolysis and renal failure precipitated by hepatitis E virus in G6PD Deficient patient: a case report," *JPMA. The Journal of the Pakistan Medical Association*, vol. 68, pp. 1397–1399, 2018.

[34] A. Wing-Yan and S. Chan, "Association between glucose 6-phosphate dehydrogenase (G6PD) deficiency and fatal outcome," *Singapore Medical Journal*, vol. 53, no. 2, pp. 148-149, 2012.

[35] L. Kamani, H. Shaikh, and A. K. Khemchandani, "Fulminant hepatic failure in glucose-6-phosphate dehydrogenase (G6PD) deficient patients caused by hepatitis E infection: a single disease with different spectrums," *Cureus*, vol. 12, no. 12, Article ID e12276, 2020.

10

Successful Treatment of Crizotinib-Induced Fulminant Liver Failure: A Case Report and Review of Literature

Kyle Kreitman, Satheesh P. Nair, and Jiten P. Kothadia

MUH James D. Eason Transplant Institute, University of Tennessee Health Sciences Center, 1265 Union Avenue, 4 Shorb Tower, Memphis, TN 38104, USA

Correspondence should be addressed to Jiten P. Kothadia; kothadia.jiten@gmail.com

Academic Editor: Mauro Vigano

Crizotinib is a first-line tyrosine kinase inhibitor used for the treatment of metastatic lung cancer. Crizotinib-induced hepatotoxicity is a rare event. We report a case of a 46-year-old female with a history of metastatic lung cancer who presented with acute liver failure after being on crizotinib for two months. The medication was discontinued, and she was treated with N-acetylcysteine for seven days. Her liver function tests returned to normal limits after 26 days after admission. The precise mechanism and risk factors of crizotinib-induced hepatotoxicity remain unknown. Physicians should be aware of the potentially lethal side effect caused by crizotinib.

1. Introduction

Lung cancer is the second most common cancer in both men and women. It is the leading cause of cancer death, with about 142670 deaths a year in the United States [1]. There are approximately 1.3 million new patients diagnosed worldwide each year. Non-small-cell lung cancer (NSCLC) accounts for 85% of lung cancer patients. Of those diagnosed with NSCLC, 4–7% are positive for the anaplastic lymphoma kinase (ALK) gene rearrangement [2]. Targeting the ALK gene rearrangement has been shown to be more effective in patients with advanced NSCLC when compared to standard chemotherapy, and it is the first-line therapy for these patients [3].

Crizotinib is a tyrosine kinase inhibitor that targets ALK, mesenchymal epithelial transition factor (MET), and ROS1 proto-oncogene receptor tyrosine kinase (ROS1) [4]. The FDA has approved crizotinib as the first-line agent for the treatment of ALK-positive NSCLC. Common side effects of crizotinib include vision changes, fatigue, anorexia, diarrhea, nausea, vomiting, fatigue, dizziness, and upper respiratory tract infection [5, 6]. Elevated liver function tests have been reported with crizotinib treatment, which usually resolves with cessation of the drug or dose adjustment. Although rare, crizotinib-induced severe hepatotoxicity with fatal outcome occurred in 0.1% of patients in clinical trials [5]. Review of the literature extracted 12 cases of crizotinib-induced liver injury, with 66% (8/12) mortality. We report a case of crizotinib-induced fulminant liver failure which was treated with discontinuation of the drug and N-acetylcysteine with complete recovery.

2. Case Report

A 46-year-old African American female with a past medical history significant for metastatic NSCLC, ovarian vein thrombosis, and gastroesophageal reflux disease (GERD) presented to our hospital with a primary complaint of intermittent right upper quadrant pain over a two-week duration. Her symptoms were associated with nausea, generalized weakness, jaundice, dark urine, and mild dyspnea on exertion. The patient denied any history of alcohol use, smoking, illicit drug use, family history of liver disease, or history of recent travel outside of the United States. She was not sexually active.

Regarding her history of lung cancer, she was diagnosed to have stage IV metastatic adenocarcinoma of the lung (T2aN3M1c, Stage IVB) approximately nine months ago. At the time of diagnosis, she was noted to have intracranial, skeletal, and lung metastases along with generalized lymphadenopathy. The patient was started on chemotherapy regimen with carboplatin and paclitaxel in March 2019. The chemotherapy was subsequently discontinued as the molecular analysis of the lung cancer specimen showed a ROS1 gene rearrangement. She was started on treatment with crizotinib 250 mg twice daily (PO). Four weeks after initiation of crizotinib, her transaminases were noted to be elevated and treatment was discontinued. Few weeks after discontinuation of crizotinib, her liver function tests returned to normal. She was restarted on crizotinib at a lower dose of 200 mg twice daily with close monitoring of liver function tests every 2 weeks. On day 14, her AST was 60 U/L (15–37) and ALT was 55 U/L (16–61) with normal total bilirubin and alkaline phosphatase, and crizotinib was continued. However, 4 weeks after reinitiation of crizotinib, she presented to the emergency room with jaundice.

On physical exam, she had scleral icterus and right upper quadrant tenderness but without guarding, rebound, or rigidity. She was alert and oriented, without any focal deficits and asterixis.

Liver function tests at the time of admission showed AST 4093 U/L (15–37), ALT 3653 U/L (16–61), total bilirubin 5.8 mg/dL (0.2–1), conjugated bilirubin 4.5 mg/dL, and alkaline phosphatase 358 U/L (45–117). International normalized ratio (INR) was 10 (0.8–1). The white blood cell count was 4.0×10^3/microL (4.2–10.2). The platelet count was 349×10^3/microL (150–400). Her model for end-stage liver disease (MELD) score was 39. Serologic studies for hepatitis A, hepatitis B, hepatitis C, hepatitis E, human immunodeficiency virus (HIV), treponema pallidum, cytomegalovirus, Epstein–Barr virus, herpes simplex virus, and parvovirus were negative. Her autoimmune markers including antinuclear antibody, anti-smooth muscle antibodies, anti-mitochondrial antibody, IgG levels, and anti-liver kidney microsomal 1 antibody were all negative. Serum ceruloplasmin, alpha-fetoprotein, and alpha-1 antitrypsin levels were within normal limits. A computed tomography (CT) scan of the chest, abdomen, and pelvis was performed that showed persistent airspace opacities throughout both lungs, bilateral bronchial wall thickening, and diffuse bony (skeletal) metastatic disease. The liver was described in normal morphology and size and normal bile ducts with patent hepatic vasculature.

The clinical history and lab work-up were suggestive of crizotinib-associated hepatotoxicity. The patient's updated RUCAM (Roussel Uclaf Causality Assessment Method) score came out to be 8 points, which is consistent with probable drug-induced liver injury. The crizotinib was discontinued, and she was started on intravenous (IV) N-acetylcysteine (NAC) continuous infusion (100 mg/kg). She was given vitamin K 10 mg daily for three days for coagulopathy. Her liver chemistry continued to downtrend with discontinuation of crizotinib and with continuous NAC infusion for a total of 7 days. Liver biopsy was not obtained due to significant improvement of liver function tests on discontinuation of crizotinib along with intravenous NAC. The patient was discharged after eight days. Her liver test came back within normal limits 26 days after the presentation (Figure1).

3. Discussion

Crizotinib is a multitarget tyrosine kinase inhibitor of ALK, MET, and ROS1 [4]. Food and Drug Administration (FDA) has approved crizotinib for the treatment of patients with metastatic NSCLC whose tumors are ALK or ROS1-positive [3–5]. This report describes a case of crizotinib-induced fulminant hepatitis with recovery. Other potential causes of liver failure such as viral hepatitis, hepatic metastasis, alcoholic liver disease, or other drug-induced liver injury were excluded.

Crizotinib has been known to usually cause mild elevations in liver function tests although the exact mechanism is poorly understood [7]. The drug is metabolized in the liver by CYP3A4, and it is thought that liver injury may be due to the accumulation of toxic metabolites or immune-related mechanism [7]. The symptoms of drug-induced hepatitis are generally nonspecific; thus, the diagnosis is often delayed [7].

Hepatotoxicity was a common adverse event in patients using crizotinib in phase III studies [3, 6]. Grade 3-4 transaminase elevations occurred within the first two months of crizotinib treatment, but very rarely was there jaundice or elevations in the bilirubin and alkaline phosphatase. In the majority of patients, transaminases elevations were reversible with medication interruption or reinitiation with a lower dose and rarely required permanent discontinuation [3, 6]. Most patients, who do develop drug-induced liver injury secondary to crizotinib, are asymptomatic. However, among all the patients treated with crizotinib across clinical trials, 0.1% of patients died from acute liver failure [5]. According to prescribing information on crizotinib, monitoring of liver function test every two weeks during the first two months of treatment, then once a month, and as clinically indicated is recommended [5]. Our patient was closely monitored, and crizotinib dose was reduced to 200 mg twice daily as per recommendations. Also, she was completely asymptomatic until six weeks after the initiation of treatment with crizotinib. The dose-independent and sporadic nature of hepatotoxicity is highly suggestive of an idiosyncratic mechanism [8]. Thus, monitoring of the liver function test as per manufacturer recommendations is not sufficient to prevent idiosyncratic crizotinib-induced fulminant hepatotoxicity. The specific risk factors for crizotinib-induced hepatotoxicity are not well known. Sato et al. [9] described several factors associated with an increased risk of crizotinib-induced severe hepatotoxicity. These include CYP3A inducers or inhibitors, a history of chronic hepatitis C, collagen disorders, and antidiabetic drugs. In a retrospective study, Jung et al. [10] found that concomitant use of H2-antagonist and the presence of chronic liver disease were the factors associated with increased risk of crizotinib-induced hepatotoxicity.

On review of literature, there are only 12 cases of crizotinib-induced hepatotoxicity reported (Table 1) [7–9, 11–18]. Of these 12 patients, 8 died due to progressive liver failure in spite of discontinuation of the drug. The

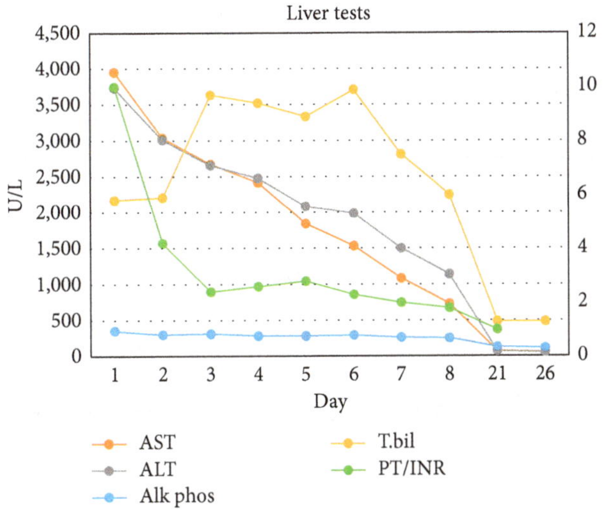

FIGURE 1: Changes in liver tests during hospitalization are plotted from admission at day 1 to day 26.

TABLE 1: Summary of patients with crizotinib-induced hepatotoxicity, characteristics, presentation, pattern of liver injury, and clinical outcome.

Year	Author	Number of cases	Age	Sex	Dosage	Duration of crizotinib exposure	Presenting symptoms	Pattern of liver injury	Mortality	Treatment	RUCAM score
2013	Ripault et al. [11]	1	69	F	500 mg qday	60 days	Fatigue	Hepatocellular	0	Withdrawal of medication with resolution	9
2014	Sato et al. [9]	1	54	F	400 mg qday	29 days	Epigastric pain	Hepatocellular	1	Withdrawal of the medication, steroids, plasma exchange	8
2016	Sassier et al. [12]	2	30, 62	M, F	250 mg/ day	10 days, 30 days	None	Hepatocellular	0	Withdrawal of medication with resolution	7, 8
2016	Adhikari et al. [8]	1	56	M	250 mg BID	39 days	Fatigue, nausea/ vomiting	Hepatocellular	1	NAC, mannitol, withdrawal of the medication, lactulose/ rifaximin/ LOLA/abx	9
2016	Van Geel et al. [7]	1	62	F	250 mg BID	24 days	Confusion	Hepatocellular	1	Supportive, withdrawal of the medication	8
2017	Brown et al. [13]	1	56	F	250 mg BID	6 weeks	Fatigue, weakness, darkening urine	Hepatocellular	1	NAC, withdrawal of the medication	NA
2017	Yasuda et al. [14]	1	51	F	250 mg BID	16 days	Abdominal pain, nausea, diarrhea	Hepatocellular	1	Steroids, supportive, withdrawal of the medication	6
2018	Charville et al. [15]	1	26	F	500 mg qday	10 weeks	Abdominal pain, jaundice	Hepatocellular	0	Withdrawal of medication with resolution, N-acetylcysteine	8

Table 1: Continued.

Year	Author	Number of cases	Age	Sex	Dosage	Duration of crizotinib exposure	Presenting symptoms	Pattern of liver injury	Mortality	Treatment	RUCAM score
2018	Kesler et al. [16]	1	69	F	250 mg BID	4 weeks	Weakness, lightheadedness and hypotension	Hepatocellular	1	Withdrawal of the medication, lactulose/ rifaximin/ antibiotics	NA
2019	Zhang et al. [17]	1	37	M	250 mg BID	55 days	Dyspnea, abdominal pain	Hepatocellular	1	Withdrawal of the medication, lactulose/ rifaximin/ antibiotics	8
2019	Ota et al. [18]	1	66	F	250 mg BID	23 days	Fever, fatigue	Mixed	0	Withdrawal of the medication with resolution	7
2019	Kreitman et al. (Present case)	1	46	F	200 mg BID	8 weeks	Fatigue, abdominal pain, jaundice	Hepatocellular	0	Withdrawal of the medication, NAC	8

M, male; F, female; NA, not applicable (cannot be calculated).

patients were treated with supportive treatments, lactulose and rifaximin for HE, mannitol for cerebral edema, broad-spectrum antibiotics, steroids, and in one instance plasma exchange. 2 out of the 8 patients received NAC; however, it was unclear timing and dose of NAC therapy. 4 patients recovered with resolution of hepatitis, and 3 of the patients improved with just the cessation of the medication. Our patient received NAC upon admission and for 7 days with subsequent improvement in her LFTs.

NAC is a thiol-containing agent that prevents hepatic damage by scavenging free oxygen radicals and replenishing glutathione stores [19, 20]. It has anti-inflammatory, antioxidant, inotropic, and vasodilating properties that may help limit the toxicities from crizotinib [21, 22]. The literature is not very clear about the benefit of using NAC in non-acetaminophen-induced acute liver failure (NAI-ALF). However, it has been suggested that there is benefit when administered early in the course of DILI or at the onset of hepatic encephalopathy [23]. We recommend that NAC should be considered in any patient that presents with suspected crizotinib-induced liver failure/ hepatitis. NAC works as a glutathione precursor, and it has anti-inflammatory and antioxidant properties that may be helpful in limiting the toxic metabolite that results from crizotinib toxicity. NAC has a very low side-effect profile, and the potential benefit of the medication exceeds the risk.

4. Conclusions

This case highlights the potentially lethal side effect of crizotinib. Hopefully, postmarketing monitoring and data analysis will help in identifying the risk factors for DILI with this agent. Early use of NAC seems to be beneficial and should be considered.

Authors' Contributions

Kyle Krietman was involved in drafting the case report and the acquisition of available literature. Jiten P. Kothadia was involved in study conception and design, drafting the case report, and critical revision of the manuscript for important intellectual content. Satheesh P. Nair reviewed the manuscript.

References

[1] R. L. Siegel, K. D. Miller, and A. Jemal, "Cancer statistics, 2019," *CA: A Cancer Journal for Clinicians*, vol. 69, no. 1, pp. 7–34, 2019.

[2] P. L. Chia, T. John, A. Dobrovic, and P. Mitchell, "Prevalence and natural history of ALK positive non-small-cell lung cancer and the clinical impact of targeted therapy with ALK inhibitors," *Clinical Epidemiology*, vol. 6, pp. 423–432, 2014.

[3] A. T. Shaw, D.-W. Kim, K. Nakagawa et al., "Crizotinib versus chemotherapy in advanced ALK-positive lung cancer," *New England Journal of Medicine*, vol. 368, no. 25, pp. 2385–2394, 2013.

[4] A. T. Shaw, S.-H. I. Ou, Y.-J. Bang et al., "Crizotinib in ROS1-rearranged non-small-cell lung cancer," *New England Journal of Medicine*, vol. 371, no. 21, pp. 1963–1971, 2014.

[5] Food and Drug Administration, *Prescribing Information XALKORI® (crizotinib)*, Food and Drug Administration, Silver Spring, MD, USA, 2013.

[6] B. J. Solomon, T. Mok, D.-W. Kim et al., "First-line crizotinib versus chemotherapy in ALK-positive lung cancer," *New England Journal of Medicine*, vol. 371, no. 23, pp. 2167–2177, 2014.

[7] R. M. J. M. van Geel, J. J. M. A. Hendrikx, J. E. Vahl et al., "Crizotinib-induced fatal fulminant liver failure," *Lung Cancer*, vol. 93, pp. 17–19, 2016.

[8] N. Adhikari, P. Kumar, B. P. Venkatesulu et al., "Crizotinib-induced fulminant hepatic failure: a rare adverse event," *Journal of Global Oncology*, vol. 4, pp. 1–4, 2018.

[9] Y. Sato, D. Fujimoto, Y. Shibata et al., "Fulminant hepatitis following crizotinib administration for ALK-positive non-small-cell lung carcinoma," *Japanese Journal of Clinical Oncology*, vol. 44, no. 9, pp. 872–875, 2014.

[10] D. Jung, J. M. Han, J. Yee, J. Y. Kim, and H. S. Gwak, "Factors affecting crizotinib-induced hepatotoxicity in non-small cell lung cancer patients," *Medical Oncology*, vol. 35, no. 12, p. 154, 2018.

[11] M.-P. Ripault, V. Pinzani, V. Fayolle, G.-P. Pageaux, and D. Larrey, "Crizotinib-induced acute hepatitis: first case with relapse after reintroduction with reduced dose," *Clinics and Research in Hepatology and Gastroenterology*, vol. 37, no. 1, pp. e21–e23, 2013.

[12] M. Sassier, B. Mennecier, A. Gschwend et al., "Successful treatment with ceritinib after crizotinib induced hepatitis," *Lung Cancer*, vol. 95, pp. 15-16, 2016.

[13] P. R. Brown, O. Sadiq, K. Umanath, and S.-M. Jafri, "Crizotinib-induced fulminant liver failure: 2331," *American Journal of Gastroenterology*, vol. 112, Article ID S1273, 2017.

[14] Y. Yasuda, Y. Nishikawa, Y. Sakamor et al., "Successful oral desensitization with crizotinib after crizotinib-induced hepatitis in an anaplastic lymphoma kinase-rearranged non-small-cell lung cancer patient: a case report," *Molecular and Clinical Oncology*, vol. 7, no. 2, pp. 295–297, 2017.

[15] G. W. Charville, S. K. Padda, R. K. Sibley, A. Puthillath, and P. Y. Kwo, "Resolution of crizotinib-associated fulminant hepatitis following cessation of treatment," *Case Reports in Hepatology*, vol. 2018, Article ID 3413592, 5 pages, 2018.

[16] A. M. Kesler and J. C. Cowdell, "A fatal case of crizotinib induced fulminant liver failure," *Journal of Hospital Medicine*, vol. 13, no. 4, 2018.

[17] Y. Zhang, Y.-Y. Xu, Y. Chen, J.-N. Li, and Y. Wang, "Crizotinib-induced acute fatal liver failure in an Asian ALK-positive lung adenocarcinoma patient with liver metastasis: a case report," *World Journal of Clinical Cases*, vol. 7, no. 9, pp. 1080–1086, 2019.

[18] T. Ota, N. Masuda, K. Matsui et al., "Successful desensitization with crizotinib after crizotinib-induced liver injury in ROS1-rearranged lung adenocarcinoma," *Internal Medicine*, vol. 58, no. 18, pp. 2554–2618, 2019.

[19] I. A. Cotgreave, "N-acetylcysteine: pharmacological considerations and experimental and clinical applications," *Advances in Pharmacology*, vol. 38, pp. 205–227, 1997.

[20] P. Harrison, J. Wendon, and R. Williams, "Evidence of increased guanylate cyclase activation by acetylcysteine in fulminant hepatic failure," *Hepatology*, vol. 23, no. 5, pp. 1067–1072, 1996.

[21] T. Nabi, S. Nabi, N. Rafiq, and A. Shah, "Role of N-acetylcysteine treatment in non-acetaminophen-induced acute liver failure: a prospective study," *Saudi Journal of Gastroenterology*, vol. 23, no. 3, pp. 169–175, 2017.

[22] P. M. Harrison, J. A. Wendon, A. E. S. Gimson, G. J. M. Alexander, and R. Williams, "Improvement by acetylcysteine of hemodynamics and oxygen transport in fulminant hepatic failure," *New England Journal of Medicine*, vol. 324, no. 26, pp. 1852–1857, 1991.

[23] W. M. Lee, L. S. Hynan, L. Rossaro et al., "Intravenous N-acetylcysteine improves transplant-free survival in early stage non-acetaminophen acute liver failure," *Gastroenterology*, vol. 137, no. 3, pp. 856–864, 2009.

11

Clarithromycin-Associated Acute Liver Failure Leading to Fatal, Massive Upper Gastrointestinal Hemorrhage from Profound Coagulopathy: Case Report and Systematic Literature Review

Ahmed I. Edhi,[1] Seifeldin Hakim,[1] Christienne Shams,[2] Damanpreet Bedi,[3] Mitual Amin,[4] and Mitchell S. Cappell[1,5]

[1]*Division of Gastroenterology & Hepatology, Department of Medicine, William Beaumont Hospital, 3535 W Thirteen Mile Rd, Royal Oak, MI 48073, USA*
[2]*Department of Medicine, William Beaumont Hospital, Oakland University William Beaumont School of Medicine, 3535 W Thirteen Mile Rd, Royal Oak, MI 48073, USA*
[3]*Transplant Surgery, Department of Surgery, William Beaumont School of Medicine, 3601 W Thirteen Mile Rd, Royal Oak, MI 48073, USA*
[4]*Department of Pathology, William Beaumont Hospital, Oakland University William Beaumont School of Medicine, 3601 W Thirteen Mile Rd, Royal Oak, MI 48073, USA*
[5]*Division of Gastroenterology & Hepatology, Department of Medicine, Oakland University William Beaumont School of Medicine, 3535 W Thirteen Mile Rd, Royal Oak, MI 48073, USA*

Correspondence should be addressed to Mitchell S. Cappell; mitchell.cappell@beaumont.edu

Academic Editor: Sorabh Kapoor

While erythromycin has caused numerous cases of acute liver failure (ALF), clarithromycin, a similar macrolide antibiotic, has caused only six reported cases of ALF. A new case of clarithromycin-associated ALF is reported with hepatic histopathology and exclusion of other etiologies by extensive workup, and the syndrome of clarithromycin-associated ALF is better characterized by systematic review. A 60-year-old nonalcoholic man, with normal baseline liver function tests, was admitted with diffuse abdominal pain and AST = 499 U/L and ALT = 539 U/L, six days after completing a 7-day course of clarithromycin 500 mg twice daily for suspected upper respiratory infection. AST and ALT each rose to about 1,000 U/L on day-2 of admission, and rose to ≥6,000 U/L on day-3, with development of severe hepatic encephalopathy and severe coagulopathy. Planned liver biopsy was cancelled due to coagulopathies. Extensive evaluation for infectious, immunologic, and metabolic causes of liver disease was negative. Abdominal computerized tomography and abdominal ultrasound with Doppler were unremarkable. The patient developed massive, acute upper gastrointestinal bleeding associated with coagulopathies. Esophagogastroduodenoscopy was planned after massive blood product transfusions, but the patient rapidly expired from hemorrhagic shock. Autopsy revealed a golden-brown heavy liver with massive hepatic necrosis and sinusoidal congestion. Rise of AST/ALT to about 1,000 U/L each was temporally incompatible with shock liver because this rise preceded the hemorrhagic shock, but the subsequent AST/ALT rise to ≥6,000 U/L each may have had a component of shock liver. The six previously reported cases were limited by failure to exclude hepatitis E (4), lack of liver biopsy (2), and uninterpretable liver biopsy (1) and by confounding potential etiologies including disulfiram, israpidine, or recent acetaminophen use (3), clarithromycin overdose (1), active alcohol use (1), and severe heart failure (1). Review of 6 previously reported and current case of clarithromycin-associated ALF revealed that patients had AST and ALT values in the thousands. Five patients died and 2 survived.

1. Introduction

Acute liver failure (ALF) refers to severe acute liver injury with encephalopathy and impaired liver synthetic function developing within 4 weeks in a patient with prior normal liver function or well-compensated liver disease [1]. ALF is commonly due to drug-induced liver injury (DILI), with implicated drugs in the United States including acetaminophen overdose (46%), idiosyncratic reactions to various drugs (12%), and occasionally (14% of cases) in which a drug is a possible cause of ALF of uncertain origin [2]. Clarithromycin is a macrolide antibiotic widely used to treat respiratory, skin, or soft tissue infections and infections by *Mycobacterium avium* complex or *Helicobacter pylori*.While erythromycin, a related macrolide antibiotic, has caused numerous cases of ALF [3, 4], comprehensive literature review revealed only 6 reported cases of clarithromycin-induced ALF [5–10], in addition to moderate liver injury with moderately elevated liver enzymes and cholestatic hepatitis ascribed to clarithromycin [11, 12]. A case of ALF secondary to clarithromycin is reported, and the syndrome is systematically reviewed.

2. Methods

Systematic literature search on liver injury from clarithromycin using PubMed and Medline with the following medical subject headings/keywords: [("liver injury") OR ("drug induced liver injury") OR ("DILI") OR ("acute hepatic failure") OR ("fulminant liver failure") OR ("acute liver failure")] AND [("clarithromycin")] and by reviewing sections on DILI in medical, hepatology, or pathology textbooks. All articles, including case reports, were reviewed. Two authors independently performed literature searches, independently reviewed prior case reports, and reconciled differences to minimize errors. Two authors abstracted the case report from the electronic medical record and reconciled differences to reduce errors.

3. Case Report

A 60-year-old nonalcoholic man with no known liver disease who was chronically administered the following drugs: albuterol and budesonide-formoterol inhalers for asthma; levothyroxine 100 mcg once daily for hypothyroidism; and amlodipine 5 mg once daily, metoprolol 25 mg once daily, and lisinopril 20 mg twice daily for hypertension, presented with atypical chest pain, dyspnea, and productive cough. Physical examination revealed normal vital signs, bilateral wheezing in both lung fields, and no hepatosplenomegaly or stigmata of chronic liver disease. Serial cardiac enzymes and electrocardiograms were within normal limits. Chest roentgenogram revealed no pulmonic consolidation or infiltrates. Laboratory analysis revealed leukocytosis, normal hemoglobin and platelet counts, and normal blood urea nitrogen and creatinine levels. Liver function tests were initially normal, except for an alanine aminotransferase (ALT) level of 72 U/L (Table 1, column 2). He was diagnosed with asthma exacerbation secondary to upper respiratory tract infection and treated with clarithromycin 500 mg twice daily orally for 7 days; intravenous corticosteroids, which were subsequently converted to a tapering dose of oral prednisone; and resumption of home medications. He was discharged on hospital day 6 when his symptoms subsided after completing 3 days of clarithromycin therapy.

Ten days after discharge and 6 days after completing a seven-day course of clarithromycin, the patient represented with diffuse abdominal pain for 4 days. Physical examination revealed blood pressure of 147/92 mmHg; otherwise normal vital signs; a soft, distended, diffusely tender abdomen with hypoactive bowel sounds and no rebound tenderness or guarding; and no stigmata of chronic liver disease. There was mild leukocytosis and normal hemoglobin level, while the aminotransferase levels were significantly elevated, and international normalized ratio (INR) was 0.9 (Table 1, column 3). The lactic acid was 0.6 mmol/L (normal: 0.5–2.2 mmol/L), ammonia was 22 μmol/L (normal 11–35 μmol/L), and acetaminophen level was <4.0 μg/ml. The next day vital signs were stable, with no change in abdominal exam. The AST and ALT levels rose to >1,000 U/L, and lactate dehydrogenase was 4,200 U/L. Extensive tests for viral hepatitis, including anti-HAV, anti-HBs, anti-HBc, HBs antigen, anti-HCV, HCV-RNA, and anti-HEV, were negative, as were tests for human immunodeficiency virus, cytomegalovirus, and Herpes simplex virus. Blood cultures were sterile. The autoimmune hepatitis panel, including anti-nuclear antibody (ANA), anti-mitochondrial antibody (AMA), anti-smooth muscle antibody (ASMA), anti-liver-kidney microsomal (LKM) antibodies, and total immunoglobulin, was negative or within normal limits. Tests for genetic hemochromatosis were negative. Ceruloplasmin level was normal. Slit-lamp ophthalmologic examination did not reveal Kayser-Fleischer rings. Abdominal computerized tomography (CT) with IV contrast and abdominal ultrasound with Doppler studies were unremarkable. Echocardiography was normal.

On day 3, the patient was transferred to an intensive care unit because of altered mental status, asterixis, and ammonia of 96 μmol/L, findings consistent with grade III hepatic encephalopathy. The AST and ALT rose to ≥6,000 U/L (Table 1, column 5), and the hemoglobin declined to 5.5 g/dL, with severe melena from acute upper gastrointestinal bleeding and development of borderline hypotension (Supplementary Table 1). Bleeding was associated with 35,000 platelets/μL, prothrombin time >100 seconds, activated partial thromboplastin time >124 seconds, D-dimer >9,999 ng/ml, and fibrinogen <35 mg/dL. Massive blood products were transfused. EGD, planned because of acute melena, and liver biopsy, planned for worsening liver failure, were both postponed due to hemodynamic instability and coagulopathy. Despite aggressive resuscitation, the patient rapidly deteriorated, suffered cardiac arrest, and expired.

The family consented to autopsy confined to liver, kidneys, lungs, and pancreas. Liver postmortem examination grossly revealed a golden-brown soft liver weighing 1,980 gm. Histopathologic hepatic examination revealed massive hepatocyte necrosis, occasional sparing of periportal hepatocytes, and diffuse sinusoidal congestion (Figures 1

Table 1: Trend of liver function tests.

Laboratory value (normal laboratory range and units)	First hospitalization (16 days prior to 2nd admission)	Day 1 second hospitalization (6 days after completing 7-day course of clarithromycin)	Day 2	Day 3	Day 4
Leukocyte count (3,500–10,100/μL)	15,000/μL	12,200/μL			
Hemoglobin (13.5–17.0 g/dL)	13.6 g/dL	14.5 g/dL		5.5 g/dL	
Platelets (150,000–400,000/μL)	209,000/μL	129,000/μL		35,000/μL	
Aspartate aminotransferase (10–37 U/L)	39 U/L	499 U/L	1,119 U/L	9,470 U/L	10,820 U/L
Alanine aminotransferase (9–47 U/L)	72 U/L	539 U/L	1,110 U/L	6,420 U/L	7,210 U/L
Alkaline phosphatase (30–110 U/L)	55 U/L	127 U/L	171 U/L	358 U/L	202 U/L
Albumin (3.5–4.9 g/dL)	3.5 g/dL	3.4 g/dL	3.6 g/dL	2.9 g/dL	2.6 g/dL
Total bilirubin (0.3–1.2 mg/dL)	1.0 mg/dL	1.0 mg/dL	0.6 mg/dL	2.3 mg/dL	1.9 mg/dL
Direct bilirubin (0.0–0.4 mg/dL)	NA	NA	NA	1.8 mg/dL	1.3 mg/dL
INR (0.9–1.2)	NA	0.9		>9.0	>9.0

INR, international normalized ratio; NA, not applicable.

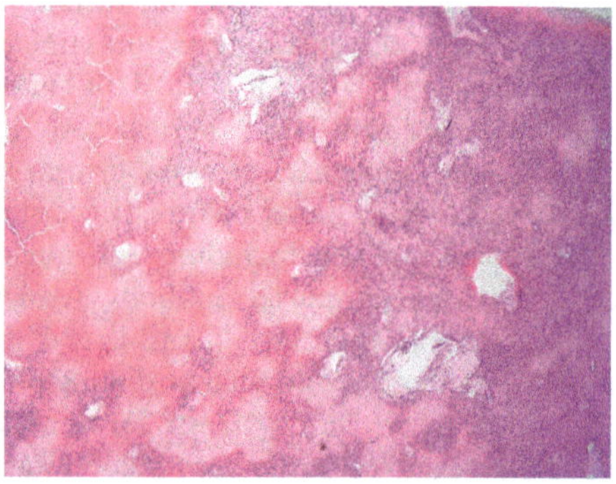

Figure 1: Low power photomicrograph of hematoxylin and eosin stain of liver section obtained at autopsy shows geographic areas of necrosis and marked sinusoidal congestion.

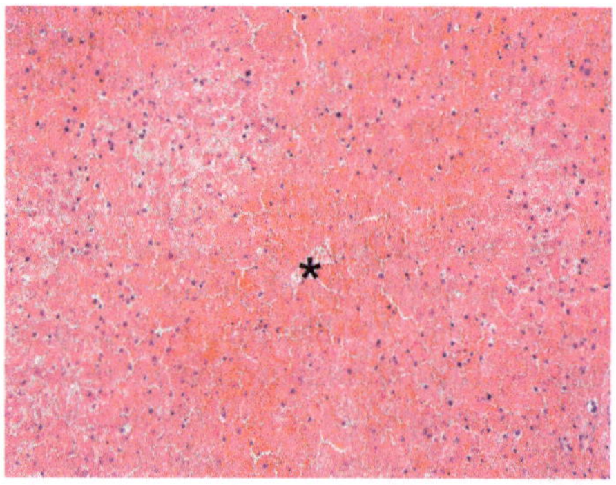

Figure 2: High power photomicrograph of hematoxylin and eosin stain of liver section obtained at autopsy shows a central vein (*) with adjacent marked sinusoidal congestion and extensive hepatocyte necrosis.

and 2). No lobular or portal inflammation, fibrosis, viral cytopathic effect, thromboemboli, or malignancy was evident. Immunohistochemistry revealed no Herpes simplex virus types 1 and 2 or cytomegalovirus.

4. Discussion

DILI accounts for approximately 10% of acute hepatitis, but is the most common cause of ALF in the United States and the most frequent reason for drug withdrawal from the marketplace [13]. DILI is classified as predictable, as for acetaminophen, or idiosyncratic, as for amoxicillin/clavulanate. DILI is also classified according to the liver injury pattern as (1) hepatocellular (primarily elevated ALT and AST), (2) cholestatic (primarily elevated alkaline phosphatase), and (3) mixed (elevated AST, ALT, and alkaline phosphatase).

This patient developed ALF 10 days after initiating clarithromycin therapy. Other causes of ALF including viral, ischemic, autoimmune, and Wilson's disease and hemochromatosis were excluded. Echocardiography revealed a normal ejection fraction. The rise of AST and ALT to about 1,000 U/L each on second hospitalization day 2 preceded the hypotension from hemorrhagic shock which began 1 day later (AST and ALT rised to >6,000 U/L each; Table 1, Supplementary Table 1). The initial rise in AST and ALT could not be attributed to shock liver, but the sharp rise in AST and ALT on day 3 might have been partly due to hepatic ischemia, from massive upper gastrointestinal hemorrhage associated with profound coagulopathy from hepatic failure. This may have contributed to finding hepatic necrosis at autopsy. Concomitant medications were unlikely causes of ALF because they were all chronically administered, except for prednisone which is not believed to cause ALF and has been previously used to treat one case of severe clarithromycin-induced hepatotoxicity [14]. Although renal insufficiency promotes clarithromycin-induced hepatotoxicity [15], the patient had normal renal function throughout the course of clarithromycin therapy.

Clarithromycin is synthesized by substituting a methoxy group for the C-6 hydroxyl group of erythromycin to improve oral bioavailability and gastrointestinal

Table 2: Reported cases of fulminant liver failure associated with clarithromycin.

Author, year	Shaheen and Grimm, 1996 [5]	Christopher et al., 2002 [6]	Masia et al., 2002 [7]	Tietz et al., 2003 [8]	Albataineh and Siddiqui, 2007 [9]	Maggi et al., 2012 [10]	Current case
Age (in years), gender. Symptoms and signs on admission	25, M. Nausea, dark urine, and acholic stools. Afebrile, deep jaundice, and right upper quadrant tenderness.	40, F. Weakness, nausea, abdominal pain, and pyrexia. Had right upper quadrant tenderness.	47, M. Generalized maculopapular rash and malaise, high fever, blood pressure 90/60 mmHg, pulse 130/min, jaundice, and edematous extremities.	58, F. Nausea, jaundice, and diarrhea. Nontender liver palpable 2 cm below right costal margin, and bilateral trace ankle edema.	39, M. Right upper quadrant pain, recurrent emesis, and confusion 1 day after starting clarithromycin.	23, M. Diarrhea, vomiting, and fever starting after taking clarithromycin. Took overdose of clarithromycin 2 gm as initial dose.	60, M. Epigastric abdominal pain. Diffusely tender abdomen, hypoactive bowel sounds, and no stigmata of chronic liver disease.
Previous medical history	Noncontributory.	Hemodialysis for end-stage kidney disease, anemia, hypertension, pancreatitis, and pulmonary sarcoid without corticosteroid use. Status-post AV fistula and total abdominal hysterectomy, and cholecystectomy.	Receiving disulfiram for 1 month for chronic alcoholism. Received acetaminophen 1,500 mg/day together with clarithromycin.	Hypertension and mitral valve prolapse with regurgitation. Repair of lumbar disk herniation.	Congestive heart failure (ejection fraction of 10%), hypertension, and heavy alcohol use.	Schizoaffective psychosis treated with amisulpride, orphenadrine, and lithium carbonate. Two prior episodes of transient mild aminotransferase elevations.	Asthma treated with albuterol and budesonide, hypertension treated with amlodipine, metoprolol, and lisinopril, and hyperthyroidism treated with levothyroxine (all these medicines administered chronically)
Peak key liver laboratory values and imaging tests	AST 3,510 U/L ALT 4,790 U/L ALP 225 U/L TB 32 mg/dL, PT 30.9 s (no peripheral eosinophilia)	AST 2,255 U/L, ALT 1,974 U/L, ALP 1,095 U/L, TB 33.4 mg/dL, PT 21 s (eosinophil count: 430/μL)	AST 1,149 U/L, ALT 2,603 U/L, ALP 240 U/L, TB 15.29 mg/dL, PT 21 s (no peripheral eosinophilia).	AST 23,166 U/L, ALT 13,853 U/L, ALP 258 U/L, TB 4.6 mg/dL, INR 5.7. Abdominal ultrasound: Enlarged and hyperechoic liver.	AST >6,000 U/L, ALT >4,000 U/L, PT 22 s. Abdominal ultrasound: Diffuse fatty liver, severe hepatomegaly.	AST 2,007 U/L, ALT 4,065 U/L, TB 10.0 mg/dL, INR 1.9	AST 10,820 U/L, ALT 7,210 U/L, ALP 358 U/L, TB 1.7 mg/dL, PT > 100 s. Abdominal ultrasound and CT: unremarkable liver. (No peripheral eosinophilia).
Reason for clarithromycin use; illness onset after starting clarithromycin therapy	Sinusitis, 9 days	Upper respiratory infection; 10 days	Pyrexia, odynophagia, and malaise for 7 days	Dry cough, fevers, and right lower lung infiltrate on chest radiograph; 4 days	Productive cough, dyspnea, pleuritic chest pain, left upper lobe infiltrate on chest radiograph. 1 day.	Sore throat. 8 days	Atypical chest pain, dyspnea, and productive cough. No pulmonic infiltrate on chest radiograph. 13 days after starting 7-day course of clarithromycin therapy.

Table 2: Continued.

Author, year	Shaheen and Grimm, 1996 [5]	Christopher et al., 2002 [6]	Masia et al., 2002 [7]	Tietz et al., 2003 [8]	Albataineh and Siddiqui, 2007 [9]	Maggi et al., 2012 [10]	Current case
Liver histologic findings	Explanted liver: massive hepatocyte necrosis, bile duct proliferation and areas of nodular regeneration.	Transjugular liver biopsy: moderate cholestasis, microvesicular steatosis, and eosinophilic infiltration.	No liver biopsy.	Diffuse, confluent necrosis involving centrilobular and midzonal areas.	Patient refused liver biopsy.	Autopsy showed marked cholestasis. Unable to fully assess microscopic hepatic structure due to advanced autolysis because autopsy performed 40 days after death.	At autopsy: diffuse sinusoidal congestion, massive hepatocyte necrosis, with occasional sparing of periportal hepatocytes.
Outcome	Underwent liver transplant after developing hepatic encephalopathy, and rising liver function tests. Died postoperatively from intracranial hemorrhage.	Developed progressive hepatic encephalopathy, and liver and pulmonary failure.	Transferred to liver transplant center for evaluation. However, rapidly died from septic shock.	Transferred to liver transplant center for evaluation. Developed severe leukocytosis, hepatic encephalopathy, very high aminotransferase levels and INR of 5.7. Recovered after stopping all medications.	After rapid worsening of liver failure when taking clarithromycin, liver function rapidly recovered towards normal when discontinuing clarithromycin.	Died from intracranial bleed (as shown by head CT). Bleeding related to coagulopathy from acute liver failure.	Rapidly expired from hemorrhagic shock from massive acute upper gastrointestinal bleeding, associated with profound coagulopathy. Planned liver biopsy could not be performed because of profound coagulopathy (see autopsy).
Confounding factors in liver injury	Took <5 gm/day of acetaminophen until 9 days before onset of symptoms. Serum acetaminophen level of zero on admission. Rarely drank alcohol. No serologic testing for hepatitis E.	Negative extensive workup for metabolic and infectious causes of liver disease. Normal ERCP findings. No recent acetaminophen use. No prior alcoholism. Extensive list of chronically used medications before instituting clarithromycin therapy.	Negative extensive workup for metabolic and infectious causes of liver disease. Disulfiram implicated as a cofactor in liver injury; disulfiram is a cytochrome P450 enzyme inhibitor which may increase clarithromycin levels. Taking acetaminophen 1,500 mg/day. No serologic testing for hepatitis E.	Recent trip to India. Social drinker of alcohol. Suffering from left-sided heart failure treated with atenolol. Also, receiving israpidine when developed liver failure.	Possible ischemic hepatitis from heart failure (ejection fraction = 10%); heavy alcohol use; started ceftriaxone concomitant with clarithromycin. Extensive workup found no other metabolic or infectious causes of acute liver failure. No serologic testing for hepatitis E.	Took four times normal initial dose of clarithromycin. Taking antipsychotic medications. Extensive workup found no other metabolic or infectious causes of acute liver failure. No serologic testing for hepatitis E. Liver histology at autopsy of limited value due to advanced autolysis because autopsy performed 40 days after death	Taking several other drugs for various diseases, but all of these drugs were chronically taken without prior toxicity. Extremely extensive workup found no other metabolic or infectious cause of acute liver failure. Had terminal hypotension from massive gastrointestinal hemorrhage in last 24 hrs (after having AST and ALT levels about 1,000 U/L each on the previous day).

AST, aspartate aminotransferase; ALT, alanine aminotransferase; ALP, alkaline phosphatase; TB, total bilirubin; PT, prothrombin time; INR, international normalized ratio; F, female; M, male; N/A, not applicable.

tolerance [16]. ALF has been reported secondary to other macrolides, especially erythromycin and roxithromycin [3, 4, 17, 18]. Clarithromycin is generally well tolerated, with dose reduction required in patients with renal insufficiency [15]. Clarithromycin-induced hepatotoxicity is attributed to (1) dose-related hepatotoxicity with elevated liver enzymes with ≥2 gm/day of clarithromycin in the elderly [19] and (2) possible idiosyncratic or hypersensitivity reactions with no evident dose-dependent relationship [11].

The epidemiology, presenting symptoms, signs, liver function tests, clarithromycin use, outcome, and confounding factors in the prior six cases of ALF associated with clarithromycin and the currently reported case are summarized in Table 2 [5–10]. Review of these 7 patients show that 5 were males (71%), on average were 41.7 ± 14.5 (SD) years old, and had onset of ALF 7.0 ± 3.4 days after onset of clarithromycin use. All patients had peak AST and ALT levels >1,000 U/L. Peak alkaline phosphatase levels ranged from 220–358 U/L, except 1 patient had a level of 1,095 U/L. Peak total bilirubin ranged from 1.7–33.4 mg/dL. All patients had predominantly hepatocellular injury, except that one patient had mixed hepatocellular and cholestatic injury [6]. All patients had significant coagulopathies (peak INR ≥1.9). In four patients having interpretable liver biopsies, performed premortem during ALF or postmortem, findings included moderate to massive hepatic necrosis in 3 and one each with bile duct proliferation, focal nodular regeneration, microvesicular steatosis, eosinophilic infiltration, or diffuse sinusoidal congestion.

Histopathologic analysis of the current patient's liver revealed diffuse hepatocellular necrosis, consistent with prior reported cases and idiosyncratic DILI as previously reported [20], but had no eosinophilic infiltrates characteristic of certain DILI pathology. Two prior patients also lacked eosinophilic infiltrates [5, 8]. Prominent eosinophilic infiltrates can suggest drug-induced hypersensitivity, but rarely occur in idiosyncratic drug reactions. No histopathologic findings are pathognomonic of DILI; a high index of clinical suspicion and compatible histopathologic findings are required for the diagnosis.

This review suffers from limitations of the 6 previously reported cases, including lack of liver biopsy (2) [7, 9], uninterpretable liver biopsy (1) [10], and administration of confounding potentially hepatotoxic drugs (3), including disulfiram [7], israpidine [8], or acetaminophen [5]. Other confounding variables included alcoholism (1) [7], heart failure (1) [9], and clarithromycin overdose (1) [10]. Also, hepatitis E, which can mimic DILI, [21] was not excluded in 4 prior cases [5, 7, 9, 10]. This work is also subject to limitations as one retrospectively reported case. The clinical picture of clarithromycin-induced hepatotoxicity might have been modified by terminal ischemic hepatitis from massive gastrointestinal bleeding during his last 24 hours of life that produced very high AST and ALT levels. However, the AST and ALT rise to about 1,000 U/L each one day earlier was associated with normal blood pressure readings and cannot be ascribed to shock liver/hepatic ischemia.

5. Conclusions

A 60-year-old nonalcoholic man, with normal baseline liver function tests, was admitted with diffuse abdominal pain and AST = 499 U/L and ALT = 539 U/L, 6 days after completing a 7-day course of clarithromycin 500 mg twice daily. AST and ALT each rose to ≥6,000 U/L two days later, accompanied by severe hepatic encephalopathy and coagulopathy. Extensive workup revealed no infectious, metabolic, or immunologic etiology of liver failure. The patient died soon thereafter from hemorrhagic shock from massive upper gastrointestinal bleeding and coagulopathy. Postmortem histopathologic hepatic examination revealed massive hepatocyte necrosis and diffuse sinusoidal congestion. Systematic review of 6 prior reported cases and this case of clarithromycin-associated ALF promotes further understanding of this syndrome.

Disclosure

Dr. Cappell, as a consultant of the United States Food and Drug Administration (FDA) Advisory Committee for Gastrointestinal Drugs, affirms that this paper does not discuss any proprietary confidential pharmaceutical data submitted to the FDA. Dr. Cappell was also until 2 years ago a member of the speaker's bureau for AstraZeneca and Daiichi Sankyo, co-marketers of Movantik. This work does not discuss any drug manufactured or marketed by AstraZeneca or Daiichi Sankyo.

Authors' Contributions

Dr. Edhi and Dr. Cappell are the primary authors. Dr. Edhi and Dr. Hakim wrote early drafts of the case report and discussion sections. Dr. Cappell as a mentor edited the case report section and wrote the bulk of the other sections. Dr. Amin performed all the microscopic pathology and wrote the pathologic sections of the paper. Dr. Shams and Dr. Bedi participated in the patient care.

Supplementary Materials

Supplementary Table 1 reports the daily blood pressure recordings every morning on the first hospitalization and reports all the blood pressure recordings for the second hospitalization. This table demonstrates that the blood pressure throughout the first hospitalization was stable (and not hypotensive) and throughout the second hospitalization was stable (not hypotensive) until late in the evening of day 3 of the second hospitalization 16 hours before the patient's demise. These recordings demonstrate that the patient developed hypotension from hemorrhagic shock as a terminal event (associated with profound coagulopathy) after suffering acute liver failure associated with clarithromycin. Therefore, the hypotension did not directly cause the acute liver failure but was a consequence of the acute liver failure. (*Supplementary Materials*)

References

[1] W. M. Lee, R. T. Stravitz, and A. M. Larson, "Introduction to the revised American Association for the Study of Liver Diseases Position Paper on acute liver failure 2011," *Hepatology*, vol. 55, no. 3, pp. 965–967, 2012.

[2] W. M. Lee, R. H. Squires, S. L. Nyberg, E. Doo, and J. H. Hoofnagle, "Acute liver failure: summary of a workshop," *Hepatology*, vol. 47, no. 4, pp. 1401–1415, 2008.

[3] C. F. Gholson and G. H. Warren, "Fulminant hepatic failure associated with intravenous erythromycin lactobionate," *Archives of Internal Medicine*, vol. 150, no. 1, pp. 215-216, 1990.

[4] J. L. Carson, B. L. Strom, A. Duff et al., "Acute liver disease associated with erythromycins, sulfonamides, and tetracyclines," *Annals of Internal Medicine*, vol. 119, no. 7, pp. 576–583, 1993.

[5] N. Shaheen and I. S. Grimm, "Fulminant hepatic failure associated with clarithromycin," *The American Journal of Gastroenterology*, vol. 91, no. 2, pp. 394-395, 1996.

[6] K. Christopher, P. A. Hyatt, C. Horkan, and P. C. Yodice, "Clarithromycin use preceding fulminant hepatic failure," *The American Journal of Gastroenterology*, vol. 97, no. 2, pp. 489-490, 2002.

[7] M. Masiá, F. Gutiérrez, A. Jimeno et al., "Fulminant hepatitis and fatal toxic epidermal necrolysis (Lyell disease) coincident with clarithromycin administration in an alcoholic patient receiving disulfiram therapy," *Archives of Internal Medicine*, vol. 162, no. 4, pp. 474–476, 2002.

[8] A. Tietz, M. H. Heim, U. Eriksson, S. Marsch, L. Terracciano, and S. Krähenbühl, "Fulminant liver failure associated with clarithromycin," *Annals of Pharmacotherapy*, vol. 37, no. 1, pp. 57–60, 2003.

[9] H. Albataineh and F. Siddiqui, "Acute liver failure secondary to clarithromycin. A case report and a literature review," *Practical Gastroenterology*, vol. 31, no. 7, p. 87, 2007.

[10] P. Maggi, B. Solarino, P. Cassano et al., "Fatal fulminant hepatitis following administration of clarithromycin in a patient chronically treated with antipsycotic drugs," *Immunopharmacology and Immunotoxicology*, vol. 35, no. 1, pp. 191–194, 2013.

[11] W. W. Yew, C. H. Chau, J. Lee, and C. W. Leung, "Cholestatic hepatitis in a patient who received clarithromycin therapy for a *Mycobacterium chelonae* lung infection," *Clinical Infectious Diseases*, vol. 18, no. 6, pp. 1025-1026, 1994.

[12] J. C. Fox, R. S. Szyjkowski, S. O. Sanderson, and R. A. Levine, "Progressive cholestatic liver disease associated with clarithromycin treatment," *The Journal of Clinical Pharmacology*, vol. 42, no. 6, pp. 676–680, 2002.

[13] H. J. Zimmerman, "Drug-induced liver disease," *Clinics in Liver Disease*, vol. 4, no. 1, pp. 73–96, 2000.

[14] A. Giannattasio, M. D'ambrosi, M. Volpicelli, and R. Iorio, "Steroid therapy for a case of severe drug-induced cholestasis," *Annals of Pharmacotherapy*, vol. 40, no. 6, pp. 1196–1199, 2006.

[15] D. R. P. Guay, D. R. Patterson, N. Seipman, and J. C. Craft, "Overview of the tolerability profile of clarithromycin in preclinical and clinical trials," *Drug Safety*, vol. 8, no. 5, pp. 350–364, 1993.

[16] S. C. Piscitelli, L. H. Danziger, and K. A. Rodvold, "Clarithromycin and azithromycin: new macrolide antibiotics," *Clinical Pharmacy*, vol. 11, no. 2, pp. 137–152, 1992.

[17] A. Dubois, N. Nakache, C. Raffanel, and J. L. Balmes, "Acute cholestatic hepatitis after ingestion of roxithromycin," *Gastroentérologie Clinique et Biologique*, vol. 13, no. 3, pp. 317-318, 1989.

[18] F. M. Pedersen, L. Bathum, and C. Fenger, "Acute hepatitis and roxithromycin," *The Lancet*, vol. 341, no. 8839, pp. 251-252, 1993.

[19] R. J. Wallace, B. A. Brown, and D. E. Griffith, "Drug intolerance to high-dose clarithromycin among elderly patients," *Diagnostic Microbiology and Infectious Disease*, vol. 16, no. 3, pp. 215–221, 1993.

[20] J. H. Lefkowitch, "The pathology of acute liver failure," *Advances in Anatomic Pathology*, vol. 23, no. 3, pp. 144–158, 2016.

[21] P. Grewal and J. Ahmad, "Beware of HCV and HEV in patients with suspected drug-induced liver injury," *Current Hepatology Reports*, vol. 17, no. 3, pp. 270–275, 2018.

12

Ruptured Multifocal Hepatic Aneurysms in a Woman with Systemic Lupus Erythematosus Successfully Treated with Transcatheter Arterial Embolization: A Case Report and Literature Review

Sz-Iuan Shiu,[1,2] **Su Ann Yong**,[3] **Kuo-Lung Lai**,[4] **Chih-Wei Tseng**,[4] **Chen-Yu Wang**,[2] **Bor-Jen Lee**,[2] **and Yi-Hsing Chen**[4,5]

[1]*Division of Gastroenterology and Hepatology, Department of Internal Medicine, Taichung Veterans General Hospital, Taichung, Taiwan*
[2]*Department of Critical Care Medicine, Taichung Veterans General Hospital, Taichung, Taiwan*
[3]*China Medical University, Taichung, Taiwan*
[4]*Division of Allergy, Immunology and Rheumatology, Department of Internal Medicine, Taichung Veterans General Hospital, Taichung, Taiwan*
[5]*Faculty of Medicine, National Yang-Ming University, Taipei, Taiwan*

Correspondence should be addressed to Yi-Hsing Chen; ysanne@vghtc.gov.tw

Academic Editor: Hiromasa Ohira

To present a first reported case of ruptured multifocal hepatic aneurysms in a woman with systemic lupus erythematosus (SLE) who was treated successfully with transcatheter arterial embolization (TAE) in literature, similar cases in the previous English literature were also reviewed and analyzed to summarize the clinical manifestations, management, and outcome in these patients. The data were gathered from the medical record and literature reviews were searched from PudMed. In our review, patients with SLE-related hepatic aneurysms were often middle-aged females. Most of them presented with acute abdominal pain and hypotension. The overall mortality rate was 50%, but it was lower (12.5%) in patients who received TAE. Both TAE and surgical intervention are used to treat SLE-related hepatic aneurysms. Our review raised concerns about early detection, diagnosis, and prompt intervention of possible hepatic aneurysm rupture in patients with SLE.

1. Introduction

Hepatic aneurysms are rare with an estimated incidence of approximately 0.002%. Very few cases have been reported in patients with systemic lupus erythematosus (SLE) [1] and the pathological mechanism, optimal treatment, and prognosis in this patient population are not clear. We present a case of multifocal hepatic aneurysm rupture in a woman with SLE successfully treated with transcatheter arterial embolization (TAE).

2. Case Presentation

A 35-year-old woman presented to the emergency department (ED) complaining of sudden-onset, persistent, moderately severe, left-sided headache with focal left visual field defect followed by right limb clumsiness three hours priorly. She was diagnosed with SLE 11 years previously after developing nephritis, intermittent arthritis, thrombocytopenia, and chronic leg ulcers. She was lupus anticoagulant positive. Treated with monthly cyclophosphamide pulse therapy followed by trimonthly injections for the first two and a half years, she remained free of flares on daily maintenance therapy (azathioprine, 50 mg; hydroxychloroquine, 200 mg; prednisolone, 5 mg (0.05 mg/kg/day); and aspirin, 100 mg).

Neurological exam revealed right homonymous hemianopsia without facial palsy but with right-sided hyperesthesia and dysmetria. Brain computed tomography (CT) and magnetic resonance angiography showed acute cerebral infarction in the left posterior cerebral artery territory involving the thalamus and occipital lobe complicated by minimal left temporo-occipital subarachnoid hemorrhage. She was weakly positive for lupus anticoagulant and borderline positive for anticardiolipin antibodies.

Her symptoms gradually improved, but she developed sudden-onset, severe epigastric pain with tachycardia, hypotension, and altered level of consciousness two weeks after hospitalization. Her hemoglobin dropped from 114 to 88 g/L, and abdominal CT angiography (CTA) showed a massive subcapsular hematoma with contrast extravasation in the left lateral segment of the liver (Figure 1). Emergent angiography showed diffuse hepatic artery aneurysms bilaterally over the liver parenchyma with contrast extravasation from a left hepatic subcapsular hematoma (Figure 2). Diagnosed with hepatic aneurysm rupture, embolization of left proximal hepatic artery with Gelfoam cubes was performed. However, her tachycardia persisted, and her hemoglobin was 66 g/L the next day. Follow-up CTA showed a new hematoma over liver segment 7/8. A second superselective TAE with Gelfoam cubes was performed via branches of right hepatic artery after which her vital signs stabilized. Concerned that antiphospholipid antibodies were responsible for the vascular events, rituximab was administered (500 mg in two consecutive doses two weeks apart). Follow-up abdominal CTA three months later showed resolution of the hepatic aneurysms (Figure 3).

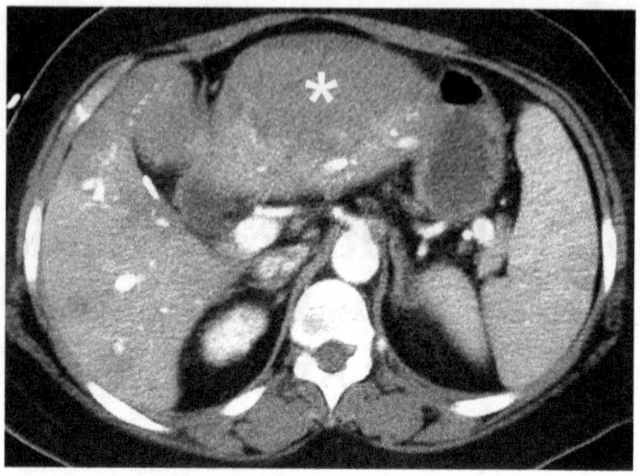

Figure 1: The computed tomographic angiography of abdomen of first time revealed subcapsular hematoma (asterisk) with contrast extravasation at left lateral segment of liver.

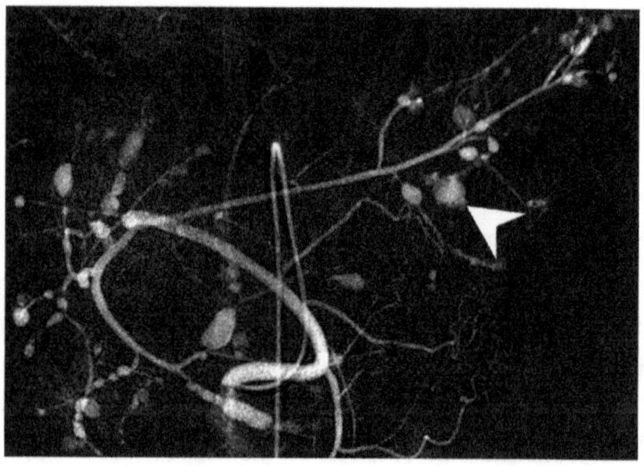

Figure 2: The angiography of abdomen revealed diffuse hepatic artery aneurysms over bilateral liver parenchyma with contrast extravasation over branches of left hepatic artery (arrowhead).

3. Discussion

Hepatic aneurysm rupture is rare but life-threatening. SLE-related hepatic aneurysms are even rarer, with only 13 reported cases in the literature [1–8]. Mean patient age at admission was approximately 34 years with a female predominance (71%) (Table 1). Mean SLE duration was 7.1 years with three-fourths of patients using continuous steroids and only 7% being hypertensive. Most patients presented with acute abdominal pain (78.6%) and hypotension (57.1%). The hepatic aneurysms were on the right lobe in 50%, left lobe in 41.6%, and bilateral lobes in 8.4%. Approximately 83% of patients had a ruptured aneurysm at presentation. The overall mortality rate was 50%, but it was lower (12.5%) in patients who received TAE. Lobectomy may be required as rescue therapy in 21.4% of patients.

The precise mechanism of hepatic aneurysm in SLE is not yet clear. Several hypotheses have been proposed including collagen degeneration, and destruction of smooth muscle and elastic fibers due to vasculitis as well as long-term steroid use [8]. Kurata et al. proposed two different pathogenic mechanisms for aortic aneurysms in lupus patients [9]. In younger patients, systemic vasculitis causes cystic medial degeneration leading to aortic dissection. In older patients on long-term glucocorticoid therapy, aneurysm formation is more likely to be caused by atherosclerosis due to aging. Our patient was relatively young, and the aneurysms resolved with treatment, so vasculitis is more likely to be the cause.

Owing to the large proportion of patients presenting with rupture as the first and only manifestation of hepatic aneurysm, the mortality rate is high, so rapid, appropriate diagnosis and management are crucial. We recommend CTA for diagnosis. Both TAE and surgical intervention are used to treat hepatic aneurysms [1, 10–13]. Choice of treatment modality depends on patient vital signs, aneurysm location, and presence of hepatic collateral circulation. TAE is preferred in patients with a patent portal vein who do not have obstructive jaundice but are a high surgical risk. Surgical intervention with vascular reconstruction is preferred in patients with obstructive jaundice and profound hypovolemic shock despite rapid resuscitation. In our case, prophylactic embolization of the main hepatic artery was performed during the second TAE to reduce intra-aneurysmal pressure, which may have contributed to shrinkage and disappearance of the aneurysms found at her three-month follow-up visit.

TABLE 1: The demographic data of patients with SLE-related hepatic aneurysms rupture in literature review.

Patient (reference)	Age	Gender	CAD risk*	Duration since SLE diagnosed (years)	Steroid use prior to admission	Presentation	Diagnostic tools	Hepatic aneurysms location	Hepatic rupture	Intervention	Outcome
Paronetto F et al., 1964	26	F	No	6	Yes	Abd pain and hypotension	Autopsy	NA	NA	Conservative therapy with transfusion	Death
Haslock I, 1974	32	F	No	14	Yes	Abd pain and hypotension	Laparotomy	Right lobe	Yes	Lobectomy	Death
Levitin PM et al., 1977	27	F	No	> 3	No	Abd pain	Laparotomy	NA	NA	Liver packing	Death
McCollum CN et al., 1979	33	F	HTN	12	Yes	Abd Pain and hypotension	Laparotomy	Left lobe	Yes	Left lateral lobectomy	Death
Trambert J et al., 1989	49	M	No	< 1	No	Abd pain	Abd CT and angiography	Left lobe	Yes	Embolization	Survival
Stratton R et al., 1999	24	F	No	3	Yes	Abd pain	Abd CT	Left lobe	No	Embolization, pulse therapy of steroid, and cyclophosphamide monthly	Survival
Huang JW et al., 1999	31	F	No	10	Yes	Hematemesis and tarry stool	Abd CT	Right lobe	Yes	Embolization	Death
Kong KO et al., 2002	21	M	No	2	Yes	Abd pain and cardiac arrest	Autopsy	Right lobe	Yes	Cardiopulmonary resuscitation	Death
Singh R et al., 2003	33	F	No	10	Yes	Abd pain and hypotension	Laparotomy	Right lobe	Yes	Laparotomy and cauterization of bleeding vessels	Death
Yamazaki K, 2004	34	M	No	13	Yes	Abd pain and hypotension	Abd CT	Left lobe	Yes	Embolization	Survival
Pollono EN et al., 2010	56	F	No	0.5	No	GI bleeding	Abd CT and angiography	Right lobe	No	Embolization	Survival
Liu C et al., 2011	31	M	No	7	Yes	Hemobilia	Angiography	Left lobe	Yes	Embolization and left lateral lobectomy	Survival
Reiter DA et al., 2013	41	F	No	NA	NA	Abd Pain and hypotension	Abd CT	Right lobe	Yes	Embolization	Survival
Our patient	35	F	No	11	Yes	Abd pain, hemobilia, and hypotension	Abd CT and angiography	Bilateral lobes	Yes	Embolization	Survival

Table 1: Continued.

Patient (reference)	Age	Gender	CAD risk*	Duration since SLE diagnosed (years)	Steroid use prior to admission	Presentation	Diagnostic tools	Hepatic aneurysms location	Hepatic rupture	Intervention	Outcome
Mean	33.8	4M10F	7%	7.1 yrs [1–14]	76.9%	78.6% abd pain; 14.3% hemobilia; 57.1% with hypotension; 28.6% with GI bleeding (including hemobilia)		50% right lobe; 41.6% left lobe; 8.4% bilateral lobe	83.3%	57.1% with embolization (mortality rate 12.5% within patients with embolization); 21.4% with lobectomy (mortality rate 67% within patients with lobectomy);	50% mortality

*HTN, hyperlipidemia, DM, PAOD, stroke.
F: female, M: male, NA: not available, HTN: hypertension, Abd: abdominal, CT: computed tomography, and GI: gastrointestinal.

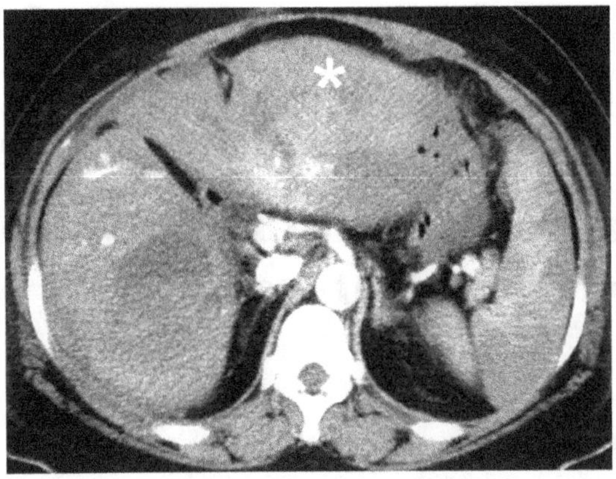

FIGURE 3: The computed tomographic angiography of abdomen 3 months later showed complete resolution of subscapular hematoma (asterisk). A residual hematoma over right lobe of liver was noted but without any clinical manifestation.

B cell depletion with the anti-CD20 monoclonal rituximab has been found to be effective in patients with SLE in several open-label cohort studies [14] and rituximab has also been suggested in refractory SLE [15]. Under the concern that hepatic aneurysm might be related to refractory SLE, we prescribed rituximab as induction and maintenance therapy for residual hepatic aneurysm after embolization. No residual hepatic aneurysm was discovered at her three-month follow-up visit.

To our knowledge, this is the first reported case of bilateral multifocal hepatic aneurysm rupture in a young woman with SLE successfully treated with TAE. It emphasizes the need for rapid diagnosis and treatment to achieve a successful clinical outcome in patients with hepatic artery aneurysm.

Authors' Contributions

Sz-Iuan Shiu and Su Ann Yong contributed equally to this work.

Acknowledgments

Evidence-based Practice and Policymaking Committee, Taichung Veterans General Hospital, Taichung, Taiwan, is acknowledged.

References

[1] D. A. Reiter, A. M. Fischman, and B. D. Shy, "Hepatic artery pseudoaneurysm rupture: a case report and review of the literature," *The Journal of Emergency Medicine*, vol. 44, no. 1, pp. 100–103, 2013.

[2] F. Paronetto, L. Deppisch, and L. R. Tuchman, "Lupus erythematosus with fatal hemorrhage into the liver and lesions resembling those of periarteritis nodosa and malignant hypertension. Immunocytochemical observations," *American Journal of Medicine*, vol. 36, no. 6, pp. 948–955, 1964.

[3] P. M. Levitin, D. Sweet, and C. M. Brunner, "Spontaneous rupture of the liver. an unusual complication of SLE," *Arthritis & Rheumatology*, vol. 20, no. 2, pp. 748–750, 1977.

[4] C. N. McCollum, M. E. Sloan, A. M. Davison, and G. R. Giles, "Ruptured hepatic aneurysm in systemic lupus erythematosus," *Annals of the Rheumatic Diseases*, vol. 38, no. 4, pp. 396–398, 1979.

[5] J. Trambert, E. Reinitz, and S. Buchbinder, "Ruptured hepatic artery aneurysms in a patient with systemic lupus erythematosus: case report," *CardioVascular and Interventional Radiology*, vol. 12, no. 1, pp. 32–34, 1989.

[6] E. N. Pollono, D. C. Madoff, S. C. Spence, and M. E. Suarez-Almazor, "Multiple hepatic artery aneurysms in a patient with systemic lupus erythematosus," *Lupus*, vol. 19, no. 1, pp. 93–95, 2010.

[7] R. Singh, Y. Menon, H. McGrath, and L. R. Espinoza, "Acute abdomen due to spontaneous organ rupture in systemic lupus erythematosus," *The American Journal of Medicine*, vol. 114, no. 2, pp. 160-161, 2003.

[8] J.-W. Huang, M.-S. Wu, T.-S. Chu, and T.-J. Tsai, "Hepatic aneurysm and portal vein thrombosis in a patient with lupus erythematosus on dialysis," *Nephrology Dialysis Transplantation* , vol. 14, no. 3, pp. 753–756, 1999.

[9] A. Kurata, T. Kawakami, J. Sato, A. Sakamoto, T. Muramatsu, and K. Nakabayashi, "Aortic aneurysms in systemic lupus erythematosus: a meta-analysis of 35 cases in the literature and two different pathogeneses," *Cardiovascular Pathology*, vol. 20, no. 1, pp. el–e7, 2011.

[10] D. P. Nathan, G. J. Wang, E. Y. Woo, R. M. Fairman, and B. M. Jackson, "Open and endovascular repair of hepatic artery aneurysm: two case reports and review of the literature," *Vascular*, vol. 19, no. 1, pp. 42–46, 2011.

[11] A. Gabelmann, J. Görich, and E. M. Merkle, "Endovascular treatment of visceral artery aneurysms," *Journal of Endovascular Therapy*, vol. 9, no. 1, pp. 38–47, 2002.

[12] N. Tulsyan, V. S. Kashyap, R. K. Greenberg et al., "The endovascular management of visceral artery aneurysms and pseudoaneurysms," *Journal of Vascular Surgery*, vol. 45, no. 2, pp. 276–283, 2007.

[13] S. S. Saltzberg, T. S. Maldonado, P. J. Lamparello et al., "Is endovascular therapy the preferred treatment for all visceral artery aneurysms?" *Annals of Vascular Surgery*, vol. 19, no. 4, pp. 507–515, 2005.

[14] J. Furtado and D. A. Isenberg, "B cell elimination in systemic lupus erythematosus," *Clinical Immunology*, vol. 146, no. 2, pp. 90–103, 2013.

[15] B. Duxbury, C. Combescure, and C. Chizzolini, "Rituximab in systemic lupus erythematosus: an updated systematic review and meta-analysis," *Lupus*, vol. 22, no. 14, pp. 1489–1503, 2013.

13

Hepatic Epithelioid Angiomyolipoma Treated with Laparoscopic Resection: Case Report and Review of the Literature

Chloe H. Williams,[1] **Kelli Hickle,**[1] **Katherine Bakke,**[1]
Sarah Jamshed,[2] **and Adel Bozorgzadeh**[1]

[1] *UMass Memorial Medical Center, Department of Surgery, Worcester, MA 01655, USA*
[2] *UMass Memorial Medical Center, Department of Pathology, Worcester, MA 01655, USA*

Correspondence should be addressed to Chloe H. Williams; chloe.williams@umassmemorial.org

Academic Editor: Dario Lorenzin

Hepatic angiomyolipoma is a rare primary liver tumor, with a radiographic appearance very similar to hepatocellular carcinoma. We present the case of a noncirrhotic patient with a liver tumor suspicious for HCC by imaging features. Liver biopsy demonstrated angiomyolipoma, and the patient successfully underwent a laparoscopic liver resection.

1. Introduction

Hepatic angiomyolipoma (AML) is a rare primary liver tumor, described only by small case series. Most cases occur in middle-aged women, who either are asymptomatic or describe vague abdominal pain. AMLs are tumors of mixed mesenchymal origin and predominantly occur in the kidney. Radiographically, hepatic AML can be difficult to differentiate from other liver tumors, particularly hepatocellular carcinoma (HCC), as they commonly appear as well-defined lesions with CT arterial phase enhancement and "washout" in the portal and delayed phases. Imaging features are not specific and can lead to a misdiagnosis of HCC if pathologic confirmation is not obtained [1]. The gold standard for the diagnosis of hepatic AML is histologic examination and immunohistochemical staining from biopsy or surgical specimen.

We present a case of epithelioid hepatic AML diagnosed preoperatively by biopsy and successfully laparoscopically resected.

2. Case Report

A 54-year-old Caucasian female with a history of cholecystectomy, obesity, and hypertension presented to the Emergency Department with acute onset right upper abdominal pain. Basic laboratories including liver function tests, complete blood count, and basic metabolic panel were unrevealing.

Outpatient workup revealed normal AFP, CA19-9, and CEA levels and negative hepatitis serologies. Ultrasound demonstrated a 2.3 cm, low-density mass in the left liver lobe. MRI showed a 3.4 cm mass with arterial phase enhancement and contrast washout in delayed sequences (Figure 1). By imaging, a diagnosis of HCC was suspected. However, as she did not have cirrhosis or other risk factors for HCC, she underwent percutaneous liver biopsy and was diagnosed with epithelioid AML.

The patient underwent laparoscopic hand-assisted left lateral hepatic segmentectomy. Our surgical approach included three trocar sites and a small midline hand port. Resection was completed using a combination of Ligasure and Cavitron Ultrasonic Surgical Aspirator (CUSA). One Jackson-Pratt drain was left at the cut edge of the liver.

Pathologic gross examination revealed a 3.0 x 2.5 x 2.0 cm mass, well-demarcated from adjacent hepatic parenchyma (Figure 2). On microscopy, an admixture of haphazardly arranged mature adipocytes, smooth muscle fascicles, and thick-walled vessels was seen, which was positive for HMB45, MelanA, MITF, and smooth muscle actin and negative for

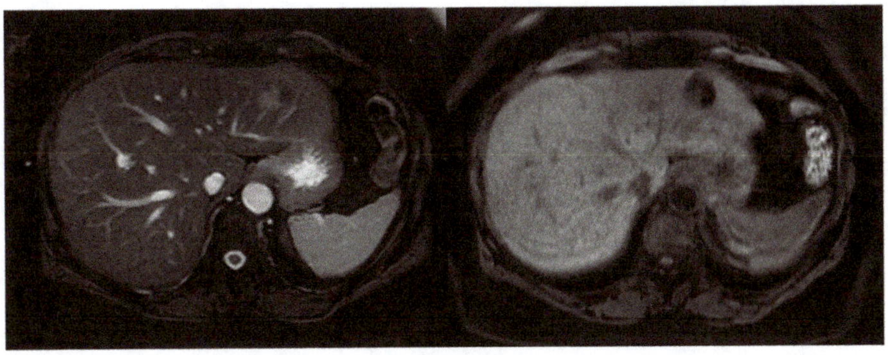

FIGURE 1: *MRI.* FIESTA (right) and T1-weighted images (left) revealed a 3.1 x 3.4 x 2 cm mass in the left lateral lobe of the liver. The lesion is hypervascular with washout of contrast on delayed post-contrast enhanced sequences.

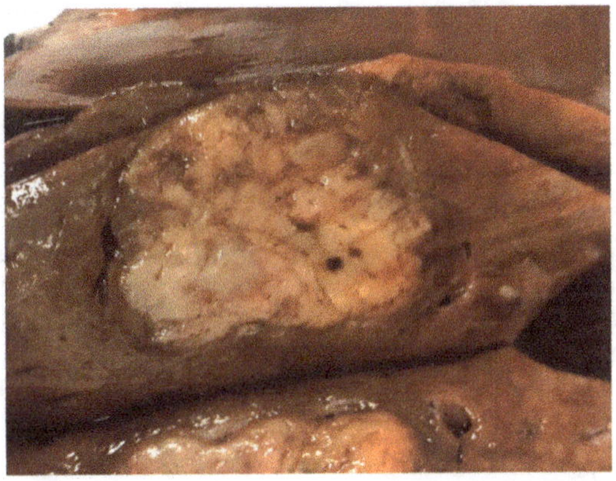

FIGURE 2: *Gross specimen.* On gross examination of the liver specimen, the cut surface of liver showed a well-demarcated, glistening, tan-yellow, lobular mass, measuring 3.0 x 2.5 x 2.0 cm. Final surgical pathology confirmed the diagnosis of epithelioid angiomyolipoma with no evidence of malignancy and 2.2 cm surgical margins.

pan-cytokeratin, HepParl, and S100, confirming the diagnosis (Figure 3). She was discharged after an uneventful hospital course.

The patient was seen in follow-up one year after her tumor resection. She was doing well and had fully returned to her presurgical level of function. 4-phase liver CT done at that time demonstrated no tumor recurrence or evidence of abdominal metastasis. LFTs were all within normal range.

3. Discussion

Hepatic AML typically presents as an incidentally found liver mass or in patients with vague abdominal discomfort, as in our case. Rarely are these tumors large enough to lead to presentation from mass effect, palpation, or rupture, though this has all been reported [2]. There is a known link associated with tuberous sclerosis of 5-15%, but this link is stronger in renal AML [3]. Hepatic epithelioid AML is rare and routinely misdiagnosed. One report identified 292 patients with hepatic AML, only 12 of which were epithelioid subtype [4].

On contrast-enhanced imaging, both hepatic AML and HCC appear hyperenhanced in the arterial phase with early washout times [5]. Several reports reveal rates of misdiagnosis of hepatic AML as HCC ranging from 25 to 80% [1, 5–7]. Because radiologic features make hepatic AML difficult to distinguish from HCC, the diagnosis of hepatic AML relies on immunohistochemical staining; HMB45 and SMA are positive, and Hep Parl and S100 are negative [8]. On histology, smooth muscle presence with variable distribution of epithelial cells, adipose cells, and blood vessels is seen.

Misdiagnosis as HCC has serious clinical and psychological implications for patients. Biopsies are not routinely performed once a radiographic diagnosis of HCC is made. Traditional treatment for HCC in a noncirrhotic patient is liver resection. However, liver transplantation is evolving as the standard of care for small HCCs due to simultaneous survival benefit and reduction in disease recurrence [9]. The diagnosis of HCC in our otherwise healthy patient was suspicious in the absence of other risk factors; therefore image-guided biopsy was performed to confirm her diagnosis. Preoperative biopsy providing accurate diagnosis in this case was useful as it allowed for comprehensive patient education and surgical planning. With liver transplant becoming an option for HCC management in many patients, misdiagnosis by imaging alone could have led to unnecessary and invasive

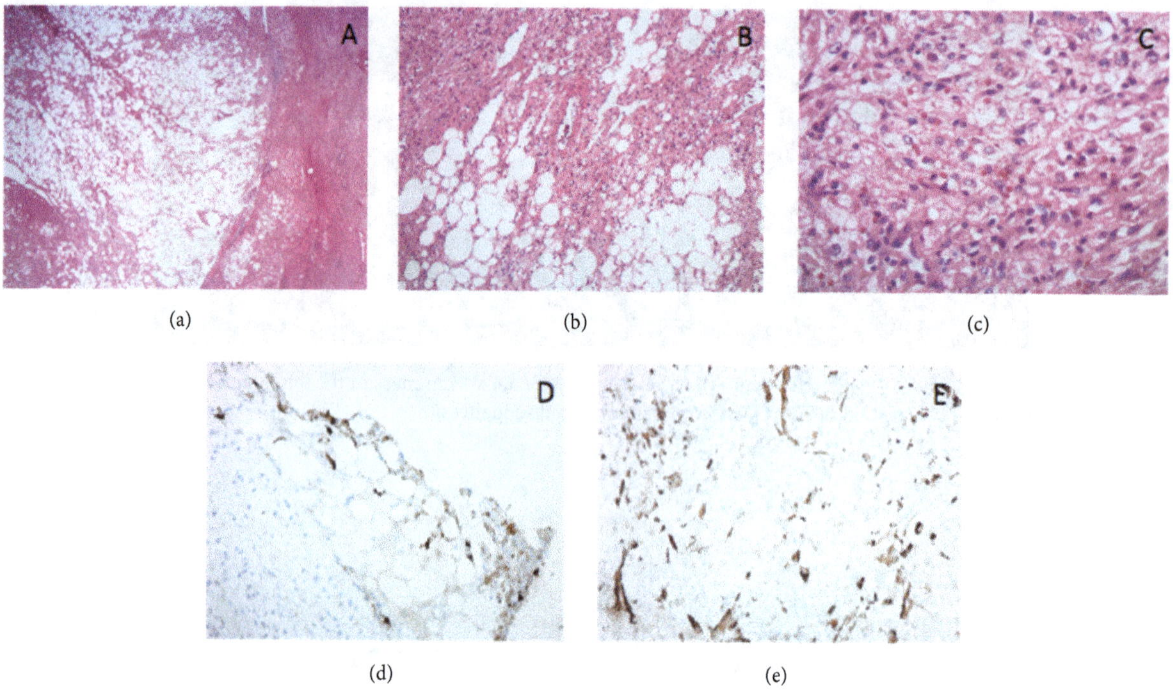

FIGURE 3: *Histopathologic features of epithelioid angiomyolipoma.* (a) Well-circumscribed mass with adjacent, mildly steatotic liver parenchyma (H&E; 20x). (b) The tumor is composed of eosinophilic cells, mature adipocytes, and thick walled vessels (center) (H&E; 100x). (c) The smooth muscle component includes a mixture of large epithelioid cells with abundant eosinophilic cytoplasm and prominent nucleoli, with interspersed smaller epithelioid cells and spindle cells (H&E; 400x). Immunohistochemistry performed on the biopsy of this lesion for HMB45 (200x) (d) and Smooth Muscle Actin (200x) (e) showed patchy, strong positivity in the lesional cells.

procedures. Due to the risk of malignant transformation or rupture of hepatic AML [10], resection is typically recommended. In select cases, a nonoperative approach with close surveillance is appropriate as mortality remains low at 0.8% [4].

Accurate preoperative diagnosis as AML allowed the patient and surgeon to come to an informed decision and to undergo the appropriate treatment of minimally invasive resection. Damaskos et al. reported the first laparoscopic resection of hepatic AML in 2017, and our case further demonstrates the safety and utility of this approach [11]. In the absence of metastatic lesions, most reports support good surgical outcomes and long-term survival for hepatic AML patients [2, 3].

We encourage clinicians to have a high index of suspicion of misdiagnosis of HCC in noncirrhotic patients without other HCC risk factors and to employ preoperative biopsy to confirm diagnosis in these cases. A correct diagnosis is crucial to tailor appropriate tumor management. HCC warrants excision in noncirrhotic patients and, increasingly, referral for transplant evaluation; hepatic AML can be treated with a laparoscopic resection as a safe, novel alternative to open surgery or clinical observation.

References

[1] C. Dai, L. P. Xue, and Y. M. Li, "Multi-slice computed tomography manifestations of hepatic epithelioid angiomyolipoma," *World Journal of Gastroenterology*, vol. 20, no. 12, pp. 3364–3368, 2014.

[2] W. Liu, Z. Meng, H. Liu et al., "Hepatic epithelioid angiomyolipoma is a rare and potentially severe but treatable tumor: a report of three cases and review of the literature," in *Oncology Letters*, vol. 11 of *3675*, p. 3669, 2016.

[3] Z. Garoufalia, N. Machairas, I. Kostakis et al., "Malignant potential of epithelioid angiomyolipomas of the liver: a case report and comprehensive review of the literature," *Molecular and Clinical Oncology*, vol. 9, pp. 226–230, 2018.

[4] A. J. Klompenhouwer, D. Verver, S. Janki et al., "Management of hepatic angiomyolipoma: A systematic review," *Liver International*, vol. 37, no. 9, pp. 1272–1280, 2017.

[5] Y. Tan, X. Xie, Y. Lin, T. Huang, and G. Huang, "Hepatic epithelioid angiomyolipoma: clinical features and imaging findings of contrast-enhanced ultrasound and CT," *Clinical Radiology*, vol. 72, no. 4, pp. 339.el–339.e6, 2017.

[6] J. Liu, C. Zhang, D. Hong et al., "Primary hepatic epithelioid angiomyolipoma: A malignant potential tumor which should be recognized," *World Journal of Gastroenterology*, vol. 22, no. 20, pp. 4908–4917, 2016.

[7] S. Ortiz and F. Tortosa, "Epithelioid angiomyolipoma of the liver: Clinicopathological correlation in a series of 4 cases," *Revista Española de Enfermedades Digestivas*, vol. 108, no. 1, pp. 27–30, 2015.

[8] H. Talati, J. Radhi, S. Popovich, and M. Marcaccio, "Hepatic epithelioid angiomyolipoma: case series," *Gastroenterology Research*, vol. 3, no. 6, pp. 293–295, 2010.

[9] G. Sapisochin and J. Bruix, "Liver transplantation for hepatocellular carcinoma: outcomes and novel surgical approaches," *Nature Reviews Gastroenterology & Hepatology*, vol. 14, no. 4, pp. 203–217, 2017.

[10] S. Tajima, A. Suzuki, and K. Suzumura, "Ruptured hepatic epithelioid angiomyolipoma: a case report and literature review," *Case Reports in Oncology*, vol. 7, no. 2, pp. 369–375, 2014.

[11] C. Damaskos, N. Garmpis, G. Anna, A. Nonnu, S. Sakellariou, G. Margonis et al., "Angiomyolipoma of the liver: a rare benign tumor treated with a laparoscopic approach for the first time," *In Vivo*, vol. 31, no. 6, pp. 1169–1173, 2017.

14

Hepatocellular Glycogen Accumulation in the Setting of Poorly Controlled Type 1 Diabetes Mellitus: Case Report and Review of the Literature

Atinuke Aluko,[1,2] Ikponmwosa Enofe,[1,2] Jacob Burch,[1,2] Julie Yam,[3] and Nazia Khan[1]

[1]*Michigan State University, Department of Internal Medicine, East Lansing, MI, USA*
[2]*Sparrow hospital, Lansing, MI, USA*
[3]*Michigan State University, Gastroenterology Fellowship, East Lansing, MI, USA*

Correspondence should be addressed to Jacob Burch; jacob.burch@sparrow.org

Academic Editor: Sorabh Kapoor

Glycogenic hepatopathy (GH) is the accumulation of glycogen in the hepatocytes and represents a rare complication in patients with diabetes mellitus (DM), most commonly type 1 DM. We present a case of a 23-year-old woman with a medical history of poorly controlled type 1 DM and gastroesophageal reflux disease (GERD) who presented with progressively worsening right-sided abdominal pain. Diagnostic workup resulted in a liver biopsy with hepatocytes that stained heavily for glycogen with no evidence of fibrosis or steatohepatitis. A diagnosis of glycogenic hepatopathy was made, and an aggressive glucose control regimen was implemented leading to resolution of symptoms and improvement in AST, ALT, and ALP. In addition to presenting this rare case, we offer a review of literature and draw important distinctions between glycogenic hepatopathy and other differential diagnoses with the aim of assisting providers in the diagnostic workup and treatment of glycogenic hepatopathy.

1. Introduction

Glycogenic hepatopathy, a rare occurrence usually seen in poorly controlled type 1 DM, is due to the accumulation of glycogen within the hepatocytes [1]. Patients with GH have an enlarged liver, elevated liver enzymes, and commonly present to the hospital with complaints of right upper abdominal pain [1–5]. It is crucial that this condition is diagnosed and differentiated from other conditions which present with similar symptoms, as GH is reversible unlike other differentials including nonalcoholic fatty liver disease (NAFLD) which is more commonly seen in type 2 DM [3]. Despite the increasing incidence of diabetes in the United States [6], the real incidence and prevalence of GH are unknown [1–5, 7–16], commonly being misdiagnosed or underdiagnosed. We present a case of a patient with poorly controlled type 1 diabetes who presented with abdominal pain, abnormal liver enzymes, and massive enlargement of the liver and was subsequently diagnosed with glycogenic hepatopathy.

2. Case Presentation

A 23-year-old woman with type 1 DM, GERD, amenorrhea (resolved) and more recently irregular menstrual periods whom presented to the emergency department with complaints of right-sided abdominal pain of 14 days duration. Pain was described as sharp in nature, intermittent, worsened by eating, and without any relieving factors. It was associated with nausea and had been progressively increasing in intensity and frequency of occurrence. She was diagnosed with type 1 DM 11 years prior, which was poorly controlled, with a mean HbA1c of 12.05% over a 2-year period. She had been admitted multiple times for DKA.

At presentation, the patient appeared well developed for her age except for a short stature and being underweight (BMI 17.54). She was tachycardic (HR 117 bpm) and tender in the right upper and lower quadrants of the abdomen without guarding or rebound tenderness. The liver was palpable 3 inches below the right costal margin. Laboratory results revealed mild DKA as evidenced by the elevated blood sugar (344 mg/dl), anion gap acidosis of 17, HCO3 of 18 mMol/L, venous pH 7.31, serum ketones < 1 : 4 dilution, and trace urine ketones. Her blood glucose reduced to 76 mg/dl after two liters of intravenous fluids. Her home insulin regimen was promptly resumed, and she did not require an insulin infusion. AST (511 mg/dl), ALT (366 mg/dl), and ALP (304 mg/dl) were elevated. Lactic acid was elevated at 8.0 mg/dL. Total bilirubin (0.4 mg/dl), albumin (4 mg/dl), INR (0.9), and platelet count (248 cells/microliter) were within normal limits. HbA1c on presentation was 11.5%. Other laboratory values including amylase and lipase were within normal limits.

Commuted tomography (CT) of the abdomen and pelvis with contrast (Figures 1 and 2) showed an enlarged liver, 26 cm in full length with mass effect on adjacent structures including the inferior vena cava, stomach, duodenum, pancreas, and hepatic flexure of the colon. Abdominal ultrasound with Doppler was negative for hepatic vein thrombosis. Of note, the patient was not on any hepatotoxic medications. Laboratory workup for causes of elevated liver enzymes including: infective workup (EBV, CMV, Hepatitis A, B, and C), iron studies (normal ferritin, decreased total iron, and iron saturation), ceruloplasmin level, serum alpha-fetoprotein, and thyroid function were all within normal limits. Celiac disease had been ruled out previously in the outpatient setting with negative tissue transglutaminase antibodies and endomysial antibody. Autoimmune workup including antinuclear antibody (ANA) titer, antismooth muscle antibody, antimitochondrial antibody, and liver/kidney microsome were all negative or within normal limits. A transthoracic echocardiogram showed normal right and left ventricular functions, with a left ventricular ejection fraction of 55–60%.

CT-guided biopsy of the liver was done due to diagnostic uncertainty and increasing AST/ALT (Table 1). Liver biopsy showed pale and swollen hepatocytes (Figure 3) with heavy glycogen staining seen on Periodic Acid Schiff (PAS) stain (Figure 4) which was absent after digestion with diastases (Figure 5). Numerous intranuclear glycogen inclusions, as well as some patchy steatosis, were noted. There were no signs of fibrosis or increased iron deposition.

A diagnosis of glycogenic hepatopathy was made. She was managed symptomatically for pain and strict glycemic control was implemented. Symptoms of abdominal pain improved, and lactic acid returned to normal (1.7 mg/dl) on hospital day 3 with adequate fluid resuscitation. The patient was discharged home on hospital day 7 (Table 1) with a more aggressive insulin regimen, and follow-ups with her primary care physician (PCP) and endocrinologist were scheduled. At discharge (day 7), AST, ALT, and ALP were 237 mg/dl, 271 mg/dl, and 200 mg/dl, respectively. Unfortunately, the patient was not compliant with follow-up and was not seen for another year at which time her HbA1C was 12.6%. Liver enzymes however were within normal limits with ALT, AST, and ALP at 20 mg/dl, 35 mg/dl, and 54 mg/dl, respectively. Repeat contrasted CT abdomen twelve months later showed persistent hepatomegaly measuring 27.8 × 21.4 × 15.5 cm (Figures 6 and 7). Liver dimensions were similar to the CT findings at initial presentation. The importance of strict glycemic control was reemphasized, and she was rescheduled for follow-up with her primary care physician and endocrinologist.

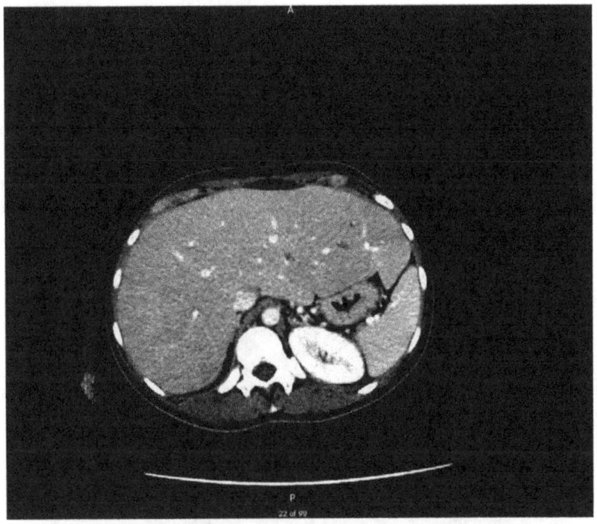

FIGURE 1: Axial commuted tomography scan, cross-sectional view showing massive hepatomegaly.

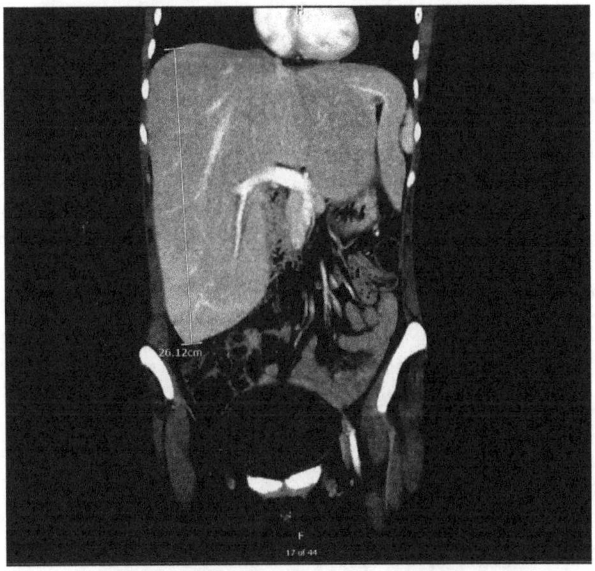

FIGURE 2: Coronal commuted tomography scan section showing an enlarged liver with maximum dimensions measuring 25.0 × 23 × 14.8 cm liver.

TABLE 1: Trends in liver enzyme during hospitalization and at follow-up a year later.

Trends in liver enzymes											
Days	0	1	2	3	4	5	6	7	14	24	365
AST	511	371	307	275	617	764	630	367	237	101	23
ALT	366	284	249	236	321	374	355	320	271	91	33

3. Discussion

Glycogenic hepatopathy (GH) is the accumulation of glycogen in the hepatocytes [1–5, 7–11]. Mauriac first described

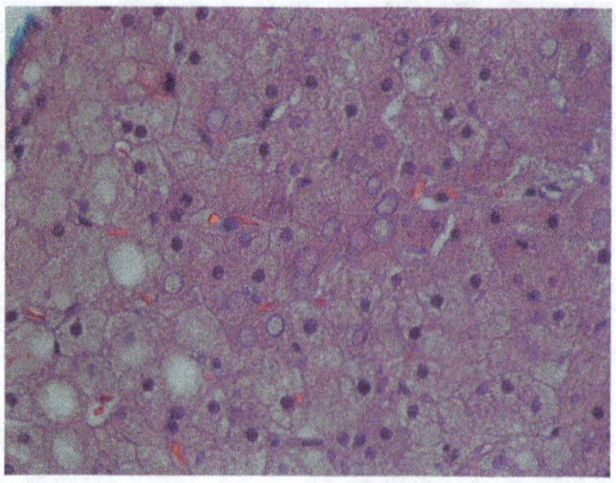

FIGURE 3: Histology of the liver showing hematoxylin and eosin (H & E) stain 40x showing pale and swollen hepatocytes.

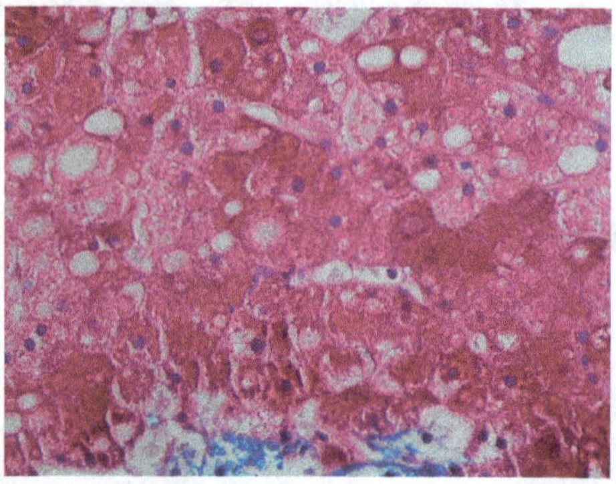

FIGURE 4: Histology of the liver with Periodic Acid Schiff (PAS) staining 40x without diastase showing hepatocytes heavily staining for glycogen.

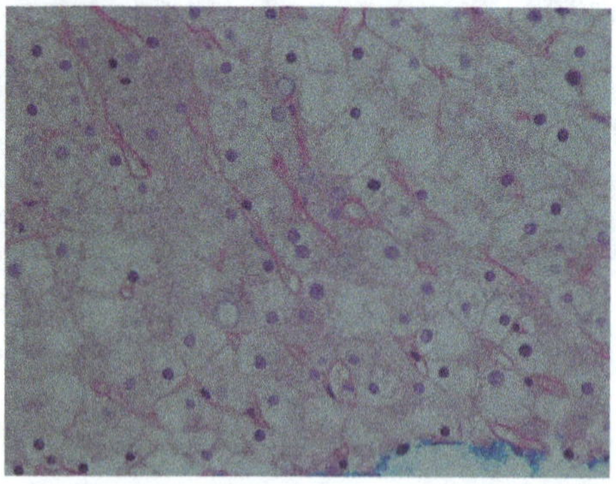

FIGURE 5: Histologic finding following periodic shift acid staining (PAS) after digestion with diastase 40x showing hepatocytes which do not stain with PAS confirming glycogen is responsible for findings.

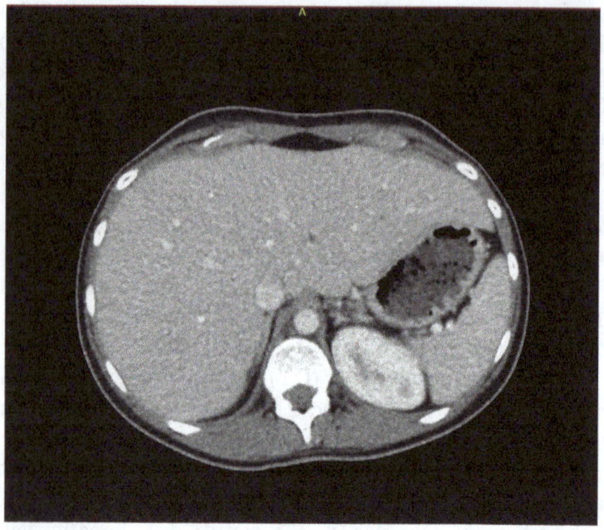

FIGURE 6: Axial commuted tomography scan, cross-sectional view showing massively enlarged liver at 12 months follow-up.

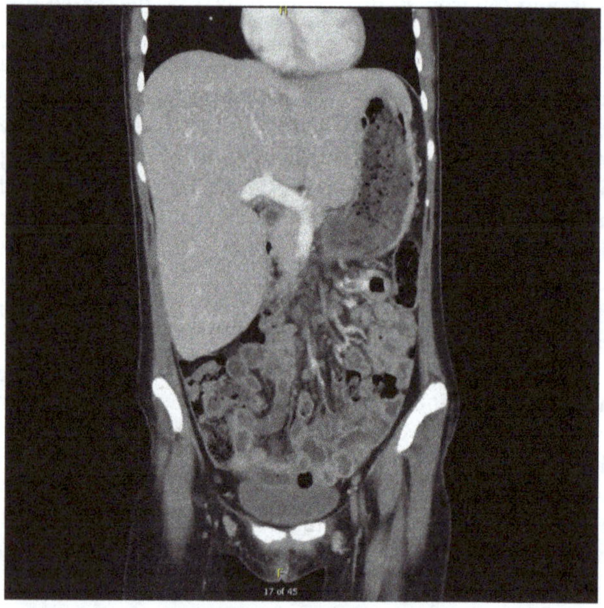

FIGURE 7: Coronal commuted tomographic scan section showing an enlarged liver with maximum dimensions measuring 25.0 × 23 × 14.8 cm at 12 months follow-up.

a syndrome in the 1930s after observing children with brittle diabetes who had reduced growth, delayed puberty, Cushing-like features, hepatomegaly, and elevated liver enzymes [5]. Over time, children and adults with brittle diabetes were noted to present with some components of Mauriac syndrome, commonly hepatomegaly and elevated liver enzymes termed glycogenic hepatopathy [7]. GH is underrecognized and often confused with fatty liver disease and nonalcoholic steatohepatitis, which is more common in type 2 diabetes.

The exact incidence and prevalence of the disease are unknown [1–5, 7–11]. Classically it is seen in longstanding, poorly controlled, type 1 diabetes (98% of cases) with a mean duration of 10.5 years and a mean HbA1c of 11.8 [1–3]. No gender predilection exists for developing GH [1, 4], and patients typically have a healthy body mass index [1–4].

The exact mechanism by which glycogen accumulates in the cytoplasm of the hepatocytes in patients with glycogenic hepatopathy is unknown. Higher glucose concentration activates the passive diffusion of glucose across the cell membrane by a noninsulin-dependent mechanism bypassing the insulin-dependent serum glucose transporter-2 (SGT-2) that acts to maintain glucose equilibrium between the extracellular and intracellular space [17]. This passive diffusion of glucose across the cell membrane by a non-insulin-dependent mechanism leads to increased glucose in the cytoplasm [17]. High levels of glucose in the cell results in more substrates for glycogen synthesis. Glucokinase present in the cytoplasm converts glucose to glucose-6-phosphate while glycogen synthetase, an enzyme also present in the cytoplasm of hepatocytes, converts glucose-6-phosphate to glycogen [8, 10]. A phosphatase activates glycogen synthase by dephosphorylation, and a high concentration of glucose and insulin modulate the activities of this phosphatase [18]. Thus, increased hepatic glycogenesis is thought to occur due to the presence of high cytoplasmic glucose concentration as well as the presence of exogenous insulin [3, 8–10]. The activation of phosphatase by increased cytoplasmic glucose and high levels of exogenous insulin rather than an alteration in the coding sequence of the glycogen phosphorylase gene better explain the increased activity of phosphatase seen in patients with GH [19].

Clinically, patients with GH may present in DKA with symptoms such as polyuria, polydipsia, dehydration, abdominal pain, nausea, and vomiting [18, 20]. They also have hepatomegaly (more than 90% of the time) [21], varying degree of elevated transaminases, and rarely elevated alkaline phosphatase. Elevated liver enzymes present with a hepatocellular pattern of injury rather than a cholestatic pattern [1, 2, 9], usually with AST greater than ALT [22]. This is likely due to enzyme leakage as a result of hepatocyte membrane injury [1, 19]. There is no histologic evidence to suggest cell death as a cause of elevated transaminases [22]. Hepatocellular injury in GH can present with mild elevations in transaminases to dramatically elevated values with some reported cases of liver enzymes up to 30 times the upper limit of normal [23–25]. Satyarengga et al. reported a case with peak AST of 3725 mg/dl and ALT 1049 mg/dl [24]. However, no cases of acute liver failure have been reported in the literature. As seen in our patient, elevation in lactic acid can occur in these patients [16]. The exact significance of this remains unknown [26]. However, some studies attribute this to reduced gluconeogenesis and lack of conversion of pyruvate to glucose [16]. Patients with GH do not have abnormalities in the synthetic function of the liver [2, 20]. There are a few cases of GH presenting with ascites without any signs of cirrhosis. The mechanism of ascites remains unclear [1]. Other laboratory abnormalities in patients with GH include a high amylase and/or lipase in patients with no clinical or radiographic evidence of acute pancreatitis [11]. The underlying mechanism of this is also unknown [11]. However, these findings of elevated lipase and amylase were not present in our patient.

A high index of suspicion is required in a patient with poorly controlled type 1 diabetes who presents with abdominal pain, hepatomegaly, and elevated liver enzymes [21]. There are, however, case reports of GH occurring in patients with type 2 diabetes with poor glycemic control [12, 13]; nondiabetics on high dose steroids [14]; a 3-year-old with dumping syndrome associated with gastrostomy feeding without glucose intolerance [15]; a patient who developed rapid onset hyperglycemia but had a HbA1c of 6.2% [27]; and a person with type 2 diabetes who attempted suicide with large dose of insulin glargine, treated with hypercaloric infusion [13].

The diagnosis of GH is made in patients in whom we have a high index of suspicion following a comprehensive history, physical examination, laboratory testing, and imaging studies. Liver biopsy is the gold standard for making a diagnosis of GH [21] but this is not always necessary. Liver biopsy should be performed in cases where the diagnosis is not definite, and other causes of hepatic dysfunction cannot be excluded [21]. Similarly, liver biopsy is reserved for patients who do not respond to treatment with tight glycemic control or have a persistent rise in liver enzymes despite improved glycemic control [28]. In evaluating diabetic patients with abdominal pain, hepatomegaly, and elevated liver enzymes in whom we suspect GH, history should include the duration of symptoms, how long the patient has had diabetes, and level of glycemic control. Abdominal imaging including ultrasound scan (US), CT, and gradient dual echo magnetic resonance imaging (MRI) are helpful non-non-invasive tools which, in addition to history and physical examination, can aid in the diagnosis of GH and reduce the need for invasive liver biopsies [21]. Sweetser and Kraichely reported the usefulness of CT to distinguish GH from fatty liver disease [29]. CT scan can differentiate higher liver densities in GH from lower densities seen in patients with fatty liver [29]. However, the use of CT scan is limited in cases where lower liver densities associated with fatty change occur in patients with GH [27] or cases with a smaller increase in liver density than expected, as seen in glycogen storage diseases [30, 31]. The use of CT scan in diagnosing GH may further be complicated by conditions that cause the liver to be hyperdense on imaging as seen in hemochromatosis and iodine deposition in the liver of patients who take amiodarone [28, 29]. Gradient dual echo MRI can distinguish fat deposition from edematous conditions, such as patients with acute liver injury, and from hepatitis both of which may appear as low-density areas on CT [32, 33]. The sensitivity of gradient dual echo MRI combined with other imaging modalities, like abdominal US and CT, increases in differentiating between GH and NASH thus reducing the need for a liver biopsy [27]. Unfortunately, our patient did not get a gradient dual echo MRI as this is not done at our center. Due to diagnostic uncertainty in our patient's presentation, a liver biopsy was done to confirm the diagnosis. Noninvasive tests like Fibro Sure have no use in the evaluation of GH or in differentiating GH from NASH [21]. The importance of differentiating these two clinical entities is necessary as their management and prognosis differ. All cases reported so far indicate that GH runs a benign [2, 10, 18, 19] and reversible course with tight glycemic control, while some cases of NASH progress to cirrhosis and hepatocellular carcinoma [34].

Histologically, accumulation of glycogen in the hepatocytes is pathognomonic. Hepatocytes are pale and swollen. There is absent to minimal inflammation and no fatty changes or spotty lobular necrosis. The architecture of the liver is preserved without any significant fibrosis. Glycogen accumulation demonstrated using PAS-diastase staining shows abundant cytoplasmic glycogen deposits which disappear after digestion with diastase [1, 20].

Liver enzymes usually normalize within 2–14 weeks of tight glycemic control, mostly achieved by subcutaneous insulin administration [10, 35, 36]. In two case reports, patients with poorly controlled type 1 diabetes and frequent episodes of hypoglycemia diagnosed with GH had a resolution of GH following pancreatic transplantation for other indications [19]. GH can recur if there is a relapse in poor glycemic control [9]. The level of glycemic control required for normalization of transaminitis and complete resolution of hepatomegaly remains unclear. However, few cases have reported decrease or normalization of liver enzymes and improvement of symptoms with a modest drop in HbA1c, without the need for aggressive insulin treatment [22, 29]. Cha et al. reported the resolution of transaminitis in patients with HbA1c above 11%. Similarly, Parmar et al. reported relief of abdominal pain and a decline in liver enzymes in their patient with a decrease in HbA1c of 0.6% (13.7% to 12.7%) [25].

In our patient, despite suboptimal glucose control, transaminitis resolved and liver enzymes were within normal limits a year later, which points towards the benign course of the disease. Follow-up repeat CT of the abdomen did not show a reduction in liver size which could be explained by the suboptimal glucose control, noncompliance with insulin regimen evident by HbA1c of 12.6%, and temporary loss to follow-up. The patient remains at risk for relapse due to inadequate glycemic control [9, 37].

4. Conclusion

Patients with GH usually present with nonspecific symptoms that may lead to a delay in diagnosis. In patients with type 1 DM with elevated liver enzymes with or without hepatomegaly, glycogenic hepatopathy should be considered as a differential diagnosis. A high index of suspicion by clinicians can lead to prompt diagnosis and potentially decrease the need for unnecessary testing in this patient population. It is important to distinguish GH from NAFLD for prognostication and management with the former following a benign cause and the latter progressing to cirrhosis in some cases. We advocate more research to understand better risk as well as potentiating and/or protective factors associated with the development of GH.

References

[1] M. Toberson, Y. Y. Chen, E. Brunt et al., "Glycogenic hepatopathy: an underrecognized hepatic complication of diabetes mellitus," *American Journal of Surgical Pathology*, vol. 30, no. 4, pp. 508–513, 2006.

[2] R. Chatila and B. A. West, "Hepatomegaly and abnormal liver tests due to glycogenosis in adults with diabetes," *Medicine*, vol. 75, no. 6, pp. 327–333, 1996.

[3] A. Abaci, O. Bekem, T. Unuvar et al., "Hepatic glycogenosis: a rare cause of hepatomegaly in type 1 diabetes mellitus," *Journal of Diabetes and Its Complications*, vol. 22, no. 5, pp. 325–328, 2008.

[4] G. S. Sayuk, J. E. Elwing, and M. Lisker-Melman, "Hepatic glycogenosis: an underrecognized source of abnormal liver function tests?" *Digestive Diseases and Sciences*, vol. 52, no. 4, pp. 936–938, 2007.

[5] P. Mauriac, "Gros ventre: hepatomegaly, troubles de las croissance chez les enfants diabetiques traits depuis plusieurs annes par l'insuline," *Gax Hebd Med Bordeaux*, vol. 26, pp. 402–410, 1930.

[6] Center for Disease Control and Prevention, *National Diabetes Statistics Report*, CDC, Atlanta, GA, USA, 2017.

[7] N. M. O. Zuckerman-Levin and N. Shehadeh, "Glycogenic hepatopathy in an adolescent with type 1 DM," in *Diabetes Case Studies*, B. Draznin, C. C. L. Wang, and D. J. Rubin, Eds., pp. 175–179, American Diabetes Association, Alexandria, VA, USA, 2015.

[8] S. S. Rogal, C. Ukomadu, B. D. Levy, and J. Loscalzo, "A sweet source of abdominal pain," *New England Journal of Medicine*, vol. 364, no. 18, pp. 1762–1767, 2011.

[9] S. Messeri, L. Messerini, F. Vizzutti, G. Laffi, and F. Marra, "Glycogenic hepatopathy associated with type 1 diabetes mellitus as a cause of recurrent liver damage," *Annals of Hepatology*, vol. 11, no. 4, pp. 554–558, 2012.

[10] C. Munns, R. McCrossin, M. Thomsett, and J. Batch, "Hepatic glycogenosis: reversible hepatomegaly in type 1 diabetes," *Journal of Paediatrics and Child Health*, vol. 36, no. 5, pp. 449–452, 2000.

[11] M. Silva, M. Marques, H. Cardoso et al., "Glycogenic hepatopathy in young adults: a case series," *Revista Espanola de Enfermedades Digestivas*, vol. 108, 2016.

[12] M. Nakamuta, M. Ohashi, K. Goto, Y. Tanabe, K. Hiroshige, and H. Nawata, "Diabetes mellitus- associated glycogen storage hepatomegaly: report of a case and review of the Japanese literature Fukuoka," *Igaku Zasshi*, vol. 84, no. 7, pp. 354–358, 1993.

[13] T. Tsujimoto, M. Takano, M. Nishiofuku et al., "Rapid onset of glycogen storage hepatomegaly in a type-2 diabetic patient after a massive dose of long-acting insulin and large doses of glucose," *Internal Medicine*, vol. 45, no. 7, pp. 469–473, 2006.

[14] T. C. Lance, H. Shiloh, and L. Dembo, "Hepatomegaly following short-term high-dose steroid therapy," *Journal of Pediatric Gastroenterology and Nutrition*, vol. 5, no. 1, pp. 41–46, 1986.

[15] J. M. Resnick, I. Zador, and D. L. Fish, "Dumping syndrome, a cause of acquired glycogenic hepatopathy," *Pediatric and Developmental Pathology*, vol. 14, no. 4, pp. 318–321, 2011.

[16] M. C. G. J. Brouwers, J. C. Ham, E. Wisse et al., "Elevated lactic levels in patients with poorly regulated type 1 diabetes and glycogenic hepatopathy: a new feature of Mauriac syndrome," *Diabetes Care*, vol. 38, no. 2, pp. e11–e12, 2015.

[17] H. R. Jeong, Y. S. Shim, Y. B. Kim, H. S. Lee, and J. S. Hwang, "Glycogenic Hepatopathy in a Korean girl with poorly controlled type 1 diabetes mellitus," *Annals of Pediatric Endocrinology & Metabolism*, vol. 19, no. 1, pp. 49–52, 2014.

[18] S. Mukewar, A. Sharma, K. A. Lackore et al., "Clinical, biochemical, and histopathology features of patients with glycogenic hepatopathy," *Clinical Gastroenterology and Hepatology*, vol. 15, no. 6, pp. 927–933, 2017.

[19] J. A. Fridell, R. Saxena, N. P. Chalasani, W. C. Goggins, J. A. Powelson, and O. W. Cummings, "Complete reversal of glycogen hepatopathy with pancreas transplantation: two cases," *Transplantation*, vol. 83, no. 1, pp. 84–86, 2007.

[20] T. Saadi, "Glycogenic hepatopathy: a rare disease that can appear and resolve rapidly in parallel with glycemic control," *Israel Medical Association Journal*, vol. 14, no. 4, pp. 269-270, 2012.

[21] J. Khoury, Y. Zohar, N. Shehadeh, and T. Saadi, "Glycogenic hepatopathy," *Hepatobiliary & Pancreatic Diseases International*, vol. 17, no. 2, pp. 113–118, 2018.

[22] J. H. Cha, S. H. Ra, Y. M. Park et al., "Three cases of glycogenic hepatopathy mimicking acute and relapsing hepatitis in type I diabetes mellitus," *Clinical and Molecular Hepatology*, vol. 19, no. 4, pp. 421–425, 2013.

[23] M. T. Julián, N. Alonso, I. Ojanguren et al., "Hepatic glycogenosis: an underdiagnosed complication of diabetes mellitus?," *World Journal of Diabetes*, vol. 6, no. 2, pp. 321–325, 2015.

[24] M. Satyarengga, Y. Zubatov, S. Frances, G. Narayanswami, and R. J. Galindo, "Glycogenic hepatopathy: a complication of uncontrolled diabetes," *AACE Clinical Case Reports*, vol. 3, no. 3, pp. e255–e259, 2017.

[25] N. Parmar, M. Atiq, L. Austin, R. A. Miller, T. Smyrk, and K. Ahmed, "Glycogenic hepatopathy: thinking outside the box," *Case Reports in Gastroenterology*, vol. 9, no. 2, pp. 221–226, 2015.

[26] M. Chen, T. Y. Kim, and A. M. Pessegueiro, "Elevated lactate levels in a non-critically ill patient," *JAMA*, vol. 313, no. 8, pp. 849-850, 2015.

[27] F. Murata, I. Horie, T. Ando et al., "A case of glycogenic hepatopathy developed in a patient with new-onset fulminant type 1 diabetes: the role of image modalities in diagnosing hepatic glycogen deposition including gradient-dual-echo MRI," *Endocrine Journal*, vol. 59, no. 8, pp. 669–676, 2012.

[28] A. Chandel, B. Scarpato, J. Camacho, M. McFarland, and S. Mok, "Glycogenic hepatopathy: resolution with minimal glucose control," *Case Reports in Hepatology*, vol. 2017, Article ID 7651387, 3 pages, 2017.

[29] S. Sweetser and R. E. Kraichely, "The bright liver of glycogenic hepatopathy," *Hepatology*, vol. 51, no. 2, pp. 711-712, 2010.

[30] J. L. Doppman, M. Cornblath, A. J. Dwyer, A. J. Adams, M. E. Girton, and J. Sidbury, "Computed tomography of the liver and kidneys in glycogen storage disease," *Journal of Computer Assisted Tomography*, vol. 6, no. 1, pp. 67–71, 1982.

[31] P. R. Biondetti, D. Fiore, and P. C. Muzzio, "Computed tomography of the liver in von Gierke's disease," *Journal of Computer Assisted Tomography*, vol. 4, no. 5, pp. 685-686, 1980.

[32] M. A. Fischer, D. Nanz, C. S. Reiner et al., "Diagnostic performance and accuracy of 3-D spoiled gradient-dual-echo MRI with water- and fat- signal separation in liver-fat quantification: comparison to liver biopsy," *Investigative Radiology*, vol. 45, no. 8, pp. 465–470, 2010.

[33] F. Springer, J. Machann, C. D. Claussen et al., "Liver fat content determined by magnetic resonance imaging and spectroscopy," *World Journal of Gastroenterology*, vol. 16, no. 13, pp. 1560–1566, 2010.

[34] P. Angulo, "Nonalcoholic fatty liver disease," *New England Journal of Medicine*, vol. 346, no. 16, pp. 1221–1231, 2002.

[35] P. Saxena, I. Turner, and R. McIndoe, "Hepatobiliary and pancreatic: glycogenic hepatopathy: a reversible condition," *Journal of Gastroenterology and Hepatology*, vol. 25, no. 3, p. 646, 2010.

[36] K. E. Imtiaz, C. Healy, S. Sharif et al., "Glycogenic hepatopathy in type 1 diabetes: an underrecognized condition," *Diabetes Care*, vol. 36, no. 1, pp. e6–e7, 2013.

[37] J. M. Sherigar, J. D. Castro, Y. M. Yin, D. Guss, and S. R. Mohanty, "Glycogenic hepatopathy: a narrative review," *World Journal of Hepatology*, vol. 10, no. 2, pp. 172–185, 2018.

15

Hepatic Cyst: An Unusual Suspect of Syncope

Mohammad K. Choudhry,[1] **Bei Xiong**,[2] **Antony Anandaraj**,[2] **and John Trillo**[1]

[1]*Department of Gastroenterology, NYCHH-Coney Island Hospital, Brooklyn, NY, USA*
[2]*Department of Medicine, NYCHHC-Coney Island Hospital, Brooklyn, NY, USA*

Correspondence should be addressed to Mohammad K. Choudhry; choudhrykhawar@gmail.com

Academic Editor: Atsushi Irisawa

The patient is a 75-year-old man with history of diabetes and hypertension who presented with syncope after experiencing sharp, 10/10 right flank and abdominal pain worsening over three weeks associated with decreased appetite. Physical examination revealed hepatomegaly and right lower quadrant (RUQ) tenderness, negative for peritoneal signs. Bloodwork showed leukocytosis (13 K/mcl), alkaline phosphatase (141 U/L), total bilirubin (2.0 mg/dL), and gamma-glutamyl transferase (172 U/L). Computed Tomography (CT) revealed multiple hepatic cysts with the largest measuring $17 \times 14 \times 18$ cm (Figure 1). Parenteral opiates provided minimal relief. Cardiac and neurologic etiologies of syncope were ruled out. The patient's course was complicated by opioid-induced delirium as his abdominal pain progressively worsened despite escalating doses of parenteral and oral analgesics. Gastroenterology and interventional radiology consulted to evaluate for Glisson's capsular stretch. Therapeutic aspiration yielded 2.5 L of serous fluid, which alleviated the patient's pain. Cytology was negative for malignancy. Opiates were titrated down. Repeat CT (Figure 2) showed cysts that were significantly reduced in size. The patient showed complete resolution of symptoms and was subsequently discharged. We present a rare case of a large hepatic cyst causing syncope. In the appropriate clinical setting, syncope with RUQ tenderness and hepatomegaly should raise the index of suspicion for hepatic cysts.

1. Background

Syncope is transient loss of consciousness with many potential causes. The evaluation of syncope typically involves a thorough history and physical exam followed by diagnostic studies to rule out possible etiologies including orthostatic hypotension, cardiac arrhythmia, structural heart diseases, neurologic, mediation side effects, psychiatric, and stress-related conditions. We present a 75-year-old male with severe pain-related vasovagal syncope due to a hepatic cyst.

2. Case Presentation

The patient is a 75-year-old man with a past medical history of type 2 diabetes mellitus and hypertension who was brought in by emergency medical services after experiencing a possible syncope due to severe right side flank pain. The patient had two witnessed syncopal episodes while waiting for the ambulance service as per the wife. He was then admitted for further evaluation of syncope.

The patient had worsening right-sided flank pain since the past 3 weeks. He described the pain as sharp, 10/10 in intensity which was also associated with a decrease in appetite. He had never experienced these symptoms in the past and denied any associated nausea, vomiting, dysuria, hematuria, fever, chills, or rigors.

On examination, he was alert and oriented to time, place, and person complaining of abdominal pain. His abdomen was soft and distended, and right lower quadrant was tender to palpate without any guarding. He also had significant hepatomegaly. Laboratory findings were indicative of leukocytosis (13), elevated alkaline phosphatase (141), total bilirubin (2.0), and GGT (172). CT head ruled out any intracranial pathologies. CT abdomen/pelvis (Figure 1) showed multiple hepatic cysts. Largest cyst was in the right lobe measuring about $17 \times 14 \times 18$ cm and others measured up to 9 cm and 4 cm in the right inferior lobe and the left

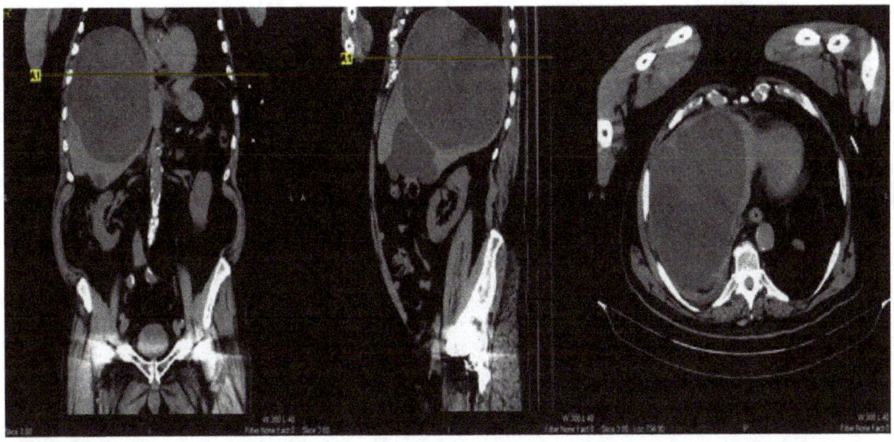

Figure 1: Initial CT abdomen/pelvis with multiple views of large hepatic cysts.

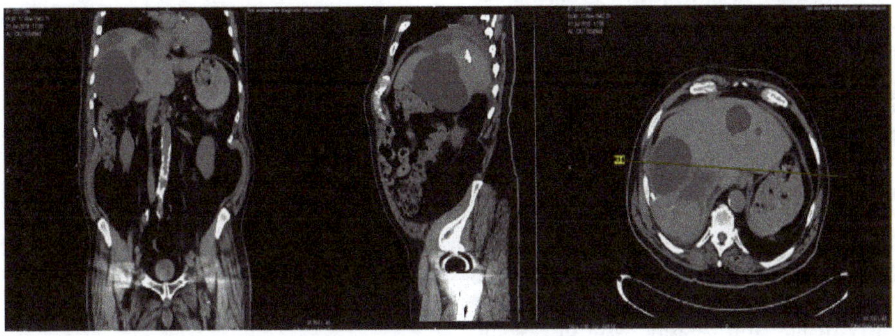

Figure 2: Postdrainage CT abdomen/pelvis showing significant reduction of the size of the cysts.

lobe, respectively. Since admission, he was started on parenteral opiates which minimally helped his pain symptoms with no further reported syncopal episodes. Additional testing including EEG, 24 hours holter monitor, and echocardiogram did not reveal any cardiac or neurologic etiologies of syncope.

During his course, his abdominal pain symptoms got worse despite escalating doses of parenteral and oral opioid pain medication, which eventually progressed to opiate induced delirium. Gastroenterology as well as interventional radiology was consulted since his symptoms were attributed to stretching of the liver capsule. A multidisciplinary decision was made after a detailed discussion about the risk of reaccumulation with the patient, and a therapeutic aspiration of the cyst was performed. 2.5 L of serous colored fluid was aspirated, and cytology was negative for malignancy. This intervention resolved his pain symptoms and opiates were titrated down as tolerated over the next few days.

A Repeat abdominal/Pelvis CT (Figure 2) showed a significantly smaller cyst measuring $8 \times 6 \times 6$ cm. In an attempt to prevent reaccumulation, sclerotherapy was offered to the patient and family, but due to the risk of iatrogenic sclerosis of the biliary system, the patient refused sclerotherapy at the time. His abdominal pain eventually resolved requiring no pain medications with significant improvement in his appetite and was discharged to the rehabilitation center.

3. Discussion

This case demonstrates a unique presentation of hepatic simple cyst-induced vasovagal syncope. Most liver cysts are incidental findings on imaging usually requiring no treatment and tend to have a benign course [6]. Our patient presented with a huge $17 \times 14 \times 18$ cm cyst with capsular stretching that led to severe pain-related vasovagal syncope due to parasympathetic activation. Even though aspiration of the cyst is not the typical intervention given the high likelihood of reaccumulation, we proceeded with the goal of therapeutic pain relief. This intervention of therapeutic CT-guided aspiration not only provided resolution of symptoms also helped with rapid taper of his opioid pain medications. Simple aspiration has a high likelihood of recurrence (10–25 percent recurrence rate), and sclerotherapy was considered in this patient to prevent reaccumulation; however, due to the high incidence of iatrogenic sclerosis, sclerotherapy was not performed. In our patient, *R* factor was suggestive of cholestasis; however clinical and radiological findings were not supportive of cholestatic injury.

Benign liver cysts occur in 4–5% of individuals with a female predominance [1]. They are usually incidental findings on imaging because no more than 10–15% of these patients have symptoms. Prevalence of simple cysts occurs more commonly in the right lobe and increases with age. More than half of individuals older than 60 years of age are likely to have one or more simple cysts. Cysts that reach giant sizes occur almost exclusively in patients greater than 50 years of age [2].

Larger cysts can lead to complications including hemorrhage, pain, rupture into the peritoneal cavity, infection, and obstruction of the biliary duct [3]. Therapeutic interventions include needle aspiration with or without injection of sclerosing agents (alcohol and minocycline hydrochloride), laparoscopic unroofing of the cyst, and liver resection [4]. It is recommended that interval (6 to 12 months) ultrasounds be utilized to monitor for reaccumulation, growth, or resolution of the hepatic cyst [5].

References

[1] C. O. Mărginean, C. Mărginean, L. Elena Meliţ, V. Ş. Săsăran, M. Poruţiu, and C. D. Mărginean, "An incidental diagnosis of a giant paraovarian cyst in a female teenager: a case report," *Medicine*, vol. 97, no. 48, Article ID e13406, 2018.

[2] N. S. Salemis, E. Georgoulis, S. Gourgiotis, and E. Tsohataridis, "Spontaneous rupture of a giant non parasitic hepatic cyst presenting as an acute surgical abdomen," *Annals of Hepatology*, vol. 6, no. 3, pp. 190–193, 2007.

[3] K. Hanazaki, M. Wakabayashi, H. Mori et al., "Hemorrhage into a simple liver cyst: diagnostic implications of a recent case," *Journal of Gastroenterology*, vol. 32, no. 6, pp. 848–851, 1997.

[4] J. P. Benhamou and Y. Menu, "Non-parasitic cystic diseases of the liver and intrahepatic biliary tree," in *Surgery of the Liver and Biliary Tract*, L. H. Blumgart, Ed., p. 1197, 2nd edition, Churchill Livingstone, New York, NY, USA, 1994.

[5] H. L. Nisenbaum and S. E. Rowling, "Ultrasound of focal hepatic lesions," *Seminars in Roentgenology*, vol. 30, no. 4, pp. 324–346, 1995.

[6] B. R. Taylor and B. Langer, "Current surgical management of hepatic cyst disease," *Advances in Surgery*, vol. 31, no. 31, pp. 127–48, 1997.

[7] A. Koratala and V. Bhatti, "An unusual cause of syncope," *Internal and Emergency Medicine*, vol. 12, no. 5, pp. 717–719, 2017 Aug.

[8] E. Belyavskiy, M. Tadic, S. Hassfeld, and B. Pieske, "A giant hepatic cyst: a rare cause of syncope," *Canadian Journal of Cardiology*, vol. 34, no. 9, pp. 1234.e1–1234.e2, 2018.

16

Acute Hepatitis Induced by Intravesical BCG Therapy: A Rare but Serious Complication

Hakima Abid ,[1,2] Mouna Figuigui ,[1,2] Sidi Adil Ibrahimi ,[1,2] Mohamed El Abkari,[1,2] Mohamed Mzyiene ,[2,3] Soufiane Ennaciri ,[2,3] Ouima Justin Ziba ,[2,3] Mohamed Jamal El Fassi ,[2,3] Layla Tahiri Elousrouti ,[2,4] and Laila Chbani[2,4]

[1]*Department of Hepato-Gastroenterology, University Hospital Hassan II-Fez, Laboratory of Human Pathology, Biomedicine and Environment, Fes, Morocco*
[2]*Faculty of Medicine and Pharmacy of Fez, Sidi Mohamed Ben Abdellah University Fez-Morocco, Fes, Morocco*
[3]*Urology Department-University Hospital Hassan II-Fez, Fes, Morocco*
[4]*Pathological Anatomy Department, University Hospital Hassan II of Fez, Fes, Morocco*

Correspondence should be addressed to Hakima Abid; abidhakima@hotmail.com

Academic Editor: Haruki Komatsu

Bacillus Calmette and Guérin (BCG), widely used as a vaccination to prevent tuberculosis, is also used as immunotherapy, by intrabladder instillation, to treat superficial bladder cancers and prevent recurrence. Complications following instillation of BCG are most often localized reactions, such as cystitis or hematuria. They can more rarely be generalized and potentially severe such as hepatitis, pneumopathies, aortitis, and localization to hematopoietic tissue. We have reported the observation of a 47-year-old patient followed up for a bladder tumor operated for transurethral resection of the bladder, then having benefited from an instillation of BCG therapy complicated by occurrence a week later of an acute hepatitis. The diagnostic time was 2 days, and the outcome was favorable with corticosteroid therapy.

1. Introduction

Bacillus Calmette and Guérin (BCG) is a living strain of *Mycobacterium bovis* of attenuated virulence. Its main uses are the vaccination for the prevention of tuberculosis and the immunotherapy of superficial urothelial cancers. Intravesical instillation is, therefore, indicated as a first-line treatment as a complementary curative treatment to endoscopic resection and for the prevention of recurrence. BCG therapy can be complicated by systemic attacks such as pneumonia, hepatitis, aortitis, bone marrow failure, spondylodiscitis [1].

2. Observation

This is a 47-year-old patient who has been a chronic tobacco user for 20 years and gave up 4 years ago. He already had a surgery for left varicocele in 2005. The history of the disease dates back to October 2020 when the patient had undergone a transurethral resection of the bladder, including the anatomopathological study of the shavings of resection returned in favor of a pTa G2 tumor. The decision was to put the patient on BCG therapy that had started 4 months after surgery. The patient had suddenly presented one day after the first instillation of the BCG a cholestatic jaundice associated with an influenza syndrome made up of asthenia and myalgia with pain in the right hypochondrium all evolving in a context of feeling feverish, chills, and asthenia. The examination has shown a conscious, afebrile, jaundiced patient with hypogastric tenderness and right hypochondrium without hepatomegaly.

Biology has revealed a disturbed liver function test with ASAT: 245 U/L (6 times the upper limit of normal (ULN)), ALAT: 487 (12 $*$ LSN), GGT: 611 U/L (8.7 LSN), PAL:

237 U/L (1.4 * LSN), total bilirubin: 64, and direct bilirubin at 41. CRP was 7.5 mg/L. Thrombocytopenia was noted at 68000 elements/mm^3. Hemoglobin was correct at 16 g/dl as well as leukocytes (5140/mm^3), PT (100%), and renal function (creatinine = 8 g/l, urea = 0.29). The liver ultrasound and abdominal CT scan were normal except a fatty liver. The serologies for hepatitis A, B, C, HIV, CMV, and EBV were negative. Protein electrophoresis and immunoglobulin weight assay were normal. There were no antimitochondria or antitissue antibodies or antineutrophilic cytoplasm (ANCA). Blood cultures remained sterile. Thus, a hepatic biopsy was performed, and the anatomopathological analysis revealed granulomatous steatohepatitis without giant cells or caseous necrosis, classified S3A2F1, made up of an inflammatory lobular infiltrate and granulomas made of epithelioid and histiocytic cells; a special staining by Masson's trichrome was performed showing portal fibrosis without septa emissions and sinusoidal fibrosis, and special reticulin staining showed retention of the reticulin pattern. Immunohistochemical complement was performed. CD 68 highlighted granulomas described above, and CK 19 demonstrated portal cholangiolar proliferation (Figure 1).

In the absence of obvious infectious or inflammatory disease, the diagnosis of granulomatous hepatitis secondary to BCG therapy was retained. The patient was put on injectable corticosteroid therapy at a dose of 1 mg/kg/day for 15 days and then degression. The clinical course was marked by the improvement of asthenia and jaundice. Assessment at the first month after the initiation of treatment has found that the patient was in good condition with a biological improvement. The treatment continued during 3 months with a remarkable clinical improvement and a total normalization of the hepatic biological assessment (Table 1).

3. Discussion

Immunotherapy by intravesical instillation of Bacillus Calmette–Guérin (BCG) is currently the most effective treatment for noninfiltrating bladder tumors. Furthermore, it is contraindicated if there is active tuberculosis or a history of local or systemic complications due to this therapy. As sometimes this is an unrecognized pathology that can occur long after instillations, it is also important to inform the patient about the possible complications to avoid any delay in treatment.

Three pathophysiological mechanisms have been described to explain the AEs of BCG therapy:

(i) Infectious: linked to the proliferation and dissemination by the hematogenous route of BCG. The innate, nonspecific immune reaction against BCG has been responsible for a local inflammatory reaction [2].

(ii) Immunoallergic: related to a type IV hypersensitivity reaction of the Gell and Coombs classification. This hypersensitivity has been explained by the production of IL10 which directs the immune reaction towards a Th2 response.

(iii) Autoimmune: linked, on the one hand, to cross-immune reactions between BCG antigens and "self-proteins" and, on the other hand, to a suppression of the regulatory immune mechanisms considered to be protective against autoimmunity [3].

The main side effects are local, such as cystitis, hematuria, prostatitis, and epididymitis. General effects are more rarely described [4]. The diagnosis of complications of BCG therapy is sometimes difficult, especially since they can occur long time afterward, up to several years after the last instillation. It is based on a set of clinical, biological, radiological, microbiological, and pathological factors and will most often be a diagnosis of elimination [5]. Any fever occurring after an instillation of BCG should raise suspicion of the diagnosis of BCGitis. It will be necessary to look for an associated organ damage by a complete clinical examination, a biological assessment (particularly renal and hepatic assessment), and a radiological assessment including at least a chest X-ray. An inflammatory syndrome is often associated. It is important to rule out active tuberculosis, another infectious process, metastases or other causes of granulomatous lesions depending on the type of organ affected [6]. The time between instillations and systemic manifestations is very variable, from a few days to several years. This may be explained by the prolonged persistence of BCG in urothelial tissue, at least 16 months after instillation [7]. Symptoms that occurred early would preferentially concern the lungs, liver, and joints, while late damage would be rather related to arterial aneurysms and spondylodiscitis [8]. As far as our patient is concerned, severe liver damage occurred two days after the first instillation while it is noted after 5 weeks in the case of Özbakkaloğlu et al. [9].

Pathological examination for a gigantocellular granuloma, most often without caseous necrosis, appears to be of major diagnostic interest. In a series of 22 patients, it enabled the diagnosis in 71% of cases, and in a review of the literature on 183 biopsied patients, an inflammatory granuloma was found in 86% of cases [7]. In our observation, we have found granulomatous hepatitis without caseous necrosis. The classical causes of this type of attack have been ruled out: autoimmune hepatitis and primary biliary cirrhosis, chronic viral hepatitis, and lymphoma.

In the presence of caseous necrosis, the specific curative treatment is that of infection with *M. bovis*, a germ that is constantly resistant to pyrazinamide, and must, therefore, combine rifampicin, isoniazid, and ethambutol as a first-line treatment. The duration of treatment is not codified as some cases are treated for 6 to 12 months [9–11]. In our patient, corticosteroid therapy was used in a good progress. It is frequently indicated in disseminated disorders, but its use is not based on studies with a sufficient level of proof to determine its usefulness, the doses to be used, or the duration of treatment. Nevertheless, its use is recommended by learned societies in the event of a systemic adverse effect, at a dosage of 0.5 to 1 mg/kg/day for 10 to 15 days maximum [10]. It should be remembered that compliance with the contraindications of BCG therapy remains major. A period of at least 15 days must be observed between tumor resection and instillation of BCG

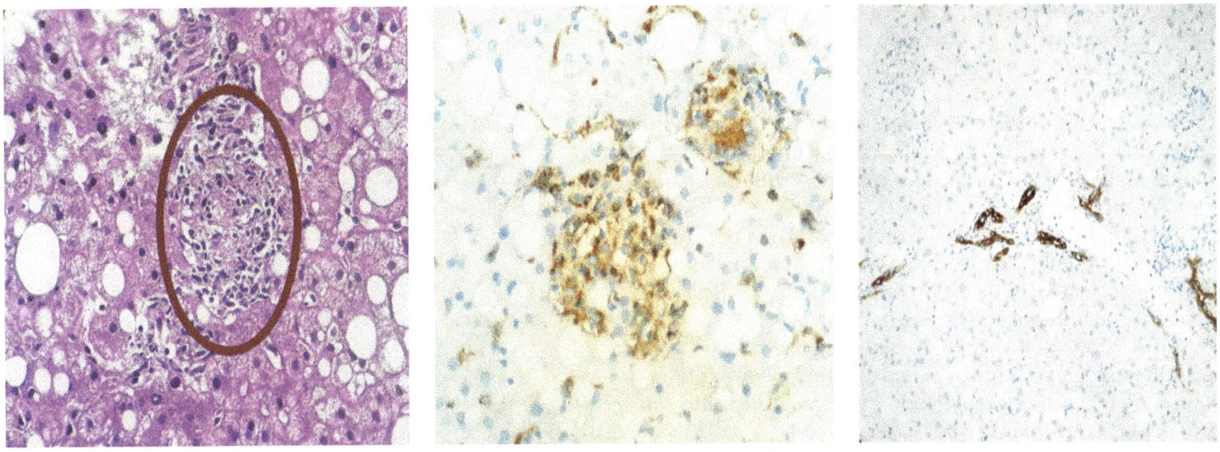

(a) (b) (c)

FIGURE 1: Histological results of the liver biopsy puncture of our patient (laboratory of pathological anatomy, CHU Hassan II of Fez). (a) Epitheloid granuloma without giant cells and without caseous necrosis (HPS * 200). (b) Anti-CD68 antibody highlighted epitheloid granulomas on immunohistochemistry. (c) Anti-CK19 antibody showed portal cholangiolar proliferation on immunohistochemistry.

TABLE 1: Results and evolution of our patient's labs.

	Two days after BCG therapy	Second day of steroids therapy	One month after steroids therapy
ASAT	6 ULN	6 ULN	1ULN
ALAT	11, 8 ULN	10, 8 ULN	1, 9 ULN
GGT	243	611	127
PAL	225	237	103
Total bilirubin	64	25	25
Direct bilirubin	41	22	19
PT	100	100	80
Platelets	68000	419000	425000

[12], which postpones the instillation in the event of traumatic catheterization, in the event of an infectious process with fever and/or positive ECBU, or in the event of local signs such as dysuria, hematuria, and urination burns.

Drug prophylaxis has been evaluated twice. Administration of isoniazid (INH) 300 mg daily for 3 days starting on the day of instillation did not show any effect on the occurrence of local and systemic side effects. Administration of ofloxacin at H6 and H18 after the first postinstillation urination showed a significant reduction in the incidence of systemic side effects (by 21.5%) and a reduction in the number of discontinuation of instillations following the instillation. Occurrence of side effects: this practice seems interesting but has not been studied any further. It is not recommended in current practice but should be considered. The reduction in the consumption of antituberculosis drugs in the treatment of complications from BCG therapy in the ofloxacin versus placebo group makes it a very interesting practice which deserves special attention [12].

4. Conclusions

Our observation illustrates a rare but serious and curable complication of intravesical BCG therapy, especially visceral diffusion in the liver. There is no specific preventive treatment to avoid such a complication, and it, therefore, appears essential to know this complication and to make an early diagnosis to limit any delay in treatment.

References

[1] A. Morales, D. Eidinger, and A. W. Bruce, "Intracavitary bacillus calmette-guerin in the treatment of superficial bladder tumors," *Journal of Urology*, vol. 116, no. 2, pp. 180–182, 1976.

[2] M. Babjuk, M. Burger, R. Zigeuner et al., "EAU guidelines on nonmuscle invasive urothelial carcinoma of the bladder," *European Urology*, vol. 64, pp. 639-753, 2013.

[3] S. Prescott, A. M. Jackson, S. J. Hawkyard, A. B. Alexandroff, and K. James, "Mechanisms of action of intravesical bacille calmette-guérin: local immune mechanisms," *Clinical Infectious Diseases*, vol. 31, no. 3, pp. S91–S93, 2000.

[4] D. Chopin, F. Saint, and B. Gattegno, "Immunothérapie endovésicale: le bacille de Calmette et Guérin," *Progrès en Urologie*, vol. 11, pp. 1067-1115, 2001.

[5] Y. Shoenfeld, A. Aron-Maor, A. Tanai, and M. Ehrenfeld, "BCG and autoimmunity: another two-edged sword," *Journal of Autoimmunity*, vol. 16, pp. 235–40, 2001.

[6] Y. Neuzillet, M. Rouprêt, H. Wallerand et al., "Diagnostic et prise en charge des événements indésirables survenant au décours des instillations endovésicales de BCG pour le

traitement des tumeurs de vessie n'infiltrant pas le muscle (TVNIM): revue du comité de cancérologie de l'Association française d'urologie," *Progrès en Urologie*, vol. 22, no. 16, pp. 989–998, 2012.

[7] L. Bowyer, R. R. Hall, J. Reading, and M. M. Marsh, "The persistence of bacille Calmette-Guerin in the bladder after intravesical treatment for bladder cancer," *British Journal of Urology*, vol. 75, no. 2, pp. 188–192, 1995.

[8] M. Pavic, E. Le Pape, P. Debourdeau et al., "Granulomatoses systémiques pseudosarcoïdosiques d'étiologie déterminée et non tuberculeuse. Étude de 67 observations," *La Revue de Médecine Interne*, vol. 29, no. 1, pp. 5–14, 2008.

[9] B. Özbakkaloğlu, Ö. Tünger, S. Sürücüoğlu, M. Lekili, and A. R. Kandiloğlu, "Granulomatous hepatitis following intravesical bacillus Calmette-Guerin therapy," *International Urology and Nephrology*, vol. 31, no. 1, pp. 49–53, 1999.

[10] S. Bouchikh, J. Stirnemann, V. Prendki et al., "Durée de traitement des tuberculoses extrapulmonaires: six mois ou plus? Analyse de la base de données TB-INFO," *La Revue de Médecine Interne*, vol. 33, no. 12, pp. 665–671, 2012.

[11] C. Q. Gao, R. Mithani, J. Leya et al., "Granulomatous hepatitis, choroiditis and aortoduodenal fistula complicating intravesical bacillus Calmette-Guérin therapy: case report," *BMC Infectious Diseases*, vol. 11, no. 1, pp. 1-6, 2011.

[12] P. D. Vegt, A. P. van der Meijden, R. Sylvester, M. Brausi, W. Höltl, and C. de Balincourt, "Does isoniazid reduce side effects of intravesical bacillus Calmette-Guérin therapy in superficial bladder cancer Interim results of European Organization for Research and Treatment of Cancer Protocol 30911," *The Journal of Urology*, vol. 157, no. 4, pp. 1246–1249, 1997.

17

Nephrotic Syndrome Induced by Lenvatinib Treatment for Hepatocellular Carcinoma

Thaninee Prasoppokakorn,[1] **Kessarin Thanapirom**,[1,2,3] **and Sombat Treeprasertsuk**[1]

[1]*Division of Gastroenterology, Department of Medicine, Faculty of Medicine, Chulalongkorn University, Bangkok, Thailand*
[2]*Center of Excellence in Liver Diseases, King Chulalongkorn Memorial Hospital, Thai Red Cross Society, Bangkok, Thailand*
[3]*Liver Fibrosis and Cirrhosis Research Unit, Chulalongkorn University, Bangkok, Thailand*

Correspondence should be addressed to Sombat Treeprasertsuk; battan5410@gmail.com

Academic Editor: Sorabh Kapoor

Lenvatinib, an oral small-molecule multiple tyrosine kinase inhibitor (TKI), has been approved for first-line therapy for unresectable hepatocellular carcinoma (HCC). Proteinuria is one of the most common adverse events associated with lenvatinib treatment. We reported a 67-year-old Thai female was diagnosed with NASH cirrhosis and HCC BCLC B with TACE refractoriness. She received 8 mg of lenvatinib for 2 weeks and began to experience worsening hypertension, bilateral pleural effusion, pedal edema, hypoalbuminemia, hypercholesterolemia, and proteinuria. After exclusion of all possible causes, lenvatinib-induced nephrotic syndrome (NS) was diagnosed. One week after discontinuing the drug, her symptoms gradually improved. To date, there have been only a handful of reported cases of lenvatinib-induced nephrotoxicity. We report herein the case of lenvatinib-induced NS in a cirrhotic patient with HCC with resolution of symptoms in a short period after drug discontinuation. In addition, we reviewed all reported cases of lenvatinib-induced nephrotoxicity.

1. Introduction

Lenvatinib is an oral small-molecule multiple tyrosine kinase inhibitor (TKI) that inhibits vascular endothelial growth factor receptor 1–3 (VEGFR1–3), fibroblast growth factor receptor (FGFR1-4), platelet-derived growth factor receptor (PDGFR), stem cell factor receptor (KIT), and rearranged during transfection (RET) [1, 2]. It has been approved for first-line therapy for unresectable hepatocellular carcinoma (HCC) [3–5]. A recent randomized controlled study showed that it was noninferior to sorafenib in terms of overall survival (OS), but was associated with: longer progression-free survival, longer time to progression, and higher objective response rate in comparison to sorafenib based on results of REFLECT trial [6]. The most common adverse events of lenvatinib are hypertension, diarrhea, decreased weight and appetite, and proteinuria. We reported herein a cirrhotic patient with unresectable HCC who received lenvatinib and developed nephrotic syndrome due to lenvatinib treatment.

2. Case Report

A 67-year-old Thai female was hospitalized due to worsening dyspnea and orthopnea for 1 week. She was previously diagnosed with nonalcoholic steatohepatitis (NASH)-related Child–Pugh A cirrhosis (6 points) and Barcelona Clinic Liver Cancer (BCLC) stage B HCC 6 months previously. Abdominal computed tomography (CT) revealed a cirrhotic liver with many arterial enhancing lesions in both hepatic lobes with rapid wash-out in portal and delayed phases. The largest tumor size of $4.0 \times 4.2 \times 4.5$ cm in segments V/VII indicated multifocal HCC with the absence of portal vein invasion and thrombosis. She received locoregional therapy for HCC by transarterial chemoembolization (TACE) 2

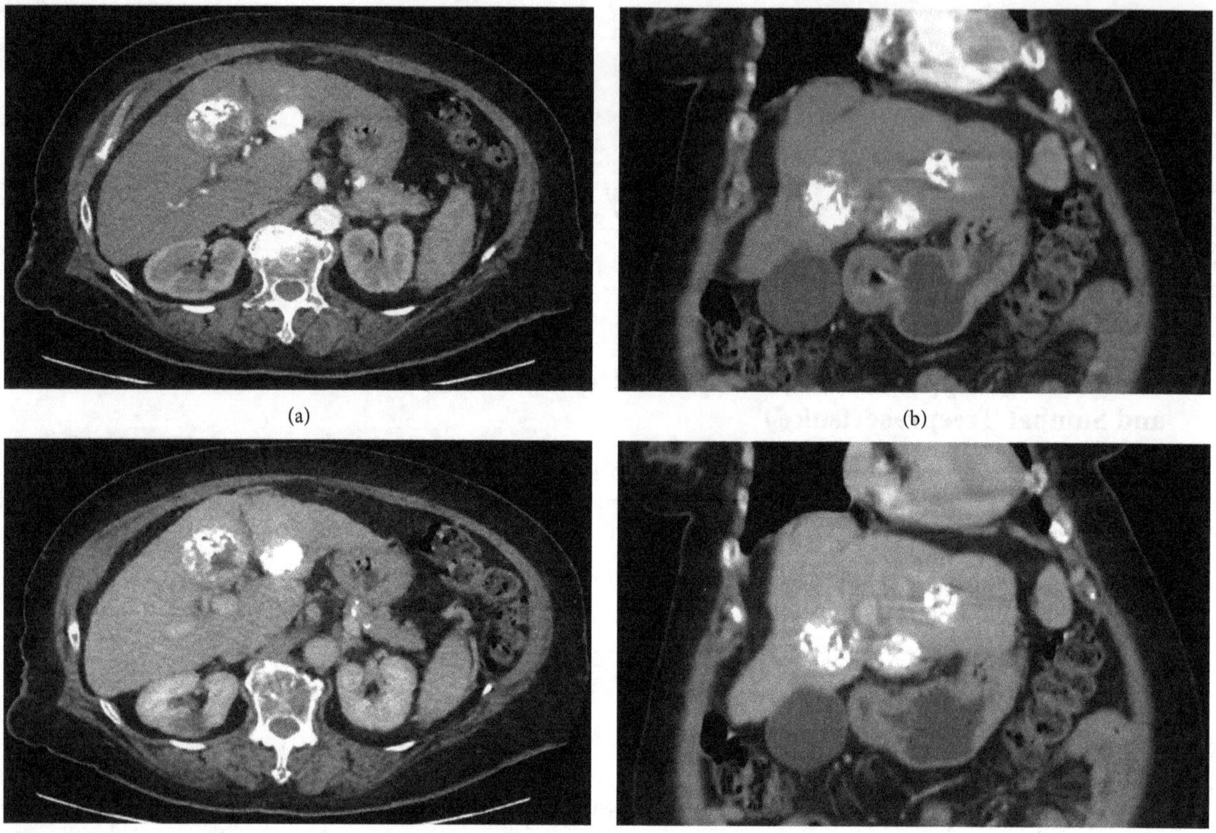

(a) (b) (c) (d)

Figure 1: Abdominal computed tomography revealing a cirrhotic liver with 3 partial lipiodol-staining masses at left hepatic lobe with remaining viable part, size 3.7 × 2.9 cm at segment III (viable part at anteroinferior aspect), 4.5 × 4.4 cm at segment IVb (viable part at right posterolateral aspect), and 2.7 × 2.5 cm at segment II (small viable part at posterior aspect) in axial and coronal view of arterial phase (a-b) and axial and coronal view of portovenous phase (c-d), respectively.

times but failed to experience significant response. CT at 1-month follow-up after TACE demonstrated a viable tumor 3.1 × 2.9 cm at hepatic segment V (Figure 1). After discussion with patient for further treatments, she was switched to systemic therapy using a molecular targeted agent. An 8 mg daily dose of lenvatinib was prescribed 2 weeks before this hospital admission. Her medical history included well-controlled hypertension, dyslipidemia, type 2 diabetes mellitus, and Graves' disease treated with radioactive iodine.

Physical examination revealed body temperature of 36.2°C, blood pressure (BP) of 190/120 mm·Hg (baseline BP 110/60), pulse rate of 110/min, respiratory rate of 24/min, puffy eye lids, decreased breath sounds and dullness on percussion at lower half of the right lung, and bilateral pedal edema.

Chest X-ray (CXR) showed moderate right pleural effusion (Figure 2(a)). Pleural fluid analysis exhibited white blood cell (WBC) of 111 cells/μL (neutrophil 28%; lymphocyte 72%), protein of 1.5 g/dL, lactate dehydrogenase of 78 U/L, and no organism on Gram stain and culture indicating transudative profile. Serum biochemical tests showed total bilirubin of 1.2 mg/dL, direct bilirubin of 0.6 mg/dL, SGOT of 50 U/L, SGPT of 34 U/L, alkaline phosphatase of 99 U/L, BUN of 29 mg/dL, creatinine of 0.9 mg/dL, eGFR of 66 mL/min/1.73 m^2, albumin of 2.0 g/dL, protein of 6.7 g/dL, LDH of 238 U/L, and cholesterol of 260 mg/dL. Urinalysis showed red blood cell and WBC of 0-1 cell/high power field (HPF) and 3^+ albumin. The 24-hour urine albumin was 7.01 g/day. The thyroid function test was normal. The diagnosis of nephrotic syndrome (NS) was definitive. After exclusion of other possible causes of NS including HIV, HBV, HCV, and autoimmune diseases, the diagnosis of lenvatinib-induced NS with worsening hypertension was made. Lenvatinib was immediately discontinued due to this serious adverse event.

One week after discontinuation of lenvatinib and supportive therapy, the patient symptoms gradually improved with a reduction of right pleural effusion (Figure 2(b)) and lowering of the urine protein creatinine ratio (UPCR) from 9.7 to 5.6 g/day after 2 weeks. After discussion with the patient and her family, the decision was made to give supportive care for her HCC for a while. Six months after stopping lenvatinib, UPCR declined to sub-nephrotic range proteinuria of 0.95 g/day as well as 24-hour urine albumin was only 0.54 g/day. Due to the patient having good performance status as well as preserved liver function, the second line systemic therapy was prescribed with 180 mg of nivolumab. The patient had well-tolerated to treatment with 7 months courses of stable disease by follow-up imaging. Besides, proteinuria was closed follow-up every outpatient visit and demonstrated no evidence of recurrence.

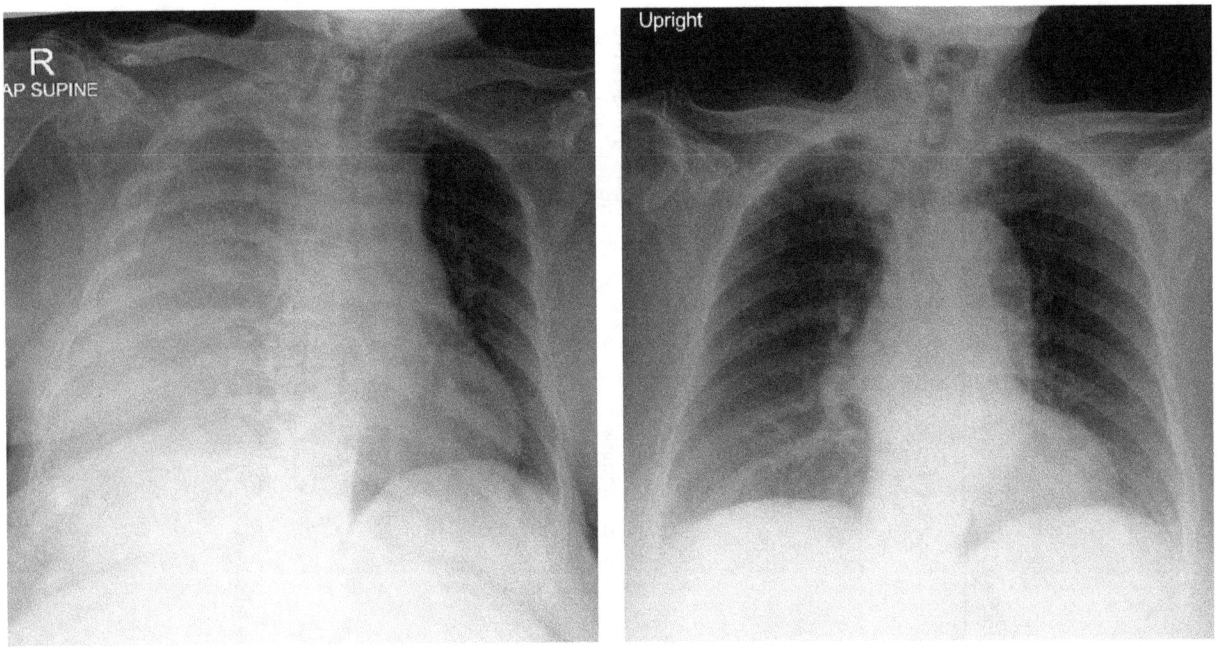

(a) (b)

FIGURE 2: Chest X-rays revealing moderate amount of right pleural effusion with pressure effect caused trachea shift to the left (a) and complete resolution of right pleural effusion after discontinuing lenvatinib for 1 week (b).

TABLE 1: Common adverse events and recommended management for lenvatinib treatment.

Adverse events	CTCAE grade	CTCAE description	Management
Proteinuria	1	0.15–1.0 g/24 h	None
	2	>1.0–3.5 g/24 h	(i) Hold lenvatinib until proteinuria resolves to ≤2.0 g/24 h (ii) Consider consult nephrology
	3	>3.5 g/24 h	(i) Hold lenvatinib until proteinuria resolves to ≤2.0 g/24 h (ii) Referral to nephrology
	4	Nephrotic syndrome	(i) Discontinue lenvatinib permanently (ii) Referral to nephrology

CTCAE, Common Terminology Criteria for Adverse Events; *g*, gram; *h*, hours.

3. Discussion

There have been very few reported cases of lenvatinib-induced nephrotoxicity published in medical journals. We reported herein a case of lenvatinib-induced NS in a cirrhotic patient with HCC, which developed within 2 weeks after beginning a course of 8 mg lenvatinib. Resolution of symptoms began soon after discontinuation of medication.

Among molecular targeted agents, lenvatinib is a TKI that inhibits many growth factors and is prescribed for the treatment of many types of cancers including thyroid cancer and HCC. The most common adverse events associated with lenvatinib include hypertension (42%), diarrhea (39%), decreased appetite (34%), decreased weight (31%), and proteinuria (25%) [6].

Preclinical studies in human HCC models have reported that lenvatinib has potent antiangiogenic activity, mainly through the pathways of VEGFR and FGFR inhibition [7]. The VEGF pathway regulates angiogenesis which is an essential event in tumor growth and metastasis which provides oxygen and nutrients to tumor cells. Targeting the VEGFR-mediated pathway can lead to starvation, hypoxia, and tumor cell death [2].

Proteinuria associated with angiogenesis inhibition is the most common renal side effect of anti-VEGF drugs with a prevalence ranging from 21 to 63% and frequently occurring with hypertension. Due to VEGFR binding in glomerular and peritubular endothelium, as well as in mesangial cells in normal conditions, this binding process plays a role in the maintenance of the glomerular basement membrane structure and proper glomerular function. The drugs block VEGFR and may induce renal abnormalities, especially in renovascular function that includes hypertension and proteinuria. Moreover, there have been reported patients developing renal thrombotic microangiopathy (TMA) cause by VEGF trap and multitargeted TKI [9]. The presentative symptoms can be mimicked with nephrotic syndrome with renal dysfunction [9]. The drugs have the potential to cause nephrotic syndrome. Potential mechanisms of lenvatinib-induced proteinuria include postexercise proteinuria-like

Table 2: A summary of all 8 patients with lenvatinib-induced renal toxicity published in English literature from 2019 to 2020.

Patient	Gender/ age (year)	Race	Cancer	Lenvatinib dose (per day)/ duration (month)	Clinical presentations	Renal function: creatinine (mg/dL)/eGFR (mL/min/1.73 m^2)	Urinalysis/24-hour protein urine (g)	Renal histological finding	Treatment	Outcome
1, 2018 [23]	F/36	Caucasian	Medullary thyroid carcinoma	24 mg/19	Worsening HT, ankle edema	Normal	NA/3.1 g	FSGS	Discontinued lenvatinib	No proteinuria in 1 year
2, 2018 [23]	F/70	Japan	Papillary thyroid carcinoma	24 mg/26	Worsening HT, legs edema	1.12/37.4	WBC <1, RBC 5–9 cells/HPF/ 3.5 g	TMA	Decreased dose to 8 mg of lenvatinib and discontinuation	Partial recovery in 2 months
3, 2018 [16]	F/79	Japan	Papillary thyroid carcinoma	10 mg/3	Worsening HT, generalized edema	1.17/34	RBC 20–29 cells/ HPF/11.8 g	FSGS	Discontinued lenvatinib	Complete recovery in 15 months
4, 2018 [22]	M/44	Caucasian	Papillary thyroid carcinoma	24 mg/6 20 mg/4 14 mg/26 10 mg/12	Worsening HT	1.90/NA	NA/3.5 g	FSGS, tubulointerstitial vascular necrosis, TMA-like pattern	Decreased dose to 10 mg of lenvatinib and discontinued	Partial recovery in 1 month
5, 2018 [22]	F/59	Caucasian	Adenoid cystic carcinoma of the minor salivary gland	24 mg/15	Acute renal failure (tubulointerstitial nephropathy by clinics)	2.81/NA	No sediment/< 1 g	Not performed	Discontinued lenvatinib. Prednisolone 40 mg taper in 6 months	Renal function improved in 10 days
6, 2018 [24]	M/67	Caucasian	Papillary thyroid carcinoma	24 mg/9	Worsening HT and renal function	2.46/26.0	NA/NA	Not performed	Discontinued lenvatinib	Partial recovery in 8 months
7, 2020 [25]	M/56	Taiwan	Papillary thyroid carcinoma	20 mg/1	Worsening HT, legs edema	0.56/115	Trace hematuria/ 9.9 g	Not performed	Decreased dose to 10 mg of lenvatinib and discontinued with sorafenib replacement	Partial recovery in 5 months
8 (our case), 2020	F/67	Thai	Hepatocellular carcinoma	8/0.5	Worsening HT, bilateral pleural effusion, legs edema	0.9/66	WBC 0–1, RBC 0–1 cells/HPF/ 7.01 g	Not performed	Discontinued lenvatinib	Partial recovery in 1 week

FSGS, focal segmental glomerulosclerosis; TMA, thrombotic microangiopathy; HT, hypertension; AEs, adverse events; WBC, white blood cells; RBC, red blood cells; F, female; *M*, male; NA, not applicable.

syndrome, perturbation of podocyte-endothelial VEGF axis signaling, podocyte protein junction downregulation, subacute glomerular thrombotic microangiopathy, and additional pathogenic factors such as hypertensive injury [10]. The exact mechanism and factors associated with the occurrence and severity of proteinuria are unknown [11, 12]. According to the reported studies in patients with thyroid cancer, lenvatinib-induced proteinuria can be observed at any time after drug initiation. The mean duration of the development of renal adverse effects after lenvatinib initiation was 43 (range 5–799) days [13–16]. Management should be dose reduced to minimize the risk of renal adverse events or complete drug discontinuation. Data showed that patients can recover within 9 weeks after stopping lenvatinib [14].

The maximum recommended dose of lenvatinib for HCC treatment is 12 mg per day, whereas 24 mg per day can be prescribed for radioiodine-refractory thyroid cancer [13]. The half-dose reduction of lenvatinib for HCC treatment may be due to the fact that lenvatinib is metabolized in the liver [17].

Management of adverse events includes supportive care, dose modification, and discontinuation of lenvatinib in cases with grade 4 adverse events. Clinical practice management of adverse events from lenvatinib-induced proteinuria according to the Common Terminology Criteria for Adverse Events (CTCAE) are listed in Table 1 [12, 17–20]. Regarding proteinuria, lenvatinib can induce renal failure defined as a decline of eGFR in the long-term analysis. They might be associated with glomerular damage, with secondary proteinuria and tubular injury, especially with long-term lenvatinib used duration over 2 years [21, 22].

Our patient rapidly developed NS just 2 weeks after lenvatinib treatment which was faster than other reported cases. Multiple patient comorbidities, including longstanding hypertension, diabetes, dyslipidemia, old age, and decompensated cirrhosis, likely predisposed the patient for the rapid development of NS. The limitation of our reported patient was an absence of definite diagnosis by renal biopsy. However, despite the lack of histopathologic findings from renal parenchyma, the diagnosis of lenvatinib-induced NS was suspected due to the improvement of patient symptoms and reduction of proteinuria following discontinuation of lenvatinib within 1 week [19].

In addition, we retrospectively reported a literature review. A total of eight patients with lenvatinib-induced renal adverse effects have currently been reported in the literature (Table 2) [16, 22–25]. Cases consisted of 3 males and 5 females with the mean age of 59.8 ± 13.3 (range: 36–79) years. There were 4 Asians and 4 Caucasians. Of the eight patients, thyroid carcinoma was the most common cancer ($n = 6$, 75.0%), followed by HCC and carcinoma of the minor salivary gland ($n = 1$, 12.5%). The dosage of lenvatinib ranged from 8 to 24 mg, and the duration of treatment ranged from 0.5 to 48 months. Compared to prior reported cases, our patient received the lenvatinib with the lowest dose (8 mg) and shortest duration (2 weeks). Regarding the clinical manifestations of nephrotoxicity, worsening hypertension was the most common event ($n = 7$, 87.5%), followed by edema ($n = 5$, 62.5%), renal function decline ($n = 2$, 25.0%), and pleural effusion ($n = 1$, 12.5% in our case). The 24-hour urine protein ranged from <1 to 11.8 g/day. With respect to renal pathology, focal segmental glomerulosclerosis and thrombotic microangiopathy were noted in 3 and 1 patients, respectively, while 4 patients did not complete a renal biopsy. The management in all patients ($n = 8$, 100%) was lenvatinib discontinuation. Three patients had been failed for prior dose reduction; one patient was treated with 40 mg of prednisolone which was tapered off within 6 months, and another one was treated by sorafenib replacement. The treatment outcomes for lenvatinib-induced renal toxicity were excellent: complete resolution ($n = 2$, 25.0%) and partial resolution ($n = 6$, 75.0%). The recovery duration after the discontinued use of lenvatinib ranged from 1 week to 15 months. Our case study patient reported the shortest symptoms recovery time of 1 week.

4. Conclusion

To date, there have been only a handful of reported cases of lenvatinib-induced nephrotoxicity. We report herein the case of lenvatinib-induced NS in a cirrhotic patient with HCC with resolution of symptoms in a short period after drug discontinuation.

Abbreviations

BCLC: Barcelona Clinic Liver Cancer
BP: Blood pressure
CT: Computed tomography
CTCAE: Common Terminology Criteria for Adverse Events
CXR: Chest X-ray
eGFR: Estimated glomerular filtration rate
FGFR: Fibroblast growth factor receptor
HBV: Hepatitis B virus
HCC: Hepatocellular carcinoma
HCV: Hepatitis C virus
HIV: Human immunodeficiency virus
HPF: High power field
KIT: Stem cell factor receptor
LDH: Lactate dehydrogenase
NASH: Nonalcoholic steatohepatitis
NS: Nephrotic syndrome
OS: Overall survival
PDGFR: Platelet-derived growth factor receptor
RET: Rearranged during transfection
SGOT: Serum glutamic-oxaloacetic transaminase
SGPT: Serum glutamic pyruvic transaminase
TACE: Transarterial chemoembolization
TKI: Tyrosine kinase inhibitor
TMA: Thrombotic microangiopathy
UPCR: Urine protein creatinine ratio
VEGFR: Vascular endothelial growth factor receptor
WBC: White blood cell.

References

[1] Z. T. Al-Salama, Y. Y. Syed, and L. J. Scott, "Lenvatinib: a review in hepatocellular carcinoma," *Drugs*, vol. 79, no. 6, pp. 665–674, 2019.

[2] Y. Zhao, Y. N. Zhang, K. T. Wang, and L. Chen, "Lenvatinib for hepatocellular carcinoma: from preclinical mechanisms to anti-cancer therapy," *Biochimica et Biophysica Acta (BBA)—Reviews on Cancer*, vol. 1874, no. 1, Article ID 188391, 2020.

[3] European Association for the Study of the Liver, "Electronic address eee, European association for the study of the L. EASL clinical practice guidelines: management of hepatocellular carcinoma," *Journal of Hepatology*, vol. 69, no. 1, pp. 182–236, 2018.

[4] J. A. Marrero, L. M. Kulik, C. B. Sirlin et al., "Diagnosis, staging, and management of hepatocellular carcinoma: 2018 practice guidance by the American association for the study of liver diseases," *Hepatology*, vol. 68, no. 2, pp. 723–750, 2018.

[5] M. Omata, A. L. Cheng, N. Kokudo et al., "Asia-Pacific clinical practice guidelines on the management of hepatocellular carcinoma: a 2017 update," *Hepatol Int*, vol. 11, no. 4, pp. 317–370, 2017.

[6] M. Kudo, R. S. Finn, S. Qin et al., "Lenvatinib versus sorafenib in first-line treatment of patients with unresectable hepatocellular carcinoma: a randomised phase 3 non-inferiority trial," *The Lancet*, vol. 391, no. 10126, pp. 1163–1173, 2018.

[7] M. Matsuki, T. Hoshi, Y. Yamamoto et al., "Lenvatinib inhibits angiogenesis and tumor fibroblast growth factor signaling pathways in human hepatocellular carcinoma models," *Cancer Medicine*, vol. 7, no. 6, pp. 2641-2653, 2018.

[8] Y. Hyogo, N. Kiyota, N. Otsuki et al., "Thrombotic microangiopathy with severe proteinuria induced by lenvatinib for radioactive iodine-refractory papillary thyroid carcinoma," *Case Reports in Oncology*, vol. 11, no. 3, pp. 735–741, 2018.

[9] M. Delsante, J. M. Monroy-Trujillo, N. Carter-Monroe, D. W. Ball, and A. Z. Rosenberg, "Lenvatinib-related renal microangiopathy: a case series," *Virchows Archiv*, vol. 480, pp. 467–473, 2021.

[10] H. Izzedine, C. Massard, J. P. Spano, F. Goldwasser, D. Khayat, and J. C. Soria, "VEGF signalling inhibition-induced proteinuria: mechanisms, significance and management," *European Journal of Cancer*, vol. 46, no. 2, pp. 439–448, 2010.

[11] V. Launay-Vacher and G. Deray, "Hypertension and proteinuria: a class-effect of antiangiogenic therapies," *Anti-Cancer Drugs*, vol. 20, no. 1, pp. 81-82, 2009.

[12] M. L. C. Santos, B. B. de Brito, F. A. F. da Silva, A. C. D. S. Botelho, and F. F. de Melo, "Nephrotoxicity in cancer treatment: an overview," *World Journal of Clinical Oncology*, vol. 11, no. 4, pp. 190–204, 2020.

[13] M. Schlumberger, M. Tahara, L. J. Wirth et al., "Lenvatinib versus placebo in radioiodine-refractory thyroid cancer," *New England Journal of Medicine*, vol. 372, no. 7, pp. 621–630, 2015.

[14] R. I. Haddad, M. Schlumberger, L. J. Wirth et al., "Incidence and timing of common adverse events in Lenvatinib-treated patients from the SELECT trial and their association with survival outcomes," *Endocrine*, vol. 56, no. 1, pp. 121–128, 2017.

[15] O. V. Ancker, M. Wehland, J. Bauer, M. Infanger, and D. Grimm, "The adverse effect of hypertension in the treatment of thyroid cancer with multi-kinase inhibitors," *International Journal of Molecular Sciences*, vol. 18, no. 3, 2017.

[16] Y. Furuto, H. Hashimoto, A. Namikawa et al., "Focal segmental glomerulosclerosis lesion associated with inhibition of tyrosine kinases by lenvatinib: a case report," *BMC Nephrology*, vol. 19, no. 1, p. 273, 2018.

[17] L. Rimassa, R. Danesi, T. Pressiani, and P. Merle, "Management of adverse events associated with tyrosine kinase inhibitors: improving outcomes for patients with hepatocellular carcinoma," *Cancer Treatment Reviews*, vol. 77, pp. 20–28, 2019.

[18] E. Inc, *Lentima (Lenvatinib) Prescribing Information*, Eisai Inc, Bunkyo, Japan, 2020.

[19] M. E. Cabanillas and S. Takahashi, "Managing the adverse events associated with lenvatinib therapy in radioiodine-refractory differentiated thyroid cancer," *Seminars in Oncology*, vol. 46, no. 1, pp. 57–64, 2019.

[20] N. Dctd, "Cancer therapy evaluation program, common Terminology Criteria for adverse events," 2003, https://ctepcancergov.

[21] C. Masaki, K. Sugino, S. Kobayashi et al., "Impact of lenvatinib on renal function: long-term analysis of differentiated thyroid cancer patients," *BMC Cancer*, vol. 21, no. 1, p. 894, 2021.

[22] S. Cavalieri, L. Cosmai, A. Genderini et al., "Lenvatinib-induced renal failure: two first-time case reports and review of literature," *Expert Opinion on Drug Metabolism and Toxicology*, vol. 14, no. 4, pp. 379–385, 2018.

[23] K. Fleming, J. McGuinness, D. Kipgen, H. Glen, and P. Spiliopoulou, "A case of lenvatinib-induced focal segmental glomerulosclerosis (FSGS) in metastatic medullary thyroid cancer," *Case Reports in Oncological Medicine*, vol. 2018, Article ID 6927639, 6 pages, 2018.

[24] L. Paschke, T. Lincke, K. S. Muhlberg, W. J. Jabs, T. H. Lindner, and R. Paschke, "Anti VEGF-TKI treatment and new renal adverse events not reported in phase III trials," *European Thyroid Journal*, vol. 7, no. 6, pp. 308-312, 2018.

[25] H. Che, K. T. C. Yang, Y. S. Lin, C. Y. Hsu, Y. C. Ou, and M. C. Tung, "Improvement of lenvatinib-induced nephrotic syndrome after adaptation to sorafenib in thyroid cancer: a case report," *World Journal of Clinical Cases*, vol. 8, no. 20, pp. 4883–4894, 2020.

18

A Rare Cause of Haemorrhagic Shock: Rupture of Gastric Wall Seeding of Hepatocellular Carcinoma

Naoki Ishimaru,[1] **Hirohisa Fujikawa**,[2,3] **Kazuya Niwa**,[1] **and Yoshifumi Kobayashi**[1]

[1]*Department of Surgery, Suwa Central Hospital, 4300 Tamagawa, Chino, Nagano 3918503, Japan*
[2]*Department of Medical Education Studies, International Research Center for Medical Education, Graduate School of Medicine, The University of Tokyo, 7-3-1 Hongo, Bunkyo-ku, Tokyo 1130033, Japan*
[3]*Department of Internal Medicine, Suwa Central Hospital, 4300 Tamagawa, Chino, Nagano 3918503, Japan*

Correspondence should be addressed to Naoki Ishimaru; bone.inthe.egg@gmail.com

Academic Editor: Sorabh Kapoor

Ruptured hepatocellular carcinoma (HCC) can lead to peritoneal dissemination. However, gastric wall seeding from HCC is exceedingly rare, and little is known about its clinical course. Herein, we report a case of an 88-year-old man who presented with a four-hour history of nausea, vomiting, and upper abdominal pain. He has a history of ruptured HCC during surgery. The patient underwent an emergency laparotomy on account of haemorrhagic shock, which confirmed the diagnosis of ruptured HCC with gastric wall seeding. The findings from this study showed that the ruptured HCC can seed into the stomach wall, and the implanted lesions may rupture and lead to life-threatening haemorrhagic shock. Surgery is an effective treatment for bleeding from the implanted lesions.

1. Introduction

Although great progress has been made in the treatment of hepatocellular carcinoma (HCC) in recent years, recurrence rate is still very high even after curative therapy [1]. Extrahepatic recurrence of HCC is usually caused by haematogenous metastasis [2]. Peritoneal seeding of HCC into the gastric serosa after HCC rupture is rare [3]. Moreover, treatment strategies for cases where the seeded lesions rupture have not been well established. Herein, we describe a rare case of ruptured gastric wall seeded HCC, leading to severe haemorrhagic shock. We opted for surgery, which helped save the patient's life.

2. Case Presentation

An 88-year-old man with chronic kidney disease presented to our hospital with a four-hour history of nausea, vomiting, and upper abdominal pain. He exhibited no symptoms of hematemesis, melena, or anaemia. Fifteen months prior to presentation, he underwent surgical dissection with lateral hepatectomy due to HCC. The liver tumour ruptured during the surgical procedure. We washed the peritoneal cavity with 5 litres of normal saline to remove the tumour cells and reduce the risk of dissemination. Nine months earlier, abdominal computed tomography (CT) had revealed a nodule (10 mm) on the gastric antrum's serous surface. Three months later, the nodule size was not remarkably different, as confirmed by abdominal ultrasonography and CT. Due to the patient's advanced age and history of renal dysfunction, adjuvant chemotherapy was not administered.

He was pale on examination with blood pressure (85/55 mm Hg), pulse rate (102 bpm), and temperature (34.9°C). He had notable tenderness in the epigastrium. Laboratory investigations showed elevated white cell count (10.1×10^9/L), while other findings were unremarkable. Contrast-enhanced abdominal CT showed contrast leakage into the peritoneal cavity from a 30 mm mass on the gastric antrum's anterior wall (Figure 1). Haemorrhage was suspected, and an emergency laparotomy was performed, which revealed

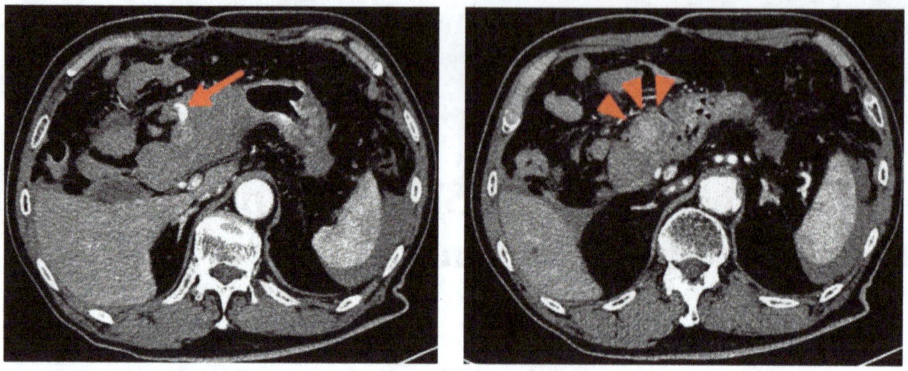

(a) (b)

Figure 1: Contrast-enhanced abdominal computed tomography showed contrast leakage ((a), arrow) into the peritoneal cavity from a hypervascular mass ((b), arrowheads, 30 mm) on the gastric antrum's anterior wall.

about 800 mL of blood in the peritoneal cavity. A gastric antrum tumour with persistent bleeding protruded from the anterior wall. The gastric serosa and tumour were resected using a vascular sealing device. We then performed wedge resection of the tumour. Since the muscularis propria of the stomach was preserved and no bleeding was observed, the gastric serosa's membrane defect was sutured.

Macroscopically, the tumour was greenish, haemorrhagic, solid, and soft and measured $30 \times 30 \times 25$ mm in size (Figure 2). Histopathological examination of the tumour revealed a moderately differentiated HCC (Figure 3). There was no indication of gastric serosa exposure to the tumour, and the surgical margins were negative. Based on these findings, a diagnosis of HCC seeding was made. The patient was discharged 18 days after surgery without any complications. According to the previous reports, postoperative chemotherapy and the use of molecular targeted drugs for hepatectomy are ineffective in preventing recurrence [4, 5]. After discussing with the patient, it was decided that adjuvant chemotherapy would not be initiated considering the published evidence, the patient's age, and poor performance status. CT surveillance is performed every 3 months since surgery; no recurrence has been observed till date (6 months since surgery).

3. Discussion

HCC can lead to peritoneal dissemination (5.6%) [6]. In this patient, a ruptured HCC had previously been implanted into the gastric wall, and this time, the implanted lesion ruptured, resulting in haemorrhagic shock. Emergency laparotomy was performed to save the patient's life.

The most common type of primary liver cancer is HCC. It usually develops in the setting of underlying chronic liver disease, especially in patients with cirrhosis due to chronic hepatitis B and/or C virus infection, excessive alcohol intake, and nonalcoholic fatty liver disease [7]. Despite treatment advancements, recurrence rate of HCC is still very high. The most frequent recurrence site is the liver. Extrahepatic metastases most commonly involve the lungs, lymph nodes, bones, and adrenal glands [2, 3, 6].

In many cases of postoperative recurrence after resection of HCC, tumour recurrence is seen in the remaining liver tissue [6]. While extrahepatic recurrence of HCC is usually caused by haematogenous metastasis, lymphatic and disseminated metastasis is rare [2]. An important HCC feature is its ability to rupture, leading to potentially life-threatening complications: haemorrhagic shock, liver failure, and peritoneal dissemination. The median survival time after HCC rupture is approximately 4-5 months [8], but dissemination of HCC is rarely a clinical problem.

The present case shows that gastric metastatic implantation can occur and the lesions can rupture. Gastric metastasis from HCC is rare [9, 10], and most of the reported cases are either caused by haematogenous metastasis or direct invasion [11]. However, in a previous autopsy case series, there were 4/181 (2.2%) cases of peritoneal seeding of HCC in the gastric serosa [3], which indicated the possibility that HCC might seed asymptomatically into the gastric serosa. This is the first case in which gastric serosa seeding by HCC was found after the HCC ruptured in the survivor. The present case is significant, and it demonstrated that seeded lesion rupture in the gastric wall can lead to fatal haemorrhagic shock. On the other hand, given the course of the prior surgery, we probably should have suspected that the 10 mm nodule that appeared on the follow-up CT might be a disseminated lesion. We should have performed an 18F-fluorodeoxyglucose positron emission tomography examination and considered early treatment.

For the treatment of extrahepatic metastases of HCC, effective molecular targeted drugs and surgery have been reported when the patient has a good Eastern Cooperative Oncology Group Performance Status and a class A Child–Pugh score [7]. The treatment for bleeding from HCC seeding has not been determined; however, the therapeutic options are transcatheter arterial embolization (TAE) and surgical haemostasis [8]. The TAE is a minimally invasive and standard treatment for intra-abdominal haemorrhage without shock. However, where TAE cannot control bleeding, the patient may risk delayed emergency haemostasis, possibly leading to worsening of haemorrhagic shock [12]. The TAE can also cause embolization site ischaemic

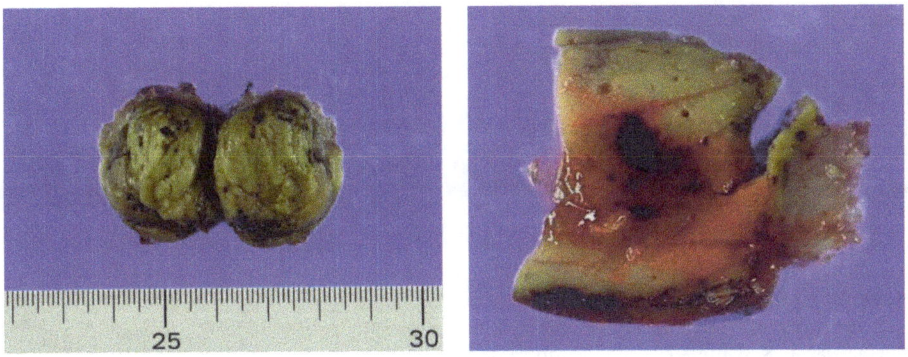

(a) (b)

FIGURE 2: Macroscopic findings. (a) Greenish and soft tumour that measured 30 × 30 × 25 mm in size. (b) The tumour was haemorrhagic solid.

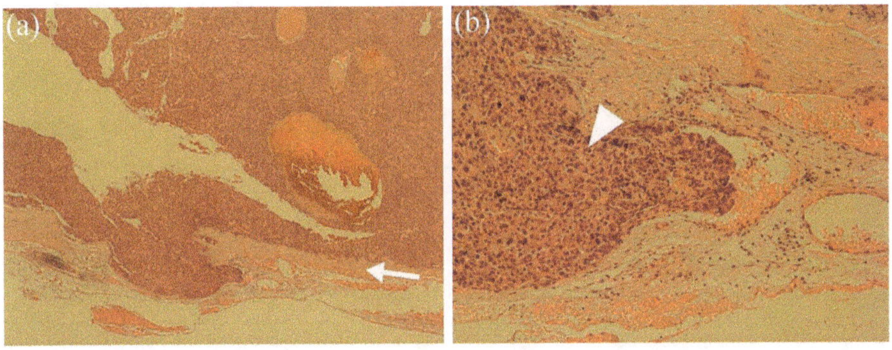

FIGURE 3: Microscopic pathological examination of the tumour. (a) There was no obvious gastric serosa (arrow) exposure of the tumour (haematoxylin and eosin stain, original magnification ×20). (b) Moderately differentiated hepatocellular carcinoma (arrowhead) (haematoxylin and eosin stain, original magnification ×100).

necrosis. In this case, since contrast-enhanced CT could not identify the vessels feeding the tumour, it was difficult to perform TAE; hence, laparotomy was performed.

4. Conclusion

In conclusion, we have reported a case of rupture of an HCC lesion seeded in the gastric wall causing haemorrhagic shock in a patient with a history of tumour rupture during HCC surgery. Emergency laparotomy saved the patient's life. HCC can cause peritoneal dissemination but rarely causes dissemination into the gastric wall. Clinicians should consider the possibility of rupture of implanted lesions. Surgery is an effective therapeutic option in cases with haemorrhagic shock due to rupture of the implanted lesions.

References

[1] D. J. Erstad and K. K. Tanabe, "Prognostic and therapeutic implications of microvascular invasion in hepatocellular carcinoma," *Annals of Surgical Oncology*, vol. 26, no. 5, pp. 1474–1493, 2019.

[2] C. N. Yeh and M. F. Chen, "Resection of peritoneal implantation of hepatocellular carcinoma after hepatic resection: risk factors and prognostic analysis," *World Journal of Surgery*, vol. 28, no. 4, pp. 382–386, 2004.

[3] S. Matsukuma and K. Sato, "Peritoneal seeding of hepatocellular carcinoma: clinicopathological characteristics of 17 autopsy cases," *Pathology International*, vol. 61, no. 6, pp. 356–362, 2011.

[4] J. Bruix, T. Takayama, V. Mazzaferro et al., "Adjuvant sorafenib for hepatocellular carcinoma after resection or ablation (STORM): a phase 3, randomised, double-blind, placebo-controlled trial," *The Lancet Oncology*, vol. 16, no. 13, pp. 1344–1354, 2015.

[5] K. Hasegawa, T. Takayama, M. Ijichi et al., "Uracil-tegafur as an adjuvant for hepatocellular carcinoma: a randomized trial," *Hepatology*, vol. 44, no. 4, pp. 891–895, 2006.

[6] H. Zhang, F. Liu, N. Wen, B. Li, and Y. Wei, "Patterns, timing, and predictors of recurrence after laparoscopic liver resection for hepatocellular carcinoma: results from a high-volume HPB center," *Surgical Endoscopy*, vol. 36, 2021.

[7] H. B. El-Serag, "Hepatocellular carcinoma," *The New England Journal of Medicine*, vol. 365, no. 12, pp. 1118–1127, 2011.

[8] F. L. Tan, Y. M. Tan, A. Y. Chung, P. C. Cheow, P. K.-H. Chow, and L. L. Ooi, "Factors affecting early mortality in spontaneous rupture of hepatocellular carcinoma," *ANZ Journal of Surgery*, vol. 76, no. 6, pp. 448–452, 2006.

[9] L. Li, W. H. Zhang, F. P. Meng et al., "Gastric metastasis of hepatocellular carcinoma with gastrointestinal bleeding after liver transplant: a case report," *Transplantation Proceedings*, vol. 47, no. 8, pp. 2544–2547, 2015.

[10] I. Oda, H. Kondo, T. Yamao et al., "Metastatic tumors to the stomach: analysis of 54 patients diagnosed at endoscopy and 347 autopsy cases," *Endoscopy*, vol. 33, no. 6, pp. 507–510, 2001.

[11] M. L. Hu, W. C. Tai, S. K. Chuah et al., "Gastric metastasis of hepatocellular carcinoma via a possible existing retrograde hematogenous pathway," *Journal of Gastroenterology and Hepatology*, vol. 25, no. 2, pp. 408–412, 2010.

[12] S. K. Sahu, Y. K. Chawla, R. K. Dhiman et al., "Rupture of hepatocellular carcinoma: a review of literature," *Journal of Clinical and Experimental Hepatology*, vol. 9, no. 2, pp. 245–256, 2019.

19

Acute Brucellosis and Cirrhosis: The Triggering Event of Fatal Liver Decompensation

Maria Kosmidou, Eleftherios Klouras, Iro Rapti, Sebastien Filippas-Ntekouan, and Haralampos Milionis

First Division of Internal Medicine, Faculty of Medicine, University of Ioannina, Ioannina, Greece

Correspondence should be addressed to Maria Kosmidou; mkosmid@uoi.gr

Academic Editor: Haruki Komatsu

Cirrhotic patients are known to be particularly susceptible to infectious complications that may vary according to regional endemic patterns. Brucellosis, a common zoonosis with worldwide distribution, exhibits a predilection for the reticuloendothelial system and thus resulting in hepatic involvement. We describe three cirrhotic patients in whom acute brucellosis and/or its treatment served as the triggering factor of hepatic decompensation, with deleterious effects. The patients suffered from alcoholic cirrhosis and culture-proven brucellosis. All patients came from an area endemic to brucellosis. The first patient exhibited a relapsing brucellosis course with progressive deterioration of his fragile liver function. The second patient progressed rapidly to jaundice, possibly partly attributed to antibiotic pharmacotoxicity, and died during liver transplantation. The third patient eventually succumbed to diffuse intravascular coagulation. Brucellosis can be a triggering event of fatal liver decompensation in cirrhotic patients. Enhancing health literacy of the patients, particularly in endemic areas, is of paramount importance for prevention of exposure to similar pathogens.

1. Introduction

Brucellosis, one of the most ubiquitous zoonotic infections worldwide [1], can induce a wide spectrum of clinical complications that range from mild, not necessitating alteration of antibiotic regimen synthesis or duration, to fortunately rare, fatal cases typically attributed to cardiac or central nervous system involvement [1]. Increasing reports incriminate brucellosis as a triggering factor on overall health derangement in patients with underlying diseases, typically as an opportunistic infection in patients with hematologic [2] or rheumatologic disorders [3]. The liver, serving as the largest organ of the reticuloendothelial system (RES) for which *Brucella* exhibits a typical predisposition, is usually affected in acute brucellosis in the form of mild biochemical alterations and/or hepatomegaly in a percentage of patients [4]. The presence of hepatic granulomas, disputed in the past in the case of the commonest species, *B. melitensis*, has been ascertained in recent years [5], although not necessarily indicating an adverse outcome. On the contrary, chronic hepatic suppurative disease remains one of the rare but therapeutically challenging forms of chronic brucellosis [6]. An etiological role of brucellosis in cirrhosis development had been supported in the early 1950s by pioneers of *Brucella* research such as Wesley Spink [7]. But, this correlation gradually regressed to isolated case reports of doubtful significance, in subsequent years. In cases of preexisting liver disease, numerous case reports have demonstrated brucellosis as a causative factor of disequilibrium development, characteristically in the form of ascites/spontaneous bacterial peritonitis (SBP) development [8–16].

Given that cirrhotic patients, in general, are predisposed through a variety of pathogenic immune disorder mechanisms to infection development, not only restricted to SBP [17], it is of paramount importance to increase these patients' health literacy in order to prevent opportunistic infections from uncommon, endemic in specific areas, pathogens such as *Vibrio vulnificus* in Southest Asia [18] or brucellosis in numerous parts of the world. The last is of further significance due to its need of protracted combined antibiotic therapy with regimens exhibiting acknowledged potential of hepatotoxicity.

Herein, we describe three cases of cirrhotic patients where acute brucellosis served as a trigger of fatal hepatic decompensation, either due to direct effect of the pathogen alone, or in combination with hepatotoxicity of the necessary antibiotic regiments used. We further underline the necessity, in face of these specific therapeutic difficulties, of raising awareness of cirrhotic patients in terms of avoidance of exposure to such pathogens.

2. Case Presentations

2.1. Patient 1. A 47-year-old male, with known alcoholic cirrhosis for the past 6 years, was admitted for persisting evening fever and abdominal dilatation. The patient abstained from alcohol since diagnosis and had a history of esophageal variceal bleeding, hepatic encephalopathy episodes, and ascites development in the past but had been ascites-free for at least 6 months prior to admission. His medical history also included insulin-dependent diabetes mellitus. He continued to work as a confectioner. On admission, clinical evaluation and subsequent imaging demonstrated massive ascites and splenomegaly, with no signs of portal thrombosis. Laboratory evaluation showed mild pancytopenia and increase C-reactive protein (CRP), while other biochemistry markers were, in general, normal. Numerous cultures were drawn from multiple sites, including bone marrow, and serology tests for various pathogens were performed. Cultures were positive for *B. melitensis*, a diagnosis further confirmed by real time-polymerase chain reaction (PCR based on direct amplification of a 207-base pair DNA sequence of a gene specific for the *Brucella* genus, BCSP31) and agglutination (Rose Bengal plate agglutination test), Wright seroagglutination test, and ELISA serology (Serion ELISA IgG/IgM/IgA antibodies to *Brucella melitensis*). The patient retrospectively admitted to consuming unpasteurized dairy products (sheep and goats) 2 months prior to admission.

Initiation of antibiotic therapy was problematic since there was a vague history of tetracycline intolerance in the past, and the underlying pathology advocated against the use of the hepatotoxic doxycycline and rifampicin and the potentially hepatorenal syndrome inducers, aminoglycosides. The remaining options were trimethoprim/sulfamethoxazole 160/800 mg twice daily and ciprofloxacin 500 mg twice daily, which were initiated as soon as diagnosis was confirmed. Defervescence was indeed achieved on day 5, albeit accompanied by renal function disorders, with a gradual increase in serum creatinine up to 2 mg/dl, with normal values (nv) of 0.6–1.2 mg/dl. On day 12, fever relapsed, accompanied by worsening pancytopenia and renal function values. Extensive diagnostic workup was performed, including further cultures and imaging and excluding any other underlying infection, and it was decided to substitute cotrimoxazole with doxycycline 100 mg twice daily, since the benefit of brucellosis therapy overruled the risk of doxycycline-hepatotoxicity at that point. Defervescence was achieved 8 days later, accompanied by partial reversal of renal function and pancytopenia. The patient was successfully discharged and referred to a transplantation center for further evaluation. Forty days after doxycycline-ciprofloxacin initiation, the patient was readmitted due to hepatic encephalopathy, worsening of ascites and pancytopenia, and low-grade fever: any underlying cause was excluded through a scrutinized workup and supportive measures initiation. Doxycycline was discontinued as a potential inducer of decompensation, and the patient was transferred to a transplantation center.

Since pulmonary hypertension had been detected, the patient was not considered a candidate for liver transplantation and he continued to rapidly deteriorate until the adverse outcome.

2.2. Patient 2. A 50-year-old man, with diagnosed alcoholic cirrhosis for the past decade, abstaining from alcohol since then, with no history of any cirrhotic complications, under no supportive treatment apart for regular follow-up, was admitted for protracted fever of two months' duration, accompanied by low backache, mild diarrhea, and abdominal distention. He had a history of splenectomy and was a shepherd. Significant ascites, accompanied by moderate pleural fluid effusion, was noted on clinical examination and subsequent imaging, the latter also demonstrating abdominal lymphadenopathy with partial central necrosis. Laboratory tests, compared to his latest follow-up, demonstrated only an increase in CRP and total and direct bilirubin. Blood cultures were positive for *B. melitensis*, a finding further confirmed by Rose Bengal plate agglutination, Wright seroagglutination test, and ELISA serology (Serion ELISA IgG/IgM/IgA antibodies to *Brucella melitensis*). The patient was treated with doxycycline 100 mg twice daily, rifampicin 600 mg daily, and ciprofloxacin 500 mg twice daily. Defervescence was achieved on day 5, accompanied though by progressive worsening of liver biochemistry indices and mild prolongation of international normalized ratio (INR) to levels of 1.34 (nv 0.8–1.2). Rifampicin dose was halved, and diuretics were added to treat ascites. Despite improvement/stabilization of other biochemical indices in later days, serum bilirubin continued to increase, reaching a plateau of total 7.2 mg/dl/direct 4.2 mg/dl and the patient was discharged, continuing treatment and follow-up as an outpatient on day 16. On day 41, the patient was readmitted with hepatic encephalopathy and jaundice. Hepatic biochemistry was steady, but total bilirubin was 16.7 mg/dl (direct bilirubin 13.6 mg/dl) and INR was 1.44. Ascites was minimal and subsequent workup excluded any underlying causes of encephalopathy. Antibiotics were discontinued as potential inducers of severe hepatotoxicity, and the patient was referred to a transplantation center due to the gradual worsening of liver function indices. He underwent liver transplantation which unfortunately had an adverse postoperative outcome.

2.3. Patient 3. A 46-year-old male with a long history of alcohol abuse was transferred to our department with a novel diagnosis of alcoholic cirrhosis. He had been admitted to another hospital with delirium tremens and rhabdomyolysis. A diagnosis of alcoholic cirrhosis was made following evaluation. During that hospitalization, mild fever was observed, which was considered as a consequence of aspiration and treated with amoxicillin-clavulanate. During hospitalization to our department for further evaluation of cirrhosis (which demonstrated extensive ascites, splenomegaly, prolongation of international normalized ratio (INR), hypoalbuminemia, and mild lower esophageal varices), low-grade fever persisted. Medical history revealed a recent, 50 days ago, trip to Spain and consumption of nonpasteurized dairy products (sheep's products).

Blood cultures were positive for *B. melitensis*, confirmed by Rose Bengal plate agglutination, Wright seroagglutination test, and ELISA serology (Serion ELISA IgG/IgM/IgA antibodies to *Brucella melitensis*). The patient was treated with doxycycline 100 mg twice daily and ciprofloxacin 500 mg twice daily, but on day 4, he exhibited rapid worsening of liver function and laboratory indices of diffuse intravascular coagulation (DIC). Discontinuation of doxycycline and subsequently ciprofloxacin, along with supportive treatment, did not reverse the rapid evolution of the syndrome towards hepatic encephalopathy, spontaneous intracranial hemorrhage, and death on day 33.

3. Discussion

In recent years, brucellosis has been recognized as a significant cause of morbidity in the developing world and also as an important parameter of travel-related medicine [1]. Numerous reports have demonstrated the emergence of disease in the developed world not only through international travel but also through dairy products' trade and immigration [1, 19]. Awareness of the disease remains limited even in regions of hyperendemicity [20]. All patients in this series were located in an endemic area from an endemic country; yet, even though employed in theoretically high-risk occupation, the first two patients did not avoid exposure through consumption of unpasteurized dairy products or direct contact, respectively. The third patient, on the other hand, is a typical example of travel-related brucellosis.

Hepatic complications are expected in brucellosis, since the liver is the largest RES organ in the human body. One should not forget that the peritoneal mononuclear phagocytic system is an integral part of RES and so it is thus not surprising that it can react by ascites formation even in previously healthy patients [21, 22], or in the context of generalized fulminant disease course [23], let alone in cirrhosis.

Treating brucellosis has always been problematic due to the pathogen's ability to survive inside human phagocytic cells and trigger relapses that can be observed even when adequate therapy is administered. Both the World Health Organization and expert therapeutic recommendations [24] stress the need for a combined protracted therapeutic regimen. In cases of preexisting liver disease though, concerns about the toxicity of the antibacterial agents active against brucellosis are further enhanced due to the need of protracted administration. Using doxycycline 100 mg twice daily and rifampicin 600 mg or 900 mg once daily for six weeks at least, and even more in cases of relapse or serious complications as spondylitis, carries an expectedly increased potential for pharmaceutical toxicity. On the other hand, using amynoglycosides in patients who have already developed cirrhotic ascites may predispose to hepatorenal syndrome and generally endanger an intravascular/extravascular volume equilibrium that is often extremely difficult to achieve in cirrhotic patients. Thus, it is difficult to administer any of the three accepted prime combinations in patients with cirrhosis and portal hypertension complications, such as doxycycline with either streptomycin or rifampicin or gentamycin. This is characteristically observed in the second patient, where the administration of both doxycycline and rifampicin may have played an important role in liver decompensation. Relevant literature on *Brucella* and SBP includes reports of successful therapy with minimal doses of rifampicin, but conclusions cannot be extrapolated from isolated cases, particularly since susceptibility of each cirrhotic patient to pharmaceutical hepatic damage cannot be prequantified. The present study focuses only on patients with an adverse outcome and does not include patients with cirrhosis, who were successfully treated with typical brucellosis regimens in our department. Furthermore, the severity of each brucellosis case is not similar, and the above-reported cases were acute, culture-positive brucellosis cases that satisfied all accepted predisposing factors to treatment relapse and failure [25]. Indeed, similar published experience varies largely regarding the outcome, since there have been reports of successful monotherapy with ofloxacin [8], of successful use of minimal dose of rifampicin with either doxycycline or ciprofloxacin [9, 10], and of prolonged courses of doxycycline for concurrent spondylitis or chronic hepatosuppurative disease [11, 12]. On the other hand, there is also published experience of adverse outcomes, similar to this series [13], with a report of interest being strikingly similar to the third patient described in the present study, with rapid deterioration and DIC development [14].

This brings us back to prevention, particularly through increasing health literacy of the patients and more specifically by acknowledging individual risk factors related to region of residence, occupation, other underlying diseases, or cause of cirrhosis [17]. Zoonoses should not be forgotten, given their global distribution and therapeutic peculiarities.

Authors' Contributions

Concept and design of the study were proposed by MK and HM. Data acquisition was performed by EK, IR, and SFN. Results were interpreted by MK, ET, IR, and SFM. Drafting of the manuscript was done by MK and HM. All authors critically revised the manuscript, approved the final version to be published, and agree to be accountable for all aspects of the work.

References

[1] M. P. Franco, M. Mulder, R. H. Gilman, and H. L. Smits, "Human brucellosis," *The Lancet Infectious Diseases*, vol. 7, no. 12, pp. 775–786, 2007.

[2] I. Sari, F. Altuntas, S. Hacioglu et al., "A multicenter retrospective study defining the clinical and hematological manifestations of brucellosis and pancytopenia in a large series: hematological malignancies, the unusual cause of pancytopenia in patients with brucellosis," *American Journal of Hematology*, vol. 83, no. 4, pp. 334–339, 2008.

[3] C. E. Papagoras, M. I. Argyropoulou, P. V. Voulgari, I. Vrabie, A. K. Zikou, and A. A. Drosos, "A case of Brucella spondylitis in a patient with psoriatic arthritis receiving infliximab," *Clinical and Experimental Rheumatology*, vol. 27, no. 1, pp. 124–127, 2009.

[4] D. Ozturk-Engin, H. Erdem, S. Gencer et al., "Liver involvement in patients with brucellosis: results of the Marmara study," *European Journal of Clinical Microbiology & Infectious Diseases*, vol. 33, no. 7, pp. 1253–1262, 2014.

[5] N. Akritidis, M. Tzivras, I. Delladetsima, S. Stefanaki, H. M. Moutsopoulos, and G. Pappas, "The liver in brucellosis," *Clinical Gastroenterology and Hepatology*, vol. 5, no. 9, pp. 1109–1112, 2007.

[6] J. Ariza, C. Pigrau, C. Canas et al., "Current understanding and management of chronic hepatosplenic suppurative brucellosis," *Clinical Infectious Diseases*, vol. 32, no. 7, pp. 1024–1033, 2001.

[7] W. W. Spink, F. W. Hoffbauer, W. W. Walker, and R. A. Green, "Histopathology of the liver in human brucellosis," *The Journal of Laboratory and Clinical Medicine*, vol. 34, no. 1, pp. 40–58, 1949.

[8] F. Demirkan, H. E. Akalin, H. Simsek, E. Özyilkan, and H. Telatar, "Spontaneous peritonitis due toBrucella melitensis in a patient with cirrhosis," *European Journal of Clinical Microbiology & Infectious Diseases*, vol. 12, no. 1, pp. 66-67, 1993.

[9] S. Gursoy, M. Baskol, O. Ozbakir, K. Guven, T. Patiroglu, and M. Yucesoy, "Spontaneous bacterial peritonitis due to Brucella," *Turkish Journal of Gastrenterology*, vol. 14, pp. 145–147, 2003.

[10] M. Guclu, T. Yakar, and M. Ali Habeoglu, "Spontaneous bacterial peritonitis and chylothorax related to Brucella infection in a cirrhotic patient," *European Journal of General Medicine*, vol. 5, pp. 201–204, 2008.

[11] S. Luk and W. K. To, "Diagnosis challenges of human brucellosis in Hong Kong: a case series inn two regional hospitals," *Hong Kong Medicinal Journal*, vol. 16, no. 4, pp. 299–303, 2010.

[12] N. R. Jacob, C. G. Rodríguez, M. A. Binaghi et al., "Brucellosis complicating chronic non-infectious disorders: diagnostic and therapeutic dilemmas," *Journal of Medical Microbiology*, vol. 57, no. 9, pp. 1161–1166, 2008.

[13] B. Kantarceken, M. M. Harputluoglu, Y. Bayndir, M. R. Bay ktar, M. Aladag, and F. Hilmioglu, "Spontaneous bacterial peritonitis due to Brucella melitensis in a cirrhotic patient," *Turkish Journal of Gastrenterology*, vol. 16, pp. 38–40, 2005.

[14] M. Dizbay, K. Hizel, S. Kilic, R. Mutluay, Y. Ozkan, and T. Karakan, "Brucella peritonitis and leucocytoclastic vasculitis due to Brucella melitensis," *Brazilian Journal of Infectious Diseases*, vol. 11, no. 4, pp. 443-444, 2007.

[15] A. Erbay, H. Bodur, E. Akinci, A. Colpan, and M. A. Cevic, "Spontaneous bacterial peritonitis due to Brucella melitensis," *Scandinavian Journal of Infectious Disesae*, vol. 35, pp. 196-197, 2001.

[16] M. Goganay, B. Aygen, M. Inan, and O. Ozbakir, "Brucella peritonitis in a cirrhotic patient with ascites," *European Journal of Medicine*, vol. 2, pp. 441-442, 1993.

[17] L. Christou, G. Pappas, and M. E. Falagas, "Bacterial infection-related morbidity and mortality in cirrhosis," *The American Journal of Gastroenterology*, vol. 102, no. 7, pp. 1510–1517, 2007.

[18] S. M. Haq and H. H. Dayal, "Chronic liver disease and consumption of raw oysters: a potentially lethal combination-a review of Vibrio vulnificus septicemia," *The American Journal of Gastroenterology*, vol. 100, no. 5, pp. 1195–1199, 2005.

[19] S. A. Dahouk, H. Neubauer, A. Hensel et al., "Changing epidemiology of human brucellosis, Germany, 1962-2005," *Emerging Infectious Disease*, vol. 13, no. 12, pp. 1895–1900, 2007.

[20] N. Zhang, H. Zhou, D. S. Huang, and P. Guan, "Brucellosis awareness and knowledge in communities worldwide: a systematic review and meta-analysis of 79 observational studies," *PLoS Neglected Tropical Diseases*, vol. 13, no. 5, Article ID e0007366, 2019.

[21] Y. Z. Demiroglu, T. Turunc, H. Aliskan, S. Colakoglu, and H. Arslan, "Primary peritonitis due to brucellosis mimicking tuberculous peritonitis," *Turkish Journal of Gastrenterology*, vol. 20, pp. 135–137, 2009.

[22] K. Bourantas, L. Christou, G. Dalekos, K. Barbati, and E. Tsianos, "A 54-year-old stockbreeder with ascites," *The Lancet*, vol. 349, no. 9057, p. 994, 1997.

[23] J. C. Garcia Casallas, W. V. Monsalve, S. C. Arias Villate, and I. M. Fino Solano, "Acute liver failure complication of brucellosis infection: a case report and review of the literature," *Journal of Medical Case Report*, vol. 12, no. 1, p. 62, 2018.

[24] R. Yousefi-Nooraie, S. Mortaz-Hejri, M. Mehrani, and P. Sadeghipour, "Antibiotics for treating brucellosis," *Cochrane Database of Systemic Reviews*, vol. 10, no. 10, Article ID CD007179, 2012.

[25] J. Ariza, M. Bosilkovski, A. Cascio et al., "Perspectives for the treatment of brucellosis in the 21st century: the Ioannina recommendations," *PLoS Medicine*, vol. 4, no. 12, p. e317, 2007.

20

Veillonella Bacteremia in Alcoholic Hepatitis

Patrick Lee,[1,2] Brandon K. K. Fields,[1,3] Tom Liang,[1,4] Michael P. Dubé,[1,5] and Seth Politano[1,2]

[1]*Keck School of Medicine, University of Southern California, Los Angeles, CA 90033, USA*
[2]*Department of Medicine, University of Southern California, Los Angeles, CA 90033, USA*
[3]*Scripps Mercy Hospital San Diego, San Diego, CA 92103, USA*
[4]*Department of Pathology, University of Southern California, Los Angeles, CA 90033, USA*
[5]*Department of Infectious Diseases, University of Southern California, Los Angeles, CA 90033, USA*

Correspondence should be addressed to Seth Politano; politano@med.usc.edu

Academic Editor: Haruki Komatsu

Veillonella species are commensal bacteria of the human oral, gut, and vaginal microbiota that are rarely identified as clinically relevant pathogens. Here, we describe a novel case of *Veillonella atypica* bacteremia in a patient with biopsy-proven alcoholic hepatitis. *Veillonella* species have been correlated with disease severity and hepatic encephalopathy in liver diseases such as autoimmune hepatitis and cirrhosis. Their abundance has also been recently observed to be increased in alcoholic hepatitis, where postinflammatory infections are known to impact mortality. This case report highlights the possible clinical manifestations that result from significant gut dysbiosis in patients with severe alcoholic hepatitis. Early identification and treatment of *Veillonella* bacteremia in susceptible populations could be crucial to survival given this organism's predilection for causing life-threatening infections, including meningitis, endocarditis, and osteomyelitis.

1. Introduction

Veillonella species is an anaerobic, Gram-negative diplococci found in the human oral, gastrointestinal, and vaginal microbiota. Although *Veillonella* is considered a commensal, it has rarely been isolated as a clinically significant pathogen in cases of osteomyelitis, endocarditis, epidural abscess, meningitis, pyelonephritis, and bacteremia [1, 2]. In this case report, we present a case of *Veillonella atypica* bacteremia without a readily identifiable source in the setting of alcoholic hepatitis. To the best of our knowledge, there have only been two previously reported cases of *Veillonella* bacteremia without a clear source of infection [2, 3].

2. Case Presentation

A 31-year-old male with a history of heavy alcohol use presented to our hospital with a 3-day history of lower extremity edema, abdominal swelling, and periumbilical pain. He reported use of 6 cans of beer daily, with the most recent use 3 days prior to admission. On presentation, the patient was alert and oriented only to person and self. His vital signs were a temperature of 38.5°C, heart rate 129 beats/minute, and blood pressure 132/74 mmHg. Physical exam was significant for scleral icterus, asterixis, systolic murmur, abdominal distention with caput medusae, palmar erythema, and spider angiomas on his chest.

Laboratory tests revealed a white blood cell (WBC) count of 11.7 K/mm^3 (with 78% neutrophils, absolute lymphocyte count 1.3 K/mm^3, and absolute monocyte count 1.0 K/mm^3), platelets 88 K/mm^3, lactate 2.1 mmol/L, alkaline phosphatase (ALP) 503 U/L, aspartate aminotransferase (AST) 172 U/L, and alanine aminotransferase (ALT) 19 U/L. Maddrey's Discriminant Function score was 35.3 (Prothrombin time 19.2 seconds and total bilirubin 6.8 mg/dL). Ascitic fluid analysis after paracentesis was negative for spontaneous bacterial peritonitis, with a nucleated cell count of 79/cumm and 23% segmented neutrophils. Further hepatitis workup yielded antinuclear antibodies positive for nuclear, speckled pattern with 1 : 1280 titer, actin antibodies IgG 57 units, and negative viral hepatitis panel for hepatitis A, B, and C. Abdominal ultrasound showed cirrhosis with hepatosplenomegaly and trace abdominal ascites.

Two sets of blood cultures obtained on hospital day 0 were negative. Intravenous ceftriaxone was started after collection of the initial blood cultures. Two additional anaerobic blood culture bottles obtained on day 2 of hospital stay were positive for *Veillonella atypica*, identified using MALDI-TOF (Figure 1). Repeat blood cultures after 2 days of intravenous ceftriaxone were negative. The infectious disease team recommended discontinuing IV ceftriaxone as repeat cultures were negative and the patient had completed a 7-day course of ceftriaxone. Transthoracic echocardiogram was negative for valvular lesions. Liver biopsy obtained on hospital day 8 demonstrated bridging fibrosis and was consistent with alcoholic hepatitis with cholestasis (Figures 2(a) and 2(b)).

Hospital course was complicated by hemodynamic instability and acute encephalopathy on day 3 and 4, where patient was tachycardic to 120 beats per minute, tachypneic to 30 shallow breaths per second, and febrile to 38.3°C. The patient's mental status was waxing and waning; there was a concern for sepsis, grade II hepatic encephalopathy, and alcohol withdrawal. Hemodynamic instability and mental status improved with IV lorazepam and lactulose, and the patient was subsequently discharged on hospital day 9. After confirmation of alcoholic hepatitis on liver biopsy, the patient started prednisolone 40 mg oral daily on day 7 after hospital discharge due to difficulty obtaining the prescription.

Patient was evaluated in outpatient hepatology clinic 7 days after prednisolone therapy (14 days after hospital discharge). Pertinent labs showed a white blood cell count of 23.9 K/mm^3, sodium of 123 mmol/L, and potassium of 2.9 mmol/L. Prothrombin time and total bilirubin had increased to 23.4 sec and 20.2 mg/dL, respectively. Calculated Lille score on day 7 of treatment was 0.577 and suggestive of treatment failure of alcoholic hepatitis. The patient was sent to the emergency room after the clinic visit for tachycardia and concern for sepsis. He was then readmitted to the hospital for further management. Repeat blood cultures and ascitic fluid culture on admission were negative. The patient was deemed a poor transplant candidate due to continued alcohol use and non-United States citizen status. After appropriate counseling, he left the hospital against medical advice to be home with family.

During a phone follow-up 3 months after discharge, the medical team was informed that the patient was deceased.

3. Discussion

In this 31-year-old male with alcoholic hepatitis, his hospital course was complicated by sepsis due to *Veillonella atypica* bacteremia. In patients with severe alcoholic hepatitis, the rates of infection range from 12 to 26% of patients, with the most common bacteria cultured being *Escherichia coli* [4]. Timing of infection was noted to be important. Infections present at admission did not impact mortality, but infections that occurred during hospitalization were associated with worse outcomes [4]. The pathophysiology of bacteremia in the setting of alcoholic hepatitis is thought to involve increased intestinal permeability secondary to the proinflammatory state, making the host more susceptible to bacterial translocation. This can result in bacteremia, with subsequent systemic inflammatory response syndrome [4].

It should be noted that although *Veillonella* is rarely a clinically significant pathogen, it has been reported in serious, potentially fatal infections, such as meningitis, pulmonary infections, endocarditis, and osteomyelitis [1, 2, 5]. However, no case reports have observed *Veillonella* bacteremia in the setting of alcoholic hepatitis. Bacterial isolates of *Veillonella atypica* from blood cultures taken on hospital day 2 were sensitive to ampicillin/sulbactam, clindamycin, imipenem, meropenem, and metronidazole and notably resistant to penicillin. Although the treatment for *Veillonella* bacteremia is not well defined, the bacteremia cleared with intravenous ceftriaxone treatment [6]. Previous case reports have discussed use of beta-lactams (notably penicillin, ampicillin, and first-generation cephalosporins), aminoglycosides, metronidazole, and clindamycin in the treatment of *Veillonella* bacteremia in the setting of endocarditis [7]. To date, there is no clear consensus on the treatment for *Veillonella* infections given the limited reports on its pathogenicity [5].

Veillonella abundance has been observed to be increased in patients with cirrhosis, autoimmune hepatitis, primary biliary cirrhosis [8], primary sclerosing cholangitis [9, 10], and alcoholic hepatitis [11]. In autoimmune hepatitis, *Veillonella dispar* was identified to be the species most significantly associated with severity of disease, correlated with serum AST [12]. *Veillonella* abundance was also found to be associated with increased systemic inflammation, endotoxemia, and more pronounced in patients with hepatic encephalopathy [13–15]. A recent study by Kim et al. observed significant gut dysbiosis, defined as a decrease in bacterial diversity and autochthonous bacteria levels, and increased *Veillonella* abundance in patients with severe alcoholic hepatitis [11]. Treatment with rifaximin in these patients improved gut dysbiosis and caused a decrease in *Veillonella* abundance [11]. Rifaximin has also been shown to decrease *Veillonella* abundance, improve endotoxemia, and improve intestinal barrier function in patients with cirrhosis complicated by hepatic encephalopathy [13]. The unique presentation of *Veillonella* bacteremia in this patient likely reflects the significant gut dysbiosis in patients with severe alcoholic hepatitis.

The role of the gut microbiota, consisting of archaea, fungi, viruses, protozoans, and bacteria such as *Veillonella*, has been described in human diseases, including obesity, diabetes, and cardiovascular diseases [16]. Recent research has demonstrated its association in liver diseases as well. Studies have observed unique gut microbiota compositions in autoimmune liver disease [8], nonalcoholic fatty liver disease (NAFLD) [17], and cirrhosis [14, 15]. Interestingly, the gut microbiota composition shifts with severity of liver disease, such as worsening fibrosis in NAFLD [17, 18]. Besides medications, such as the antibiotic rifaximin,

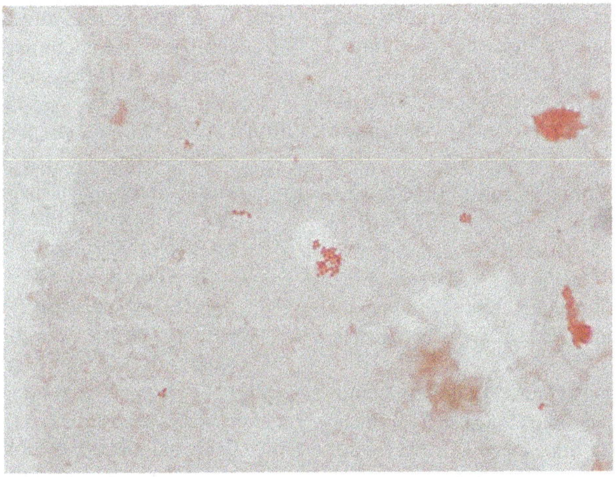

FIGURE 1: Gram stain from the anaerobic culture plate showing small Gram-negative diplococci (1000x).

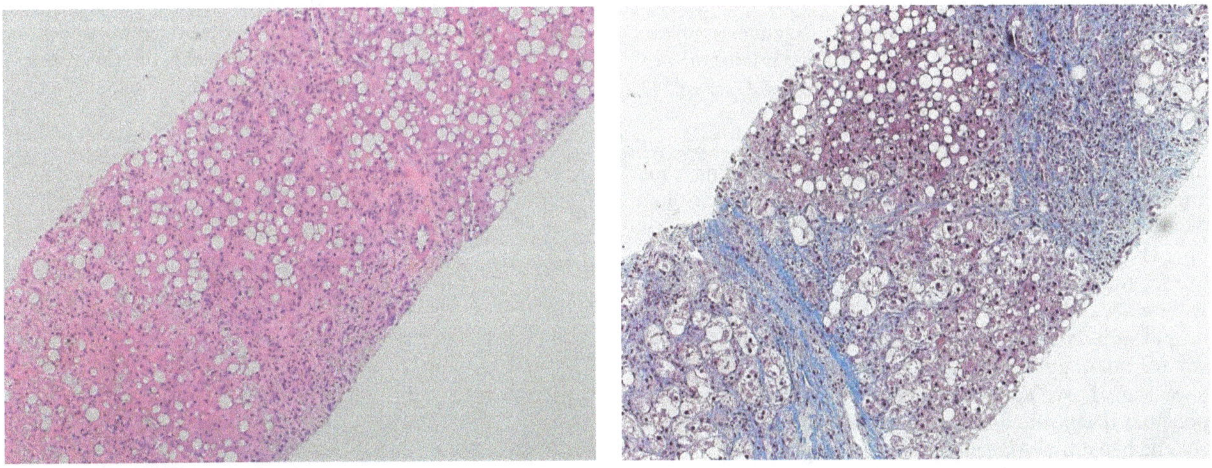

(a) (b)

FIGURE 2: (a) Liver biopsy showing portal and perivenular fibrosis with severe bridging fibrosis and alcoholic hepatitis (hematoxylin & eosin stain, 200x). (b) Trichrome stain demonstrating severe fibrosis (200x).

probiotics and fecal microbiota transplant (FMT) have been investigated as targeted therapies to alter the gut microbiota to treat certain human diseases. Recent studies have demonstrated significant improvements in survival in patients with steroid-ineligible alcoholic hepatitis treated with FMT, suggesting that FMT can be a cost-effective transition to liver transplant or augment transplant-free survival in these patients [19, 20]. Probiotics and FMT have also been shown to improve cognitive function in patients with cirrhosis complicated by hepatic encephalopathy [21, 22]. These recent studies highlight the potential for targeted therapies towards the gut microbiota to treat complications of conditions such as alcoholic hepatitis and hepatic encephalopathy.

In summary, this patient passed away from alcoholic hepatitis that was nonresponsive to steroid therapy. A Lille model score >0.45 predicts a 6-month survival of only 25% [23]. The positive results in the studies of FMT in alcoholic hepatitis demonstrate a potential alternative or adjunct to steroid therapy [19, 20]. There remains a great need for further research into alcoholic hepatitis given its high mortality, and novel therapeutic options involving immunomodulation are currently being investigated [24].

Acknowledgments

This study was funded by the Professional Education Benefit of the Committee of Interns and Residents.

References

[1] F. E. Al-Otaibi and M. M. Al-Mohizea, "Non-vertebral veillonella species septicemia and osteomyelitis in a patient with diabetes: a case report and review of the literature," *Journal of Medical Case Reports*, vol. 8, no. 1, p. 365, 2014.

[2] R. G. Fisher and M. R. Denison, "Veillonella parvula bacteremia without an underlying source," *Journal of Clinical Microbiology*, vol. 34, no. 12, pp. 3235-3236, 1996.

[3] G. Gessoni, N. Sacchetto, S. Gelmi et al., "Veillonellae: personal observation of a fatal bacteremia," *Bollettino dell'Istituto Sieroterapico Milanese*, vol. 68, pp. 193–196, 1988.

[4] A. K. Singal, V. H. Shah, and P. S. Kamath, "Infection in severe alcoholic hepatitis: yet another piece in the puzzle," *Gastroenterology*, vol. 152, no. 5, pp. 938–940, 2017.

[5] A. Bathini, C. R. Maxwell, H. Hedayat, J. Barrett, and Z. Hakma, "Case report: vertebral osteomyelitis secondary to a dental abscess," *BMC Infectious Diseases*, vol. 20, no. 1, p. 133, 2020.

[6] S. A. Roberts, K. P. Shore, S. D. Paviour, D. Holland, and A. J. Morris, "Antimicrobial susceptibility of anaerobic bacteria in New Zealand: 1999–2003," *Journal of Antimicrobial Chemotherapy*, vol. 57, no. 5, pp. 992–998, 2006.

[7] L. Saladi, C. Zeana, and M. Singh, "Native valve endocarditis due to veillonella species: a case report and review of the literature," *Case Reports in Infectious Diseases*, vol. 2017, Article ID 4896186, 3 pages, 2017.

[8] K. Abe, A. Takahashi, M. Fujita et al., "Dysbiosis of oral microbiota and its association with salivary immunological biomarkers in autoimmune liver disease," *PLoS One*, vol. 13, no. 7, Article ID e0198757, 2018.

[9] M. Kummen, K. Holm, J. A. Anmarkrud et al., "The gut microbial profile in patients with primary sclerosing cholangitis is distinct from patients with ulcerative colitis without biliary disease and healthy controls," *Gut*, vol. 66, no. 4, pp. 611–619, 2017.

[10] M. C. Rühlemann, F.-A. Heinsen, R. Zenouzi, W. Lieb, A. Franke, and C. Schramm, "Faecal microbiota profiles as diagnostic biomarkers in primary sclerosing cholangitis," *Gut*, vol. 66, no. 4, pp. 753-754, 2017.

[11] S. S. Kim, J. W. Eun, H. J. Cho et al., "Microbiome as a potential diagnostic and predictive biomarker in severe alcoholic hepatitis," *Alimentary Pharmacology & Therapeutics*, vol. 53, no. 4, pp. 540–551, 2021.

[12] Y. Wei, Y. Li, L. Yan et al., "Alterations of gut microbiome in autoimmune hepatitis," *Gut*, vol. 69, no. 3, pp. 569–577, 2020.

[13] K. Kaji, H. Takaya, S. Saikawa et al., "Rifaximin ameliorates hepatic encephalopathy and endotoxemia without affecting the gut microbiome diversity," *World Journal of Gastroenterology*, vol. 23, no. 47, pp. 8355–8366, 2017.

[14] H. Fukui, "Role of gut dysbiosis in liver diseases: what have we learned so far?" *Diseases*, vol. 7, 2019.

[15] N. Qin, F. Yang, A. Li et al., "Alterations of the human gut microbiome in liver cirrhosis," *Nature*, vol. 513, no. 7516, pp. 59–64, 2014.

[16] P. Lee, B. R. Yacyshyn, and M. B. Yacyshyn, "Gut microbiota and obesity: an opportunity to alter obesity through faecal microbiota transplant (FMT)," *Diabetes, Obesity and Metabolism*, vol. 21, no. 3, pp. 479–490, 2019.

[17] C. Caussy, A. Tripathi, G. Humphrey et al., "A gut microbiome signature for cirrhosis due to nonalcoholic fatty liver disease," *Nature Communications*, vol. 10, no. 1, p. 1406, 2019.

[18] J. Boursier, O. Mueller, M. Barret et al., "The severity of nonalcoholic fatty liver disease is associated with gut dysbiosis and shift in the metabolic function of the gut microbiota," *Hepatology*, vol. 63, no. 3, pp. 764–775, 2016.

[19] C. A. Philips, A. Pande, S. M. Shasthry et al., "Healthy donor fecal microbiota transplantation in steroid-ineligible severe alcoholic hepatitis: a pilot study," *Clinical Gastroenterology and Hepatology*, vol. 15, no. 4, pp. 600–602, 2017.

[20] C. A. Philips, N. Phadke, K. Ganesan, S. Ranade, and P. Augustine, "Corticosteroids, nutrition, pentoxifylline, or fecal microbiota transplantation for severe alcoholic hepatitis," *Indian Journal of Gastroenterology*, vol. 37, no. 3, pp. 215–225, 2018.

[21] R. K. Dhiman, B. Rana, S. Agrawal et al., "Probiotic VSL#3 reduces liver disease severity and hospitalization in patients with cirrhosis: a randomized, controlled trial," *Gastroenterology*, vol. 147, no. 6, pp. 1327–1337, 2014.

[22] J. S. Bajaj, Z. Kassam, A. Fagan et al., "Fecal microbiota transplant from a rational stool donor improves hepatic encephalopathy: a randomized clinical trial," *Hepatology*, vol. 66, no. 6, pp. 1727–1738, 2017.

[23] T. D. Sandahl, P. Jepsen, P. Ott, and H. Vilstrup, "Validation of prognostic scores for clinical use in patients with alcoholic hepatitis," *Scandinavian Journal of Gastroenterology*, vol. 46, no. 9, pp. 1127–1132, 2011.

[24] S. M. Shasthry and S. K. Sarin, "New treatment options for alcoholic hepatitis," *World Journal of Gastroenterology*, vol. 22, no. 15, pp. 3892–3906, 2016.

21

An Interesting Case of Isolated False-Reactive Hepatitis B Surface Antigen

Victoria Costa,[1] **Zhen Zhao**,[1] **Sabrina E. Racine-Brzostek**,[1] **Gadi Lalazar**,[2] **and He S. Yang**[1]

[1]*Department of Pathology and Laboratory Medicine, New York Presbyterian Hospital, Weill Cornell Medicine, New York, NY, USA*
[2]*Department of Gastroenterology and Hepatology, New York Presbyterian Hospital, Weill Cornell Medicine, New York, NY, USA*

Correspondence should be addressed to Gadi Lalazar; gal2015@med.cornell.edu and He S. Yang; hey9012@med.cornell.edu

Academic Editor: Haruki Komatsu

The standard serologic markers used to diagnose hepatitis B infection include hepatitis B surface antigen (HBsAg), hepatitis B surface antibody (anti-HBs), total hepatitis B core antibody (anti-HBc), and IgM antibody to hepatitis B core antigen (IgM anti-HBc). Different markers or combinations of markers are used to identify different phases of HBV infection and determine whether a patient has acute or chronic infection or immunity due to prior infection or vaccination or is seronegative and susceptible to future infection. Isolated HBsAg seropositivity is a peculiar serological pattern that requires investigation. Herein, we present a case of an asymptomatic female without a history of liver disease or evident risk factors for hepatitis, who underwent screening for infectious disease prior to resection of basal cell carcinoma involving her eyelid. The patient's laboratory testing showed positivity for HBsAg and the HIV 1/2 screen. To investigate, we performed serial dilutions, utilized heterophilicantibody blocking tubes, and repeated analysis using a different commercial assay (Abbott Architect i2000), all in support of a false-positive result attributed to a heterophilic antibody. Hence, we demonstrate that heterophilic antibody interference can result in isolated HBsAg positivity and recommend considering this form of interference in the differential where there is low clinical suspicion for viral infection.

1. Introduction

Hepatitis B virus (HBV) is transmitted through contact with bodily fluids, including through sexual contact, contaminated blood, or from an infected mother to her newborn. HBsAg is one of the first serum markers to appear during the course of acute HBV infection, and it is also a useful follow-up marker, since declining concentrations are observed in resolving hepatitis B virus infection. During the acute phase of infection, hepatitis B e-antigen (HBeAg) appears shortly after the appearance of HBsAg and, in some patients, disappears within several weeks as the acute infection resolves. Anti-HBc IgM antibodies are detectable at the outset of the clinical disease and gradually decline as the infection evolves. Anti-HBs antibodies become positive late in convalescence, between 6 weeks and 6 months, after HBsAg clearance. This antigen and antibody dynamic pattern occurs in the majority of HBV infections [1]. Isolated HBsAg seropositivity, where HBsAg is the only positive serologic marker within the hepatitis B panel, may be seen in the very early stage of HBV infection when HBeAg and anti-HBc IgM have not appeared yet and a patient has not shown any symptoms [1]. Transient HBsAg has also been observed in patients for up to 2 weeks after HBV vaccination [2, 3]. Other possibilities of isolated positive HBsAg may include host incompetence or HBV variants with probably mutation in the S-region [4]. In addition, it has been reported that a patient with lupus nephritis exhibited isolated HBsAg positivity [5]. Furthermore, potentially false-reactive HBsAg could be due to a range of autoimmune conditions, infection with a range of community-acquired viral or bacterial infections, and possible reactivation of latent infections such as herpes viruses or *H. pylori*.

Here, we report a case of a female patient with persistent isolated HBsAg positivity with a lack of symptoms, other serological markers, risk factors, or vaccination to explain the positivity, highly suggestive of a false-positive result requiring thorough investigation to evaluate potential interferences.

2. Case Report

A 77-year-old female with a past medical history significant for type 2 diabetes mellitus, hypertension, ischemic heart disease status after percutaneous intervention with stent placement, and cardiac ablation presented for evaluation of a positive HBsAg blood test. Several months prior to her presentation, the patient developed a basal cell carcinoma (BCC) of her right lower eyelid. During the patient's Mohs surgery, a common type of procedure performed in stages for carcinoma of the skin, to remove the BCC, a healthcare provider experienced a needle stick injury, which prompted infectious disease testing. The patient's postexposure laboratory testing revealed a positive hepatitis B surface antigen (HBsAg), a negative hepatitis B surface antibody (HBsAb), a negative hepatitis B core antibody (HBcAb), and an undetectable hepatitis B viral load (lower limit of detection 20 IU/mL), as well as a negative hepatitis A antibody and a negative hepatitis C antibody. The hepatitis panel was performed on the ADVIA Centaur XP analyzer (Siemens Healthineers, Erlangen, Germany). The HBsAg index value (IV) of this sample was 76.4 (cutoff IV = 1.0), considered to be reactive and above the threshold for confirmatory testing (IV = 50), so further testing was not performed. Hepatitis B e-antigen and antibody were sent out to a reference laboratory, and results were also negative. A rapid screening test for human immunodeficiency virus (HIV)1/2 antibodies and p24 antigen was positive (IV = 8.5, cutoff IV = 1) on the Siemens ADVIA Centaur XP, whereas the confirmatory assay (Geenius HIV 1-2 Supplemental Assay, Biorad, Hercules, CA, USA) for both HIV-1 and 2 was negative. The HIV-1 RNA qualitative test was sent out to a reference lab, and the result was negative. Liver function testing of this patient was within the normal range, including an alanine aminotransferase of <9 U/L, aspartate aminotransferase of 14 U/L, alkaline phosphatase of 80 U/L, and total bilirubin of 0.5 mg/dL.

Upon further review of the patient's history, no recognized, self-reported risk factors for viral hepatitis including unprotected sex, blood transfusions, tattoos, or intravenous drug abuse were reported. Furthermore, the patient denied personal or family history of liver disease or jaundice. Physical examination did not reveal stigmata of liver disease. Considering the patient's low risk for blood-borne infections, it was suspected that the HBsAg and HIV screening results might be false positives due to an unknown interference with the analytical assays.

The patient underwent repeat testing on the same instrument three weeks later. Both HBsAg and HIV screening tests remained positive, excluding accidental lab error or a transient contaminant as the cause of her positive results. Other hepatitis B antigens and antibodies remained negative. Both the HBsAg neutralization test and HIV 1-2 supplemental assay were negative.

Two- and four-fold dilutions of the new specimen were performed for the HBsAg. The HBsAg initial IV was 49.1 and then 19.7 with a two-fold dilution and 8.6 with a four-fold dilution. These nonlinear readings indicated the presence of an interfering substance in the specimen. Due to a suspicion of a heterophile antibody causing the interference, the samples were rerun in tubes containing a heterophilic antibody blocking reagent (Scantibodies Laboratory Inc., lot number LSFF0041B), resulting in negative HBsAg (IV < 0.10) and HIV (IV = 0.84) results. Our investigation led to the conclusion that heterophilic antibody interference may be the root cause of the false-positive HBsAg and HIV screening, especially since this antibody did not interfere with the HBsAg neutralization test and the HIV 1-2 confirmatory assay.

In order to better understand the interference of the heterophilic antibody with different testing platforms, the patient's serum specimens, with and without treatment with the heterophilic antibody blocking reagent, were sent to another laboratory which uses the Abbott Architect i2000 immunoassay analyzers (Abbott Park, Illinois, USA). Both HBsAg and HIV screening results were negative on Architect i2000, even in the absence of the heterophilic antibody blocking reagent.

The patient was retested 3 months after her Mohs surgery. The HBsAg and HIV screening tests remained positive. This study has been approved by the institutional review board (19-10020914) of Weill Cornell Medicine.

3. Discussion

Serologic testing of hepatitis B markers is vital to the diagnosis of infection and management. It is essential that these laboratory results are interpreted within the relevant clinical context. In this case, the lack of other positive serological markers and lack of risk factors or vaccination highly suggested a false-positive result early on in the workup of this patient.

This HBsAg assay is a two-site sandwich immunoassay using direct, chemiluminometric technology. The biotinylated anti-HBs mouse monoclonal antibody captures the HBsAg, forming HBsAg-antibody complexes, which are captured by the streptavidin-coated magnetic latex particles. A light signal is generated with the addition of a second acridinium-ester-labeled anti-HBs mouse monoclonal antibody. The amount of relative light units (RLUs) is directly proportional to the amount of HBsAg present in the patient sample. Heterophilic antibodies in the patient's serum are polyreactive antibodies that can bridge the two reagent antibodies and generate light signal without the presence of HBsAg. Heterophilic antibodies have been known to cause either false-positive (e.g., HIV [6]) or falsely elevated (e.g., prostate-specific antigen [7]) immunoassay results. The two-site sandwich immunoassays are particularly susceptible to this interference [8]. In light of this interference, most commercial assays over the last decade have begun incorporating blocking reagents against heterophilic antibodies in their assay reagent formulation to reduce heterophilic antibody interference, as demonstrated with the Abbott Architect immunoassay platform.

Isolated HBsAg seropositivity is a peculiar serological pattern. As such, screening results should be confirmed by an HBsAg neutralization test before the final results are reported. In this test, samples are incubated with anti-HBs antibody. If HBsAg is truly present, the anti-HBs antibody in the neutralization step blocks HBsAg, inhibiting its binding to the reagent antibodies and, consequently, reducing or eliminating its signal (positive neutralization test result) [1]. False-positive HIV 1/2/p24 screening results can also be identified by the HIV 1/2 supplemental assay which detects and differentiates individual antibodies to HIV-1 and HIV-2 in blood, as suggested by the current Centers for Disease Control and Prevention (CDC) recommendation for laboratory testing for the diagnosis of HIV infection [9].

False positivity for HBsAg has been reported in the presence of tumors, with a similar case of isolated HBsAg positivity identified in a patient with a parathyroid adenoma [2]. Our case is the first reported case in the literature of an isolated positive HBsAg in the setting of basal cell carcinoma. However, whether the presence of the heterophile antibody is due to the basal cell carcinoma, as was initially suspected, is unclear as the heterophilic antibody has persisted for several months based on repeatedly positive testing. The cause of this stable heterophilic antibody is unknown, but there are a variety of possible causes for heterophile antibodies, such as infection, transfusion, or systemic disease. Epstein–Barr Virus (EBV) infection, as an example, often causes heterophilic antibodies that persist at low levels for up to 1 year [10]. Our main limitation here is our inability to specifically identify the reason for this persistent heterophilic antibody in this isolated scenario. It may be worthwhile to evaluate for the disappearance of the antibody in this patient on repeating laboratory testing for a prolonged length of time if possible. Determining the accuracy of HBV testing is essential, particularly for certain patient groups such as dialysis patients or those who are screened for viral infection prior to administration of immune suppressive therapy, chemotherapy, or organ transplantation. For example, patients with rheumatoid arthritis are screened for HBV before beginning rituximab therapy, and HBV serology cross reactivity with rheumatoid factors has been reported. Both the laboratory and clinicians need to be aware of the possibility of false-positive screening as these results can have serious implications, such as causing potentially effective treatment strategies to be avoided, social stigma, or initiating additional testing for contacts and family members [11].

Overall, in these cases with isolated HBsAg positivity and low clinical suspicion for hepatitis infection, one should consider following a systematic trouble-shooting algorithm, including repeat testing, especially using a different commercial assay. This case demonstrates the importance of collaboration and open discussion between the clinician and the laboratory to recognize potential discrepancies of laboratory testing in the context of clinical correlation, all leading to better patient care.

Authors' Contributions

Each author contributed significantly to the submitted manuscript in accordance with the definitions set forth by the International Committee of Medical Journal Editors. HSL, GL, and VC contributed to conception, manuscript drafting, data analysis, figure design, critical revision, and submission.

Acknowledgments

The authors thank Marybeth Romana for running the HBsAg and HIV testing and sending specimens to another laboratory.

References

[1] R. A. d. A. Pondé, "The underlying mechanisms for the "isolated positivity for the hepatitis B surface antigen (HBsAg)" serological profile," *Medical Microbiology and Immunology*, vol. 200, no. 1, pp. 13–22, 2010.

[2] D. M. Tang, T. Heller, and C. Koh, "The many faces of positive hepatitis B surface antigen," *Hepatology*, vol. 64, no. 4, pp. 1379–1381, 2016.

[3] R. D. Nerenz, C. C. Felty, and M. A. Cervinski, "The curious case of an isolated positive hepatitis B surface antigen result," *Clinical Chemistry*, vol. 65, no. 3, pp. 499-500, 2019.

[4] J.-S. Wu, S.-L. Nii, W.-H. Chou et al., "Implications of isolated HBsAg positivity: hepatitis B virus variant and immune incompetence," *Journal of Gastroenterology and Hepatology*, vol. 8, no. S1, pp. S123–S127, 1993.

[5] P. Kiely, V. C. Hoad, and E. M. Wood, "False positive viral marker results in blood donors and their unintended consequences," *Vox Sanguinis*, vol. 113, no. 6, pp. 530–539, 2018.

[6] D. V. Spencer, F. S. Nolte, and Y. Zhu, "Heterophilic antibody interference causing false-positive rapid human immunodeficiency virus antibody testing," *Clinica Chimica Acta; International Journal of Clinical Chemistry*, vol. 399, no. 1-2, pp. 121-122, 2009.

[7] C. M. Preissner, L. A. Dodge, D. J. O'Kane, R. J. Singh, and S. K. Grebe, "Prevalence of heterophilic antibody interference in eight automated tumor marker immunoassays," *Clinical Chemistry*, vol. 51, no. 1, pp. 208–210, 2005.

[8] J. Tate and G. Ward, "Interference in immunoassay," *Clinical Biochemistry Review*, vol. 25, no. 2, pp. 105–120, 2004.

[9] Centers for Disease Control and Prevention, "Quick reference guide: recommended laboratory HIV testing algorithm for serum or plasma specimens," 2018, https://stacks.cdc.gov/view/cdc/50872.%202021.

[10] N. Stuempfig, *Monospot Test*, StatPearls, Treasure Island, FL, USA, 2019, https://www.ncbi.nlm.nih.gov/books/NBK539739/.

[11] L. B. Rebecca, P. Brendan, M. Stuart, and T. Ben, "False-positive Hepatitis B serology due to suspected cross-reactivity in a patient with rheumatoid arthritis," *Rheumatology*, vol. 54, no. S1, p. i50, 2015.

22

Escalation to Barbiturate-Induced Coma for Refractory Seizures after Liver Transplantation

Brittany Miles,[1] Muhammad Mujtaba,[2] Shehzad Merwat,[2] Rupak Kulkarni,[1] Jeffrey Fair,[1] and Michael Kueht[1]

[1]*Department of Surgery, Division of Transplant Surgery, UTMB Galveston=University of Texas Medical Branch, Galveston, TX, USA*
[2]*Department of Internal Medicine, Division of Transplant Medicine, UTMB Galveston=University of Texas Medical Branch, Galveston, TX, USA*

Correspondence should be addressed to Brittany Miles; brlmiles@utmb.edu

Academic Editor: Haruki Komatsu

Seizures after liver transplantation were previously thought to be a reliable harbinger of catastrophe, but more recent studies have found seizure activity to be relatively common, and most cases do not result in a poor outcome. Generalized seizures are the most common, and they typically occur de novo within the first two weeks after transplantation. The underlying cause for seizure activity in these patients may be complex, with potential etiologies including metabolic, infectious, cerebrovascular, and medication-induced causes. Identification of the underlying cause and the use of antiepileptic drugs (AEDs) is crucial for minimizing risk to the patient's neurologic and overall health. In this report, we present the case of a patient with refractory seizures unresponsive to conventional treatment, requiring prolonged barbiturate burst suppression with ventilator support. Seizure activity eventually ceased, and the patient made a full recovery.

1. Introduction

Seizures after liver transplantation were previously thought to be a reliable harbinger of catastrophe, but more recent studies have found seizure activity to be relatively common (up to 42% in some case series), and most cases do not result in a poor outcome [1, 2]. Generalized seizures are the most common, and they usually occur de novo within the first two weeks after transplantation [3]. The underlying causes for seizure activity in these patients may be complex, with potential etiologies including metabolic, infectious, cerebrovascular, and medication-induced origins [4]. Calcineurin inhibitors, which are commonly used in transplant patients for immunosuppression, are associated with Posterior Reversible Encephalopathy Syndrome (PRES), which is associated with neurologic symptoms in addition to characteristic MRI findings [5]. Identification of the underlying cause and the use of antiepileptic drugs (AEDs) is crucial for minimizing risk to the patient's neurologic and overall health. In this report, we present the case of a patient with refractory seizures unresponsive to conventional treatment, requiring prolonged barbiturate burst suppression with ventilator support. Seizure activity eventually ceased, and the patient made a full recovery.

2. Case Presentation

A 36-year-old male with a four-year history of alcohol abuse and an MELD score of 29 (See Appendix) presented for liver transplantation. At the time of evaluation, he had abstained from alcohol for more than 90 days, but his jaundice and coagulopathy persisted. He had a remote history of seizures but had been without any seizure events for more than 20 years and had not been taking antiepileptic medication during that time. Ten years prior, he underwent treatment for hydrocodone and buprenorphine use. He had been recently hospitalized for hepatic encephalopathy, and imaging showed signs of portal hypertension and chronic liver

Table 1: Outpatient medications at the time of liver transplant.

Medication	Dose (mg)	Route	Frequency
Alprazolam	0.5	PO	TID
Dextroamphetamine-amphetamine	20	PO	Daily
Fluconazole	200	PO	Daily

disease, including ascites, splenomegaly, and perigastric varices. Outpatient medications were as indicated in Table 1.

The donor of the blood-type-compatible allograft was a teenager who succumbed to head trauma. The only biochemical abnormality was a mild unconjugated hyperbilirubinemia (T. bili: 2.1, D. bili 0.3, and I. bili 1.8 mg/dL), and serologies were positive for anti-CMV IgG and anti-EBV IgG. The recipient underwent orthotopic liver transplantation utilizing a piggy-back cavoplasty technique with an operative time of 5 hours and 31 mins. Blood product requirements included two units of packed red blood cells, four of fresh frozen plasma, and two units of platelets. Vasopressors were used with a maximum norepinephrine dosage of 0.05 mcg/kg/min.

He was extubated within 12 hours of the operation and was taking clear liquids by postoperative day (POD) 2. Pain control initially required a significant amount of intravenous narcotic that was successfully weaned to oral medications by day five. The tacrolimus dosage was decreased on POD 5 due to tremor, and on POD 6, he was noted to have had four episodes of unresponsiveness, head deviation, and generalized shaking, each lasting approximately one minute. There was no incontinence or notable postictal state associated with these episodes, but they were determined to be focal seizures according to current guidelines [6, 7]. He was transferred to the ICU for monitoring and remained asymptomatic for the next 48 hours.

On POD 8, he again had focal seizures presenting as unresponsiveness with frothy oral secretions. Fosphenytoin was loaded with 20 mg/kg, and continuous electroencephalography (EEG) monitoring was begun. Over the next 24 hours, EEG revealed 8 focal seizures in the right frontotemporal and frontocentral regions that were not accompanied by convulsions. Levetiracetam was begun at 1000 mg BID. Epileptiform activity persisted on EEG, indicating progression to status epilepticus; levetiracetam was increased to 1500 mg BID, and lacosamide 200 mg q12 was added. On POD 13, seizure activity with left-sided localization remained present on EEG and gabapentin 600 mg TID and clobazam 5 mg BID were added for a total of four antiepileptic medications. Imaging of the head including Magnetic Resonance Imaging (MRI) and Computed Tomography (CT) was unrevealing aside from nonspecific scattered foci of T2/FLAIR signal abnormality in the bilateral cerebral white matter. Lumbar puncture revealed clear cerebrospinal fluid with normal glucose and protein with a single leukocyte per microliter. The use of propofol and phenobarbital for burst suppression (requiring endotracheal intubation) was initiated on POD 14, as shown in Figure 1.

The differential diagnosis list included posterior reversible encephalopathy syndrome (PRES), autoimmune/infectious causes, and benzodiazepine withdrawal.

3. Differential Diagnosis

3.1. Posterior Reversible Encephalopathy Syndrome (PRES). Posterior Reversible Encephalopathy Syndrome (PRES) is a rare but very serious condition that can occur from the use of immunosuppressive agents used to prevent transplant rejection in both hematopoietic and solid organ transplant patients [5]. It typically presents as seizures, altered sensorium, visual abnormalities, or other neurologic changes affecting the occipital area of the brain, and imaging studies typically show changes consistent with vasogenic edema [8]. Although most often associated with calcineurin inhibitors, cases of PRES have also been reported with mycophenolate during the treatment of patients with systemic lupus erythematosis [9]. Our patient underwent multiple computed tomography (CT) head and magnetic resonance imaging (MRI) scans during his hospital course, and none showed any findings to support PRES as the underlying cause for his seizures.

3.2. Autoimmune/Infectious. Autoimmune encephalitis is another possible cause for refractory seizures, although it is most frequently described in bone marrow transplant patients and often presents with autoantibodies that can be found in patients' cerebrospinal fluid or sera [10, 11]. Such patients also tend to have characteristic findings on MRI, which may vary depending on the autoantibody involved [12]. Our patient did not exhibit signs of encephalitis on imaging studies. Additionally, his cerebrospinal fluid (CSF) analysis was analyzed twice and found to be negative for organisms and PMNs, in addition to having unremarkable autoimmune and serologic studies. The patient was also on multiple medications for immunosuppression due to the recent liver transplantation, which also contributed to this being an unlikely source of seizure activity.

3.3. Benzodiazepine Withdrawal. Withdrawal from benzodiazepines is another possibility for the development of seizure activity in this patient, although the greatest likelihood of seizure development occurs in patients taking high doses or short-acting benzodiazepines [13, 14]. This patient was taking alprazolam and chlordiazepoxide prior to liver transplantation, and it is possible that the discontinuation of those medications could have contributed to the development of seizure activity. However, benzodiazepine withdrawal is typically easily controlled by reintroduction of benzodiazepine [15]. In our patient's case, persistent seizure activity was seen despite the reintroduction of benzodiazepine therapy and required the dramatic intervention of burst suppression for seizure control.

On POD 13, the patient was receiving the 4-drug combination of gabapentin, lacosamide, clobazam, and levetiracetam, and frequent epileptiform activity was still present. Generalized convulsive status epilepticus (GSCE) can be treated with anesthetic-dose barbiturates, so the patient was started on phenobarbital and placed on a

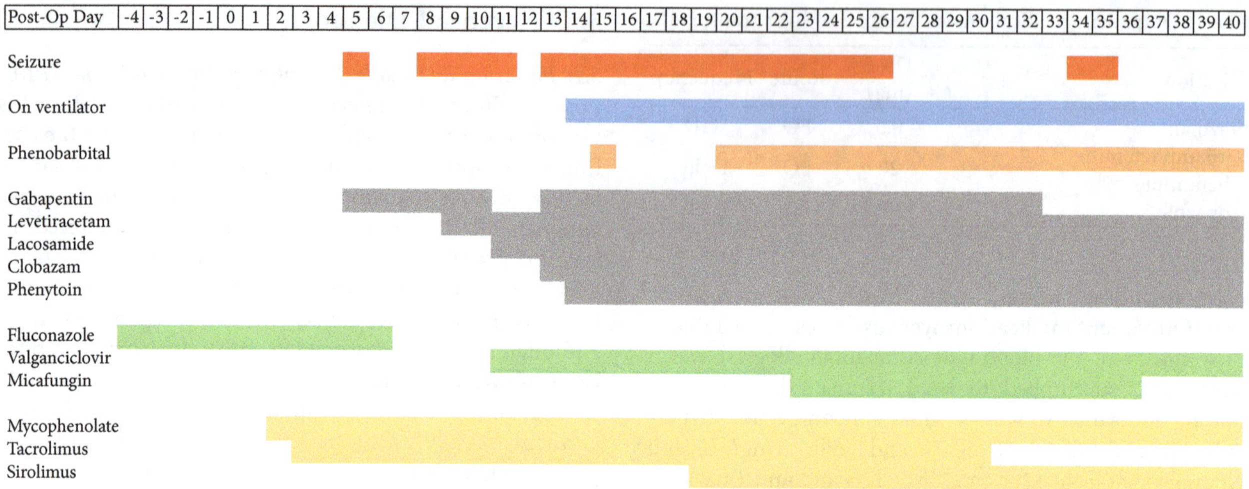

Figure 1: Timeline of seizures, medications, and ventilator use.

ventilator [16, 17]. He underwent tracheostomy after seven days of mechanical ventilation. To balance calcineurin inhibitor exposure with the needs of early posttransplant immunosuppression, sirolimus was added and tacrolimus was weaned off (see Figure 1). The patient's seizures ultimately ceased on POD 27, after 13 days of intensive barbiturate suppression. Gabapentin was discontinued on POD 32, and the final episodes of seizure activity occurred on POD 34 and 35. On postop day 40, the patient was weaned off the ventilator and no further seizure activity was noted. Although neurologic complications from prolonged barbiturate coma for refractory status epilepticus are common (33–78% of patients treated with this method), this patient primarily suffered sequelae of deconditioning including bilateral foot drop and left wrist weakness requiring splinting [18]. These improved with therapy, and he was walking prior to discharge. His cognitive function experienced a full recovery. He was discharged from the hospital on POD 72 with a plan to gradually wean the antiepileptics over the course of one year.

4. Discussion

Seizure activity after liver transplantation is a complex entity that can be a harbinger of catastrophe or can be easily treated. In this case, because the patient had preservation of liver function during these events, it was believed that the underlying cause of focal seizures progressing to bilateral convulsive status epilepticus was likely reversible. A thorough search for anatomic and infectious etiologies failed to reveal a cause, and so, a prolonged course of neurologic suppression was undertaken with the hope that if the other organ systems remained intact, the seizure threshold equilibrium would be reset. Although we may never know the underlying cause that led to refractory seizures in this patient, a possible theory is that the patient's right frontotemporal nidus of seizure activity was a previously dormant lesion that was unmasked by multifactorial causes including illness and seizure-threshold-lowering medications. Nevertheless, it is clear from this case that the use of burst suppression via barbiturate-induced coma was ultimately effective and resulted in the control of seizure activity after almost 2 weeks of intensive treatment.

Abbreviations

AED: Antiepileptic drug
BID: Twice a day dosing
CMV: Cytomegalovirus
CSF: Cerebrospinal fluid
CT: Computed tomography
D. bili: Direct bilirubin
EBV: Epstein–Barr virus
EEG: Electroencephalography
FLAIR: Fluid-attenuated inversion recovery
GCSE: Generalized convulsive status epilepticus
I. bili: Indirect bilirubin
ICU: Intensive care unit
Kg: Kilogram
Mcg: Microgram
MELD: Model for end-stage liver disease
Min: Minute
MRI: Magnetic resonance imaging
POD: Postoperative day
PRES: Posterior reversible encephalopathy syndrome
T. bili: Total bilirubin.

Appendix

MELD score of 29: Na: 143 mmol/L, INR: 3.2, Cr: 0.56 mg/dL, and T. Bili: 11.8 mg/dL.

Acknowledgments

The authors thank the UTMB epilepsy program headed by Todd Masel, MD, for assisting this case.

References

[1] E. Derle, S. Kibaroğlu, S. Kibaroğlu et al., "Seizure as a neurologic complication after liver transplant," *Experimental and Clinical Transplantation*, vol. 13, no. 1, pp. 323–326, 2015.

[2] E. F. M. Wijdicks, D. J. Plevak, R. H. Wiesner, and J. L. Steers, "Causes and outcome of seizures in liver transplant recipients," *Neurology*, vol. 47, no. 6, pp. 1523–1525, 1996.

[3] Z. K. Wszolek and R. E. Steg, "Seizures after liver transplantation," *Liver Transplantation & Surgery*, vol. 1, no. 5, pp. 334–339, 1995.

[4] P. W. Shepard and E. K. St Louis, "Seizure treatment in transplant patients," *Current Treatment Options in Neurology*, vol. 14, no. 4, pp. 332–347, 2012.

[5] T. Song, Z. Rao, Q. Tan et al., "Calcineurin inhibitors associated posterior reversible encephalopathy syndrome in solid organ transplantation," *Medicine*, vol. 95, no. 14, p. e3173, 2016.

[6] R. S. Fisher, J. H. Cross, C. D'Souza et al., "Instruction manual for the ILAE 2017 operational classification of seizure types," *Epilepsia*, vol. 58, no. 4, pp. 531–542, 2017.

[7] E. Trinka, H. Cock, D. Hesdorffer et al., "A definition and classification of status epilepticus - report of the ILAE task force on classification of status epilepticus," *Epilepsia*, vol. 56, no. 10, pp. 1515–1523, 2015.

[8] J. M. M. Gijtenbeek, M. J. Van Den Bent, and C. J. Vecht, "Cyclosporine neurotoxicity: a review," *Journal of Neurology*, vol. 246, no. 5, pp. 339–346, 1999.

[9] B. Khajuria, M. Khajuria, and Y. Agrawal, "Mycophenolate-induced posterior reversible encephalopathy syndrome," *American Journal of Therapeutics*, vol. 23, no. 4, pp. e1072–e1073, 2016.

[10] G. S. Rathore, K. S. Leung, and E. Muscal, "Autoimmune encephalitis following bone marrow transplantation," *Pediatric Neurology*, vol. 53, no. 3, pp. 253–256, 2015.

[11] A. Vogrig, B. Joubert, N. André-Obadia, G. L. Gigli, S. Rheims, and J. Honnorat, "Seizure specificities in patients with antibody-mediated autoimmune encephalitis," *Epilepsia*, vol. 60, no. 8, pp. 1508–1525, 2019.

[12] J. Guerin, R. E. Watson, C. M. Carr, G. B. Liebo, and A. L. Kotsenas, "Autoimmune epilepsy: findings on MRI and FDG-PET," *British Journal of Radiology*, vol. 92, no. 1093, p. 20170869, 2019.

[13] H. Petursson, "The benzodiazepine withdrawal syndrome," *Addiction*, vol. 89, no. 11, pp. 1455–1459, 1994.

[14] C. M. Arroyo-Novoa, M. I. Figueroa-Ramos, and K. A. Puntillo, "Opioid and benzodiazepine iatrogenic withdrawal syndrome in patients in the intensive Care unit," *AACN Advanced Critical Care*, vol. 30, no. 4, pp. 353–364, 2019.

[15] G. Chouinard, "Issues in the clinical use of benzodiazepines: potency, withdrawal, and rebound," *Journal of Clinical Psychiatry*, vol. 65, no. 5, pp. 7–12, 2004.

[16] H. Meierkord, P. Boon, B. Engelsen et al., "EFNS guideline on the management of status epilepticus in adults," *European Journal of Neurology*, vol. 17, no. 3, pp. 348–355, 2010.

[17] S. E. Nelson and P. N. Varelas, "Status epilepticus, refractory status epilepticus, and super-refractory status epilepticus," *Continuum: Lifelong Learning in Neurology*, vol. 24, no. 6, pp. 1683–1707, 2018.

[18] C. R. Newey, D. Wisco, P. Nattanmai, and A. Sarwal, "Observed medical and surgical complications of prolonged barbiturate coma for refractory status epilepticus," *Therapeutic Advances in Drug Safety*, vol. 7, no. 5, pp. 195–203, 2016.

23

Ruptured Subcapsular Liver Hematoma: A Rare Complication of HELLP Syndrome

Pratishtha Singh, Kayle Warren, and Victor Collier

Department of Internal Medicine, Grand Strand Medical Center, Myrtle Beach, SC, USA

Correspondence should be addressed to Pratishtha Singh; pratishtha.singh@hcahealthcare.com

Academic Editor: Mauro Vigano

Subcapsular liver hematoma (SLH) is a rare complication of HELLP (hemolysis, elevated liver enzymes, low platelets) syndrome. We report a previously healthy 16-year-old female presenting with pre-eclampsia requiring emergent C-section, who developed immediate postoperative bleeding and abdominal distention. Abdominal computed tomography angiography (CTA) revealed a large encapsulated liver hematoma with active extravasation. The patient was successfully treated with a multidisciplinary approach with medical and surgical management.

1. Introduction

HELLP syndrome is a complication associated with pre-eclampsia. The overall incidence of HELLP is 0.2–0.6% of all pregnancies and occurs in 4–12% of cases with severe pre-eclampsia [1]. SLH results from spontaneous bleeding between Glisson's capsule and the liver parenchyma and was first reported as a complication of pregnancy in 1844. It was attributed to the patient wrapping a handkerchief around her body to obtain relief from "gastrodynia" leading to a traumatic rupture [2]. SLH has been reported in less than 2% of pregnancies complicated by HELLP [3]. Incidence of SLH with rupture in pregnancies varies from 1/40,000 to 1/250,000 [4] and is associated with an increased maternal mortality rate of 18–86% [5]. Pathogenesis of SLH is not fully understood; however, it is likely related to microangiopathy developed during pregnancy, combined with endothelial dysfunction resulting in an inappropriate activation of the coagulation cascade [6]. Vascular injury can cause hemolysis and blood flow obstruction due to fibrin deposits in the hepatic sinusoids, which increase liver enzymes and aid in formation of SLH [6]. The right hepatic lobe is the most commonly affected lobe and is involved in 75% of cases [7]. SLH complicating HELLP syndrome should be suspected in patients with signs and symptoms, including anorexia, nausea, vomiting, epigastric or right upper quadrant pain, and dyspnea. Rupture should be suspected in the setting of hemodynamic instability. This case report highlights a patient with Grade IV SLH that was managed in an intensive care unit (ICU) with radiological and surgical interventions.

2. Case Report

A 16-year-old female, gravida 1, para 0, at 36-week gestation presented to the hospital with pre-eclampsia requiring emergent C-section with delivery of twins. Within hours of delivery, the patient was noted to be hypotensive with systolic blood pressure in 70's with slow vaginal bleeding and progressive abdominal distension. One hour after c-section, hemoglobin was 4.5 gm/dL and platelets 58,000/mm^3. Because of severe anemia and evidence of hypovolemic shock, she was taken to the operating room for an exploratory laparotomy, which revealed hemoperitoneum and a large encapsulated liver hematoma. No other evidence of bleeding elsewhere was noted. She was transfused 4 units (U) of packed red blood cells (pRBC), 2 U fresh frozen plasma (FFP), and 1 U platelets (plt) in the perioperative period. After initial stabilization, she was transferred to our level I trauma center for interventional radiology and further surgical evaluation for possible arterial embolization and hepatic resection if indicated. On arrival, vital signs were remarkable for a heart rate of 104 beats per minute and blood pressure of 156/88 mmHg. The patient was mechanically ventilated and sedated from her initial laparotomy prior to transfer. The lungs were clear to auscultation bilaterally. Her abdomen was open with a wound vacuum in place accompanied by bloody drainage. Laboratory findings revealed aspartate aminotransaminase (AST), 7429 U/L; serum alanine aminotransaminase (ALT), 3345 U/L; serum lactate dehydrogenase (LDH), >12,000 U/L; creatinine, 1.8 mg/dl; white blood cell, 18,700/mm^3; hemoglobin (Hb), 10.6 mg/dL; platelet count, 79,000/mm^3; fibrinogen, 173 mg/dL; PT, 16.6 seconds; D-dimer, >3000; and fibrin split product of 10. CTA of the abdomen and pelvis showed a large right hepatic subcapsular hematoma measuring 14 cm × 3.6 cm with active arterial extravasation (Figure 1). Mass effect from the right-sided subcapsular hematoma caused compression of the right hepatic lobe, with associated decreased perfusion. Emergent Gelfoam and coil embolization of the right hepatic artery was performed by interventional radiology. This was subsequently followed by exploratory laparotomy with unroofing of the hepatic capsular hematoma. The patient received another 5 U pRBCs, 2 U FFP, 1 U plt, and prothrombin complex concentrate intraoperatively and was transferred to the intensive care unit (ICU) in critical condition. Given the derangements of liver function, accompanied by thrombocytopenia and an elevated LDH, she was ultimately diagnosed with HELLP syndrome and DIC, complicated by a Grade IV SLH. The patient was extubated on postoperative day 1, and hemoglobin normalized and LFTs started to down trend on day 2. CTA abdomen and pelvis repeated on day 4 showed improvement, and no active extravasation was noted (Figure 2). She was discharged to home on hospital day 7 with long-term follow-up with gastroenterology to monitor liver injury and for repeat imaging of the liver to monitor for resolution.

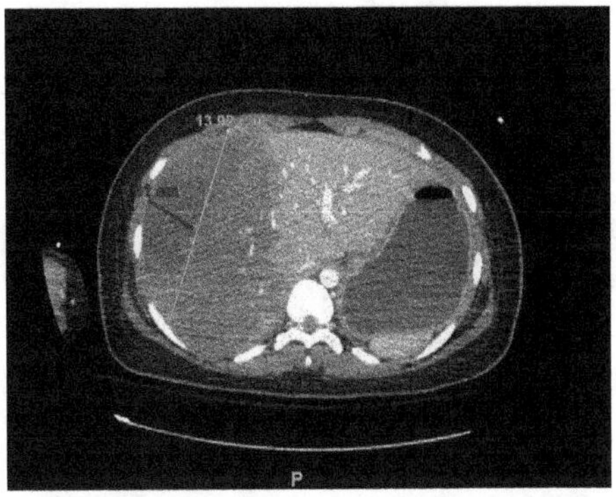

FIGURE 1: CTA abdomen on admission showing a large right hepatic subcapsular hematoma measuring 14 cm × 3.6 cm in size with active arterial extravasation.

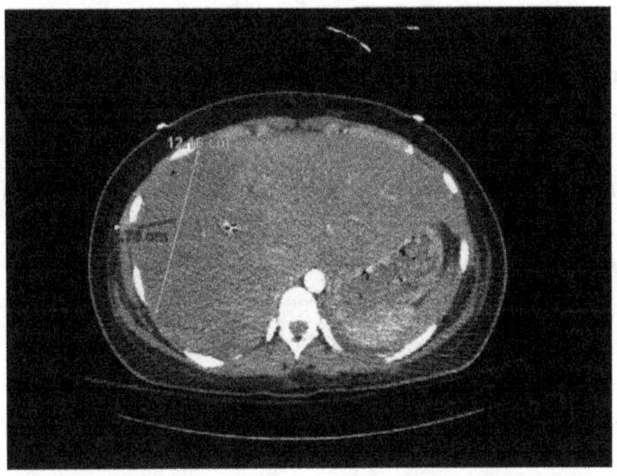

FIGURE 2: CTA abdomen on postoperative day 4 showing improvement in size and no active arterial extravasation.

3. Discussion

SLH is a rare and devastating complication of HELLP in pregnancy that requires prompt recognition and a multidisciplinary approach to ensure optimal outcomes. Some risk factors for HELLP include chronic hypertension, multiparity, advanced maternal age, and a previous history of pre-eclampsia or HELLP [8]. In addition, risk factors for pre-eclampsia include a family history, prior history of pre-eclampsia, multiple gestations, and first pregnancy [9]. Symptoms associated with SLH are generally nonspecific and include anorexia, nausea, vomiting, epigastric or right upper quadrant pain, and dyspnea [7]. Rupture may result from trauma precipitated by vomiting, abdominal palpation, transport of the patient, uterine contractions, and manual removal of the placenta [10]. It manifests as hemodynamic compromise and hypovolemic shock. The presence of the abovementioned conditions in a patient with HELLP should raise suspicion for SLH and prompt immediate imaging. Ultrasound is often the first-line modality due to access and availability; however, CT and MRI are both highly sensitive and may facilitate diagnosis as well. Imaging evidence of SLH warrants rapid transfer to a tertiary care center. Medical management is first line for hemodynamically stable patients and encompasses close monitoring of hemodynamic status and coagulation parameters, serial imaging, avoidance of liver manipulation, and replacement of blood products [11]. Alternatively, surgical management including ligation of the portal vein or hepatic artery, partial liver resection, perihepatic packing, and drainage of surgical site [7, 12, 13] should be pursued if rupture occurs and the patient is hemodynamically unstable with signs and symptoms of shock. This in conjunction with radiologic intervention including embolization, and critical care support may also be required in the event of hemodynamic compromise.

4. Conclusion

SLH with HELLP syndrome is a rare complication of pre-eclampsia and should be suspected in patients with signs and symptoms including right upper quadrant pain, nausea, vomiting, and anorexia. Rupture should be suspected in the setting of hemodynamic instability. Providers should be aware of the risk factors, signs and symptoms, diagnosis, and treatment options for subcapsular liver hematoma as this condition carries a high mortality if not recognized early and treated appropriately with combined medical, obstetrical, radiology, and surgical team.

Consent

Informed consent was obtained for this case report.

Disclosure

Notice of prior presentation: vignette accepted for presentation at SGIM Annual Meeting in Birmingham, AL, on May 9, 2020; however, the meeting was turned web based due to COVID-19 and we were unable to present.

Authors' Contributions

All authors contributed equally to this manuscript. V. Collier is the article guarantor.

References

[1] J. L. Wolf, "Liver disease in pregnancy," *Medical Clinics of North America*, vol. 80, no. 5, pp. 1167–1187, 1996.

[2] J. Abercrombie, "Case of hemorrhage of the liver," *London Medical Gazette*, vol. 34, pp. 792–794, 1844.

[3] C. Wicke, P. L. Pereira, E. Neeser, I. Flesch, E. A. Rodegerdts, and H. D. Becker, "Subcapsular liver hematoma in HELLP syndrome: evaluation of diagnostic and therapeutic options-A unicenter study," *American Journal of Obstetrics and Gynecology*, vol. 190, no. 1, pp. 106–112, 2004.

[4] J. O. Nunes, M. A. Turner, and A. S. Fulcher, "Abdominal imaging features of HELLP syndrome: a 10-year retrospective review," *American Journal of Roentgenology*, vol. 185, no. 5, pp. 1205–1210, 2005.

[5] K. Haram, E. Svendsen, and U. Abildgaard, "The HELLP syndrome: clinical issues and management. A review," *BMC Pregnancy and Childbirth*, vol. 9, 2009.

[6] J. Coll, "Hepatic subcapsular hematoma occurs in of 2% of HELLP syndrome complicated pregnancies," *College of Physicians and Surgeons Pakistan*, vol. 15, no. 11, pp. 733–735, 2005.

[7] A. Distisheim and B. M. Sibai, "Diagnosis and management of HELLP syndrome complicated by liver hematoma," *Clinical Obstetrics and Gynecology*, vol. 60, no. 1, pp. 190–197, 2017.

[8] O. Malmström and N.-H. Morken, "HELLP syndrome, risk factors in first and second pregnancy: a population-based cohort study," *Acta Obstetricia et Gynecologica Scandinavica*, vol. 97, no. 6, pp. 709–716, 2018.

[9] F. English, L. Kenny, and F. McCarthy, "Risk factors and effective management of preeclampsia," *Integrated Blood Pressure Control*, vol. 8, pp. 7–12, 2015.

[10] S. Dessole, G. Capobianco, P. Virdis, G. Rubattu, E. Cosmi, and A. Porcu, "Hepatic rupture after cesarean section in a patient with HELLP syndrome: a case report and review of the literature," *Archives of Gynecology and Obstetrics*, vol. 276, no. 2, pp. 189–192, 2007.

[11] K. L. Carlson and C. L. Bader, "Ruptured subcapsular liver hematoma in pregnancy: a case report of nonsurgical management," *American Journal of Obstetrics and Gynecology*, vol. 190, no. 2, pp. 558–560, 2004.

[12] S. Wilson, A. White, A. Young, M. Davies, and S. Pollard, "The management of the surgical complications of HELLP syndrome," *The Annals of The Royal College of Surgeons of England*, vol. 96, no. 7, pp. 512–516, 2014.

[13] E. E. Moore, T. H. Cogbill, G. J. Jurkovich, S. R. Shackford, M. A. Malangoni, and H. R. Champion, "Organ injury scaline: spleen and liver," *The Journal of Trauma: Injury, Infection, and Critical Care*, vol. 38, no. 3, pp. 323-324, 1995.

24

Disulfiram-Induced Acute Liver Injury

Lucas Ramer,[1] Matthieu Tihy,[2] Nicolas Goossens,[1] Jean-Louis Frossard,[1] Laura Rubbia-Brandt,[2] and Laurent Spahr[1]

[1]*Gastroenterology and Hepatology, University Hospitals of Geneva and Faculty of Medicine, Geneva, Switzerland*
[2]*Clinical Pathology, University Hospitals of Geneva and Faculty of Medicine, Geneva, Switzerland*

Correspondence should be addressed to Laurent Spahr; laurent.spahr@hcuge.ch

Academic Editor: Melanie Deutsch

Disulfiram is a drug used to treat alcohol dependence since many years. It interferes with the metabolism of alcohol, may be associated with neurological and dermatological symptoms, and can be hepatotoxic. Due to the frequent coexistent liver test alterations due to alcohol, the true incidence of disulfiram-associated liver injury is unclear and severity of injury may vary from mildly elevated liver enzymes to fulminant hepatitis leading to death. There are several reported cases of disulfiram hepatitis in the literature. Liver histology, when available, demonstrates some degree of portal inflammation with eosinophils and hepatocyte necrosis. We present here a well-documented case of acute hepatitis due to disulfiram with typical histological lesions, favorable outcome following drug withdrawal, and a brief steroid course. The risk of hepatotoxicity should be kept in mind when prescribing disulfiram.

1. Introduction

Disulfiram is a drug prescribed in many countries as a supportive treatment for alcohol dependence, by generating unpleasant symptoms when drinking alcohol [1]. Accordingly, the mechanism of action of the drug is based on the inhibition of acetaldehyde dehydrogenase, a key enzyme in alcohol metabolism. Consequently, acetaldehyde accumulates in blood and induces symptoms including headache, flushing, nausea, and vomiting. Side effects of disulfiram include fatigue, abdominal discomfort, and sometimes serious dermatological, neurological or psychiatric manifestations [2]. Although considered a relatively safe drug from an hepatological point of view, cases of disulfiram-associated liver injury have been reported several years ago [3–7], sometimes presenting as a fulminant hepatic failure [8, 9]. Available data favor an idiosyncratic reaction occurring after several weeks of exposition, with a positive rechallenge and a causal relationship established in most cases [10]. However, description of liver injury in a biopsy is inconstant, and histological alterations are sometimes difficult to characterize due to a coexistent advanced alcoholic liver disease [3]. Thus, we present here in detail the case of an acute disulfiram-induced hepatitis including a detailed description of histological findings on a liver biopsy and a full recovery following a brief steroid treatment.

2. Case Presentation

A 47-year-old woman was referred to our department on February 9, 2020, for abnormal liver function tests. She has no relevant medical history except for an alcohol use disorder detected 3 years ago for which she was referred to an addiction specialist in mid-2019. At this time, she met the criteria for alcohol dependence and was initially managed by a combination of psychosocial support and benzodiazepines. As this strategy failed to control the ongoing alcohol misuse, pharmacotherapy using an anticraving agent was decided. At that time, liver transaminases were normal. Thus, disulfiram was started on December 18, 2019, at 200 mg daily, corresponding to half the recommended dose [2]. During the first ten days, the drug was well tolerated at this reduced dose and the patient did not declare any alcohol consumption during this period. On December 29, the posology was further reduced to 200 mg every other day due to apparition of nausea, fatigue, and abdominal discomfort. These

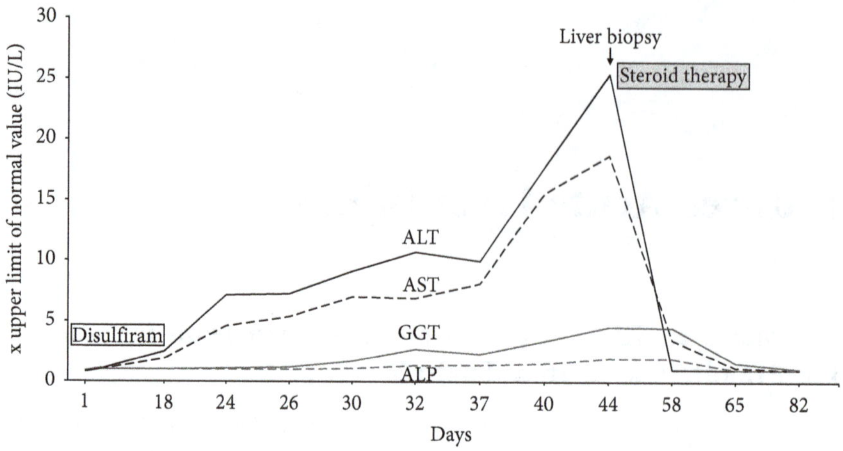

Figure 1: Graphical illustration of the course of disulfiram-induced acute hepatitis. Biological tests (AST: aspartate aminotransferase; ALT: alanine aminotransferase; GGT: gamma-glutamyl transferase; ALP: alkaline phosphatase) given as upper limit of normal value.

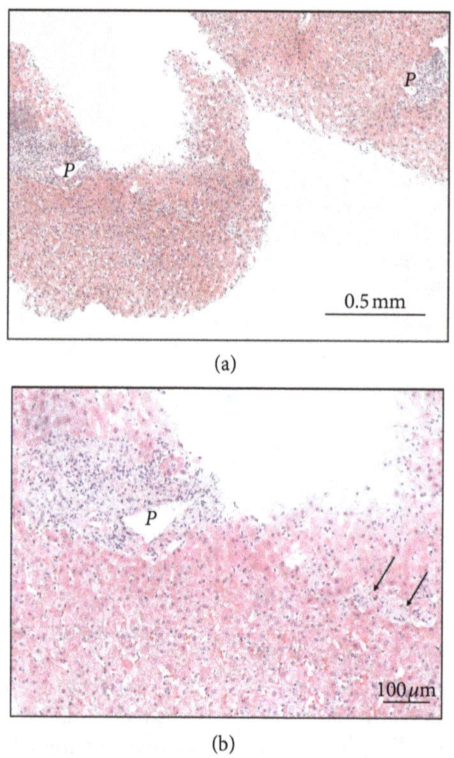

Figure 2: Histological view of the liver biopsy specimen (hematoxylin-eosin stain) showing normal architecture and no fibrosis (original magnification ×100, panel A). At a closer view (panel B, original magnification ×200), an inflammatory infiltrate is present in the portal tract P, predominantly lymphocytic, associated with scattered eosinophils. In the liver lobule, few necrotic hepatocytes and occasional micrograpulomas (arrows) are visible. Periodic acid Schiff (PAS) and Ziehl staining are negative for infections.

symptoms were considered in relation with disulfiram therapy, and serum alcohol levels were not monitored. Laboratory tests 18 days after treatment initiation revealed an elevation of AST (91 IU/L (*N*: <50)) and ALT (127 IU/L (*N*: <50), while gamma-glutamyl transferase (GGT), alkaline phosphatase (ALP) and serum bilirubin were normal. Disulfiram was then stopped. At physical examination, the patient had no signs of preexisting liver disease. At abdominal echography, the liver was slightly hyperechoic without signs of chronic liver disease. Additional blood tests showed normal INR, hemoglobin, platelets, and white blood cells with normal eosinophil count. Total IgG levels were in the normal range, while antismooth muscle and anti-actin antibodies were negative. The patient was, also, negative for hepatitis A, B, C, and E. Ceruloplasmin levels were in the normal range. She refused coadministration with other medications or illicit drugs and did not present skin rash, headache, or fever. Since disulfiram was stopped, transaminases continued to increase, as well as GGT and ALP to a lesser extent. At day 44, after initiation of disulfiram, values of ALT and AST reached 1526

IU/L and 934 IU/L, respectively, while serum bilirubin remained normal. In order to determine more precisely the etiology and severity of this acute hepatitis, we performed a liver biopsy that showed portal infiltration with lymphocytes and eosinophils, mild biliary tract dystrophy, and scattered necrotic hepatocytes in the liver lobule together with microgranulomas. There was no steatosis and no fibrosis. A diagnosis of acute drug-induced liver injury (DILI) due to disulfiram was made, as histological lesions were not consistent with alcoholic liver injury, and an alternative etiology was reasonable excluded. Figure 1 illustrates the clinical course of the hepatitis and associated biological alterations. Figure 2 illustrates histological lesions on liver biopsy.

Consistent with previously reported cases of disulfiram hepatitis [10], biological course was suggestive of an idiosyncratic reaction. Although there are no firm recommendations for steroids in acute DILI [11], we decided to initiate prednisone at a dose of 30 mg daily with gradual tapering off the dose, which was associated with a rapid diminution of transaminases and a return to completely normal values after 20 days of treatment. A strong recommendation was made to avoid reexposition to this aversion therapy.

3. Discussion

Acute liver injury due to disulfiram (tetraethylthiuram disulfide) is relatively uncommon and typically develops within 2 to 12 weeks following initiation of treatment [2, 10, 12]. The risk of severe hepatitis with liver insufficiency leading to death or liver transplantation is even less frequent, with an estimation of 1 fatal case in 30,000 treated patients per year [2]. This risk seems unrelated to the presence of an underlying liver disease, is not dose-related, and is thought to result from a hypersensitivity reaction involving P450 cytochrome enzymes [2, 11]. Using data from a Swedish registry of DILI, Björnsson et al. [10] identified 82 reports of disulfiram-induced liver injury over a 36-year period, corresponding to 1 per 1.3 million average daily dose of the drug. In Denmark, over a 5-year period, disulfiram hepatitis was the second most frequent cause of referral to a liver transplant center [13]. The true incidence of disulfiram-induced DILI is difficult to determine in a population of patients with frequent biological and histological alterations due to alcohol misuse. In alcoholic steatohepatitis, the rise in transaminases never exceeds six times the upper limit of normal value [14], while acute alcoholic microvesicular steatosis typically manifests with more elevated liver enzymes [15]. Nevertheless, when acute DILI is suspected, the pattern of injury based on the R ratio calculation of liver biological tests is useful [11]. The hepatocellular pattern of injury is more frequently reported as compared to the cholestatic pattern. To attribute liver injury to a particular drug needs to consider many items grouped under a scoring system to assess causality [16]. When using this scale in our patient, the responsibility of disulfiram in the occurrence of acute hepatitis is determined as "probable." The absence of extrahepatic manifestations including eosinophilia and no reexposition to the drug prevented to reach the state of a "definite" causal relationship.

A liver biopsy provides major information that may help to confirm, or infirm, a diagnosis of DILI. Based on reported cases, disulfiram-associated lesions include the following: portal tract inflammation mostly composed of mononuclear cells and eosinophils, mild bile ducts alterations, and necrotic and apoptotic hepatocytes in the liver lobule. These lesions were observed in our patient, together with a microgranulomatous pattern of lobular inflammation, which has not been reported in previous histological reports.

In our patient, we stopped disulfiram and initiated tapered doses of steroids in order to shorten recovery time. Corticosteroid therapy in DILI remains controversial [17], and the decision to treat depends mostly on the physician's personal experience.

Although disulfiram is not recognized nowadays as a major tool to treat alcohol dependence [18], it is described as a relatively safe treatment with no liver-related deaths reported in recent years [2, 18]. Nevertheless, the risk of hepatotoxicity needs to be kept in mind and transaminases need to be regularly monitored when starting a treatment with disulfiram. The typical pattern of injury is hepatocellular, and the fatality rate may reach 10 to 15% if jaundice complicates the course of such DILI [13]. In case of any doubt about the diagnosis of disulfiram-induced liver injury, a liver biopsy may help to confirm the diagnosis by excluding alternative causes of acute injury including alcoholic liver disease.

To conclude, we present here in detail a case of acute drug-induced liver injury resulting from a brief exposition to disulfiram, with a pattern of hepatocellular damage and a mechanism consistent with drug hypersensitivity.

Abbreviations

DILI: Drug-induced liver injury
AST: Aspartate aminotransferase
ALT: Alanine aminotransferase
GGT: Gamma-glutamyl transferase
ALP: Alkaline phosphatase.

Acknowledgments

The authors thank Françoise Jenni, addiction specialist, for sharing clinical and biological data related to the patient's history.

References

[1] M. L. G. García, S. Blasco-Algora, and C. M. Fernandez-Rodriguez, "Alcohol liver disease: a review of current therapeutic approaches to achieve long-term abstinence," *World Journal of Gastroenterology*, vol. 21, no. 28, pp. 8516–8526, 2015.

[2] J. Chick, "Safety issues concerning the use of disulfiram in treating alcohol dependence," *Drug Safety*, vol. 20, no. 5, pp. 427–435, 1999.

[3] L. Ranek and P. Buch Andreasen, "Disulfiram hepatotoxicity," *BMJ*, vol. 2, no. 6079, pp. 94–96, 1977.

[4] S. J. Morris, R. Kanner, R. O. Chiprut, and E. R. Schiff, "Disulfiram hepatitis," *Gastroenterology*, vol. 75, no. 1, pp. 100–102, 1978.
[5] L. Nassberger, "Disulfiram-induced hepatitis--report of a case and review of the literature," *Postgraduate Medical Journal*, vol. 60, no. 707, pp. 639–641, 1984.
[6] S. Kahn, J. B. Farnum, and E. Thomas, "Disulfiram-induced hepatitis," *Southern Medical Journal*, vol. 83, no. 7, pp. 833–836, 1990.
[7] X. Forns, J. Caballería, M. Bruguera et al., "Disulfiram-induced hepatitis. report of four cases and review of the literature," *Journal of Hepatology*, vol. 21, no. 5, pp. 853–857, 1994.
[8] M. Mendenhall, "Disulfiram-induced fulminant hepatic failure in an active duty soldier," *Military Medicine*, vol. 169, no. 8, pp. 671-672, 2004.
[9] R. R. Schade, J. A. Gray, A. Dekker, R. R. Varma, R. D. Shaffer, and D. H. Van Thiel, "Fulminant hepatitis associated with disulfiram. report of a case," *Archives of Internal Medicine*, vol. 143, no. 6, pp. 1271–1273, 1983.
[10] E. Björnsson, H. Nordlinder, and R. Olsson, "Clinical characteristics and prognostic markers in disulfiram-induced liver injury," *Journal of Hepatology*, vol. 44, no. 4, pp. 791–797, 2006.
[11] EASL Clinical Practice Guidelines, "Drug-induced liver injury," *Journal of Hepatology*, vol. 70, pp. 1222–1261, 2019.
[12] H. E. Poulsen, S. Loft, J. R. Andersen, and M. Andersen, "Disulfiram therapy--adverse drug reactions and interactions," *Acta Psychiatrica Scandinavica*, vol. 86, no. S369, pp. 59–65, 1992.
[13] M. Baekdal, H. Ytting, and M. Skalshøi Kjær, "Drug-induced liver injury: a cohort study on patients referred to the Danish transplant center over a five year period," *Scandinavian Journal of Gastroenterology*, vol. 52, no. 4, pp. 450–454, 2017.
[14] EASL Clinical Practice Guidelines, "Management of alcohol-related liver disease," *Journal of Hepatology*, vol. 69, pp. 154–181, 2018.
[15] T. Uchida, H. Kao, M. Quispe-Sjogren, and R. L. Peters, "Alcoholic foamy degeneration-a pattern of acute alcoholic injury of the liver," *Gastroenterology*, vol. 84, no. 4, pp. 683–692, 1983.
[16] V. A. Maria and R. M. Victorino, "Development and validation of a clinical scale for the diagnosis of drug-induced hepatitis," *Hepatology*, vol. 26, no. 3, pp. 664–669, 1997.
[17] P. F. Hu and W. F. Xie, "Corticosteroid therapy in drug-induced liver injury: pros and cons," *Journal of Digestive Diseases*, vol. 20, no. 3, pp. 122–126, 2019.
[18] J. M. A. Sinclair, S. E. Chambers, C. J. Shiles, and D. S. Baldwin, "Safety and tolerability of pharmacological treatment of alcohol dependence: comprehensive review of evidence," *Drug Safety*, vol. 39, no. 7, pp. 627–645, 2016.

25

Two Fatty Liver Conditions Masquerading as Autoimmune Hepatitis

Jonathan David Hendrie,[1] **Mary Crouse Blumer**,[1] **Hubert Henry Fenton**,[2] **and Gary Anthony Abrams**[3]

[1]*Prisma Health-Upstate, University of South Carolina School of Medicine-Greenville, Department of Medicine, 701 Grove Rd., Greenville, SC 29605, USA*
[2]*Prisma Health-Upstate, Department of Pathology, 701 Grove Rd., Greenville, SC 29605, USA*
[3]*Prisma Health-Upstate, University of South Carolina School of Medicine-Greenville Department of Medicine, Division of Gastroenterology & Liver Center, 890 W. Faris Rd., Suite 100, Greenville, SC 29605, USA*

Correspondence should be addressed to Jonathan David Hendrie; jonathan.hendrie125@gmail.com

Academic Editor: Haruki Komatsu

Acute fatty liver of pregnancy (AFLP) is a rare obstetric condition that classically presents in the third trimester or early postpartum period and can lead to liver failure and death. Only six second trimester AFLP cases have been reported in the English literature. We present the earliest case of AFLP at 15 weeks of gestation confounded by a high titer anti-nuclear antibody (ANA >1 : 1280) and concern for autoimmune hepatitis. Our patient had intrauterine fetal demise with prompt dilation and evacuation. Sepsis and multisystem organ failure ensued, and she was transferred to a liver transplant center where she expired without further intervention.

1. Introduction

Acute fatty liver of pregnancy (AFLP) is a rare and potentially fatal condition characterized by microvesicular steatosis and liver failure. The pathophysiology remains unclear, but research has implicated defective mitochondrial fatty acid oxidation as a contributing factor. AFLP typically presents in the third trimester or early postpartum period, but rare cases have been described in the second trimester [1–6]. Diagnosis is usually based on the Swansea criteria [7] in conjunction with serologic and biochemical testing although liver biopsy can be performed under certain circumstances. Treatment involves early diagnosis, prompt fetal delivery, and intensive supportive care with recovery expected over the ensuing days to weeks [8].

2. Case Report

A 41-year-old gravida 4 para 2 patient at 15 weeks and 5 days of gestation (based on ultrasound) presented to an outside hospital with decreased appetite and severe vomiting. She had WHO class III obesity (BMI 45.1 kg/m^2) but was otherwise healthy. Initial laboratory tests showed a white blood cell count (WBC) 14 k/μL, hemoglobin (Hgb) 13.7 g/dL, platelets (PLT) 354 k/μL, normal blood smear, aspartate aminotransferase (AST) 354 IU/L, alanine aminotransferase (ALT) 574 IU/L, alkaline phosphatase (ALP) 125 IU/L, and total bilirubin (TB) 4.8 mg/dL. Abdominal ultrasound and magnetic resonance cholangiopancreatography showed hepatic steatosis, pericholecystic fluid, and gallbladder wall thickening. Further workup revealed a positive anti-nuclear antibody (ANA) with 1 : 640 titer but was otherwise negative for infectious, metabolic, or serologic etiologies. She was treated with methylprednisolone and antibiotics (ceftriaxone and metronidazole) for presumed hyperemesis gravidarum and acalculous cholecystitis, respectively. By the fifth hospital day, she felt greatly improved and tolerated food by mouth; laboratory results showed AST 91 IU/L, ALT 185 IU/L, ALP 127 IU/L, and TB 7.3 mg/dL. She was discharged with a steroid taper and antiemetics.

Three days later, she presented with vomiting, pruritus, and jaundice despite medication adherence. Laboratory testing revealed WBC 18.4 k/μL, Hgb 12.1 g/dL, PLT 166 k/μL, AST 51 IU/L, ALT 88 IU/L, ALP 191 IU/L, TB 15 mg/dL, total protein 6.8 mg/dL, albumin 2.6 mg/dL, serum creatinine 1.0 mg/dL, and international normalized ratio (INR) 2.2 mg/dL. She was transferred to our facility due to her advanced age, history of preterm delivery, and hepatic decompensation. She was alert and oriented with stable vital signs on admission. Complete blood count and comprehensive metabolic panel showed comparable values to those at her outpatient visit. Human immunodeficiency virus, hepatitis B surface antigen, total core antibody, e antigen, and hepatitis C surface antibody testing were nonreactive. Extensive viral and bacterial testing was negative. She denied fever, sick contacts, or recent travel outside of the country. The patient was not taking acetaminophen, amiodarone, antiretrovirals, methotrexate, piroxicam, tetracycline, tolmetin, valproate, or other sources of drug-induced liver injury. Repeat ANA was positive with a >1 : 1280 titer; additional autoantibodies and anticardiolipin were negative.

The patient was admitted to the hospitalist service and various consultants assisted with care. An abdominal ultrasound showed hepatic steatosis and an incidental absent fetal heart rate later confirmed by fetal ultrasound on day 2. Dilation and evacuation were performed on day 3. By this point, the differential diagnosis included AFLP, hemolysis with elevated liver enzymes and low platelets (HELLP), intrahepatic cholestasis of pregnancy (IHCP), and autoimmune hepatitis (AIH). Lack of cholestasis on imaging (ultrasound and MRCP) was inconsistent with IHCP. Preeclampsia, HELLP, and AFLP were considered unlikely based on gestational age, absence of hypertension, appropriate platelet count, and normal peripheral smear. If due to AFLP, the presumption was that it should improve postpartum. However, laboratory work on day 4 showed a rising ALP 226 IU/L and TB 20.5 mg/dL. Due to her positive ANA, she was empirically treated with methylprednisolone out of concern for AIH.

Liver biopsy was performed on day 5, which yielded inadequate tissue, but was suggestive of AFLP based on microvesicular steatosis. Acute renal failure, thrombocytopenia, and disseminated intravascular coagulation (DIC) developed over days 4–7, and a repeat biopsy on day 7 revealed significant microsteatosis, macrosteatosis, ballooning hepatocytes, and a mild inflammatory infiltrate without plasma cells, interface hepatitis, rosettes, or fibrosis (Figures 1 and 2). Several hours postbiopsy, the patient became encephalopathic, rapidly decompensated, and was transferred to a liver transplant center with multisystem organ failure. She expired before further intervention.

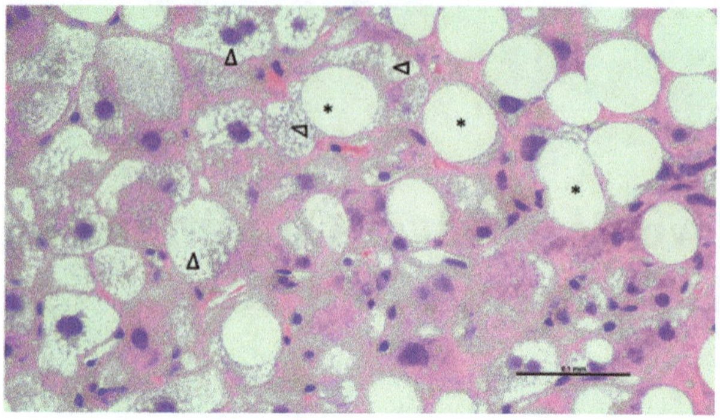

Figure 1: High power, hematoxylin and eosin (H&E) stained section of microvesicular (arrowheads) and macrovesicular (asterisk) steatosis.

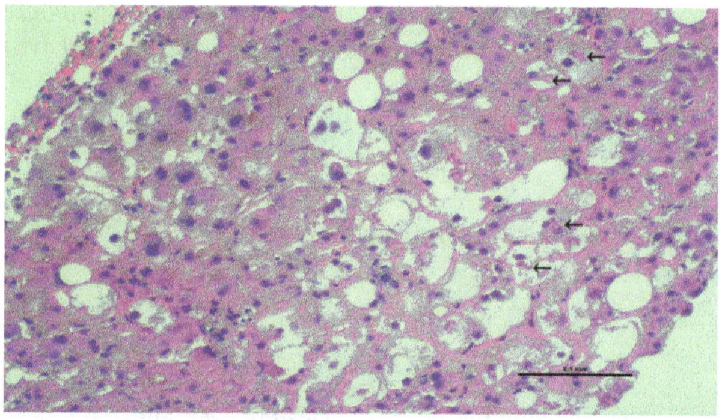

Figure 2: High power, hematoxylin and eosin (H&E) stained section showing cytoplasmic ballooning of hepatocytes with the presence of Mallory's Hyaline (arrows).

3. Discussion

There are varying reports on AFLP incidence, but most studies demonstrate a range between 1/7,000 and 1/20,000 births [9–11]. The pathophysiology is poorly defined, but dysfunction at the level of mitochondrial fatty acid (FA) oxidation is thought to play a role. Maternal-fetal FA levels are increased during pregnancy to support fetoplacental growth. One of the most well-supported theories of pathogenesis involves an inherited fetal deficiency of the long-chain 3-hydroxyacyl-coenzyme A dehydrogenase enzyme (LCHAD), which is part of a mitochondrial trifunctional protein (MTP) complex that catalyzes the β-oxidation of FA [12]. This autosomal recessive condition leads to the impairment of FA metabolism by the fetoplacental unit and subsequent buildup of toxic intermediate byproducts (i.e., long-chain metabolites) in the maternal circulation. Maternal LCHAD heterozygosity hinders the ability to clear toxins deleterious to hepatocytes [11, 13–15]. In a study of twelve women with a prior diagnosis of AFLP, eight were shown to be heterozygous for the LCHAD deficiency [16]. A separate cohort analysis found that 19% of AFLP cases had mutations in the MTP α-subunit responsible for LCHAD deficiency [13].

Most cases of AFLP occur in the third trimester or early postpartum period, but there are case reports as early as the second trimester with the earliest reported case at 18 weeks of gestation [1–6]. Clinically, AFLP leads to liver failure but is also associated with renal failure, coagulopathy, hypoglycemia, encephalopathy, and multisystem organ failure [17–19]—all of which occurred in the presented case. Presenting symptoms are often nonspecific and include fatigue, malaise, headache, nausea, vomiting, anorexia, and abdominal pain, which are obfuscated by the overlapping symptoms of mid-late pregnancy.

AFLP is a clinical diagnosis, and the Swansea criteria have been prospectively validated to aid diagnosis [7, 20, 21]. Based on these criteria, six or more of the following are required for diagnosis: vomiting, abdominal pain, polydipsia/polyuria, renal impairment, encephalopathy, coagulopathy, elevated ammonia, elevated urate, elevated bilirubin, elevated transaminases, hypoglycemia, leukocytosis, ascites or bright liver on ultrasound, and microvesicular steatosis on biopsy. A liver biopsy is rarely required for diagnosis and is often deferred due to the coagulopathic state of the patient [22] but can be justified in cases where liver function does not return to normal postpartum [23]. It is usually performed via trans-jugular approach and requires an adequate sample size of at least 2.5 centimeters with ten or more portal tracts [24–26].

Once diagnosed, management involves prompt fetal delivery and intensive supportive care with recovery expected over days to weeks [8]. Plasmapheresis initiated in the early postpartum period has demonstrated success in delaying or halting the progression of AFLP [27–30]. For patients with fulminant liver or multisystem organ failure despite the aforementioned treatments, auxiliary or orthotopic liver transplantation should be considered and has shown success [31–33]. A recent review of liver transplant outcomes in women of childbearing age showed that despite a decreased 5-year graft survival, patients transplanted for AFLP had comparable early and late survival outcomes compared to women transplanted for another reason [33].

Over the past few decades, maternal mortality in AFLP has decreased from 75–85% to 4–18% [8, 34–36]. Risk factors for adverse maternal outcomes include history of legal pregnancy termination, postpartum diagnosis, male fetus, intrauterine fetal demise, DIC, elevated serum creatinine, and prolonged prothrombin or activated partial thromboplastin time [17]. Fetal mortality is estimated at 20% [37], with negative outcomes correlated to fetal distress, prolonged partial thromboplastin time, fibrin degradation products, direct bilirubin, and decreased gestational age at delivery [3, 17]. Based on these factors, both the patient and her fetus were high risk for adverse events. Although there was diagnostic uncertainty due to the elevated ANA, our patient received the standard of care with prompt fetal delivery, biopsy, intensive supportive care, and transfer to a liver transplant center. In retrospect, plasmapheresis could have been considered but is not currently the standard of care. Whether the combination of AFLP and NAFLD portended this unfortunate outcome is unknown.

NAFLD is a general term for a group of conditions where fat accumulates in the liver of those who drink little to no alcohol. The most common condition under this umbrella term is fatty liver, which occurs when adipose accumulates in hepatocytes. Obesity is the primary risk factor for its development. In and of itself, fatty liver may not cause serious damage. However, a subgroup of patients may progress to develop nonalcoholic steatohepatitis (NASH), which is characterized by hepatocyte inflammation and liver scarring with the potential to cause cirrhosis.

Our case was challenging because AFLP has never been reported in the early second trimester and the presence of high ANA titers suggested an autoimmune etiology. To our knowledge, this is the first case that simultaneously supports two divergent fatty liver conditions: the uncommon AFLP and the very common NAFLD. AFLP seldom occurs in the second trimester, but our patient's progressive liver and renal failure, coagulopathy, hypoglycemia, encephalopathy, DIC, intrauterine fetal demise, and liver histology (characteristic diffuse microvesicular steatosis) support its diagnosis. To our knowledge, this is the earliest reported case of AFLP based on gestational age.

The concurrent diagnosis of NAFLD is supported by macrosteatosis in a patient with WHO class III obesity, as opposed to the microfat droplets of AFLP. Microvesicular steatosis is noted in 10% of NAFLD biopsies, but if present is associated with advanced fibrosis [38], which was absent in our patient. NASH is characterized by ballooning hepatocellular injury and inflammation as observed in our patient. Autoantibodies, even titers ≥1 : 640, are due to an epiphenomenon in NAFLD/NASH, and are not necessarily associated with advanced histologic features [39]. This explains the misinterpreted diagnosis of AIH, which also lacked support based on the absence of plasma cells, interface hepatitis, and rosettes.

There is an overlap between AFLP and HELLP syndrome, but there are enough factors that differentiate their diagnoses. This patient had a lactate dehydrogenase range of 586–660 U/L which is nonspecific with acute liver failure and does not necessarily point towards HELLP. The haptoglobin level was <8 mg/dL, but this was in the setting of DIC which can occur in either condition. HELLP is usually associated with elevated blood pressure, while AFLP is not [40], and the patient had no previous diagnosis of hypertension (admission blood pressure ranges: systolic 60–168 mmHg and diastolic 35–102 mmHg). Little can be drawn from these data during a prolonged hospitalization complicated by acute stress, D&E, volume overloaded requiring hemodialysis, and shock with vasopressor support. Second, acute renal failure is seen far more commonly in AFLP than HELLP (14–90% vs. 1.2–8.0%) [8–10, 19, 23, 40–43], and this patient was in fulminant renal failure requiring hemodialysis. Additional differentiating factors include hypoglycemia, encephalopathy, and coagulopathy which are described more frequently in AFLP due to hepatic insufficiency from steatosis and subsequent hepatocyte dysfunction [8–10, 19, 40–42, 44]. Throughout her hospitalization, INR ranged from 2.0 to 3.2 and she had seven hypoglycemic events (blood glucose < 70 mg/dL), even while tolerating a diet. Measurement of low antithrombin III levels has been described as useful in diagnosing AFLP but was not tested in this patient [44]. Lastly, the patient had biopsy-confirmed microvesicular steatosis which does not occur in HELLP.

In conclusion, we report that AFLP can occur in the early second trimester of pregnancy and should be in a clinician's differential diagnosis for acute liver failure regardless of gestational age. NAFLD is a common disorder associated with autoantibodies that can confound the diagnosis of liver diseases related to pregnancy.

Disclosure

The authors agree on the findings presented herein and approve this work for publication. The authors received no funding for this case report.

Authors' Contributions

Each author contributed significantly to the submitted manuscript in accordance with the definitions set forth by the International Committee of Medical Journal Editors. JDH contributed to manuscript drafting, data analysis, figure design, and submission. MCB was responsible for conception, manuscript drafting, data analysis, and critical revision. HHF assisted in manuscript drafting, data analysis, figure design, and critical revision. GAA was involved in conception, manuscript drafting, data analysis, figure design, and critical revision.

References

[1] M. Monga and A. R. Katz, "Acute fatty liver in the second trimester of pregnancy," *Primary Care Update for Ob/Gyns*, vol. 5, no. 4, p. 191, 1998.

[2] A. Yassin, W. Denguezli, A. Fessi et al., "Mild clinical presentation of acute Fatty liver in the second trimester of pregnancy," *Case Reports in Obstetrics and Gynecology*, vol. 2011, p. 402710, 2011.

[3] Y.-P. Zhang, W.-Q. Kong, S.-P. Zhou, Y.-H. Gong, and R. Zhou, "Acute fatty liver of pregnancy," *Chinese Medical Journal*, vol. 129, no. 10, pp. 1208–1214, 2016.

[4] M. Wong, F. Hills, K. Vogler, I. Zardawi, and N. Nandi, "Acute fatty liver of pregnancy from 18 Weeks' gestation," *Hepatology*, vol. 71, no. 6, pp. 2167–2169, 2020.

[5] F. Afridi, M. Feely, and R. Reddy, "Acute fatty liver disease of pregnancy in the second trimester," *Case Report Critical Care*, vol. 2020, Article ID 6705784, 5 pages, 2020.

[6] M. K. Ramadan, J. Khaza'al, D. Cha'ar, Z. Bazzi, R. Bachnak, and P. Haibeh, "Second-trimester acute fatty liver disease of pregnancy: a brief review of the literature and a case report," *Journal of Obstetrics and Gynaecology Research*, vol. 47, no. 1, pp. 34–43, 2021 Jan.

[7] C. L. Ch'ng, M. Morgan, I. Hainsworth et al., "Prospective study of liver dysfunction in pregnancy in Southwest Wales," *Gut*, vol. 51, no. 6, pp. 876–880, 2002.

[8] D. B. Nelson, N. P. Yost, and F. G. Cunningham, "Acute fatty liver of pregnancy: clinical outcomes and expected duration of recovery," *American Journal of Obstetrics and Gynecology*, vol. 209, no. 5, pp. 456.e1–7, 2013.

[9] K. Mjahed, B. Charra, D. Hamoudi, M. Noun, and L. Barrou, "Acute fatty liver of pregnancy," *Archives of Gynecology and Obstetrics*, vol. 274, no. 6, pp. 349–353, 2006.

[10] M. Knight, C. Nelson-Piercy, J. J. Kurinczuk, P. Spark, and P. Brocklehurst, "A prospective national study of acute fatty liver of pregnancy in the UK," *Gut*, vol. 57, no. 7, pp. 951–956, 2008.

[11] R. H. Lee, *Acute Fatty Liver of Pregnancy*, UpToDate, Waltham, MA, USA, 2020.

[12] J. A. Ibdah, M. J. Bennett, P. Rinaldo et al., "A fetal fatty-acid oxidation disorder as a cause of liver disease in pregnant women," *New England Journal of Medicine*, vol. 340, no. 22, pp. 1723–1731, 1999.

[13] Z. Yang, J. Yamada, Y. Zhao et al., "Prospective screening for pediatric mitochondrial trifunctional protein defects in pregnancies complicated by liver disease," *JAMA*, vol. 288, no. 17, pp. 2163–2166, 2002.

[14] R. S. Rector and J. A. Ibdah, "Fatty acid oxidation disorders: maternal health and neonatal outcomes," *Seminars in Fetal and Neonatal Medicine*, vol. 15, no. 3, pp. 122–128, 2010.

[15] S. Natarajan and J. Ibdah, "Role of 3-hydroxy fatty acid-induced hepatic lipotoxicity in acute fatty liver of pregnancy," *International Journal of Molecular Sciences*, vol. 19, no. 1, p. 322, 2018.

[16] W. R. Treem, M. E. Shoup, D. E. Hale et al., "Acute fatty liver of pregnancy, hemolysis, elevated liver enzymes, and low platelets syndrome, and long chain 3-hydroxyacyl-coenzyme A dehydrogenase deficiency," *The American Journal of Gastroenterology*, vol. 91, no. 11, pp. 2293–2300, 1996.

[17] Q. Gao, X. Qu, X. Chen et al., "Outcomes and risk factors of patients with acute fatty liver of pregnancy: a multicentre retrospective study," *Singapore Medical Journal*, vol. 59, no. 8, pp. 425–430, 2018.

[18] J. E. Hay, "Liver disease in pregnancy," *Hepatology*, vol. 47, no. 3, pp. 1067–1076, 2008.

[19] H.-H. Lau, Y.-Y. Chen, J.-P. Huang, C.-Y. Chen, T.-H. Su, and C.-P. Chen, "Acute fatty liver of pregnancy in a Taiwanese tertiary care center: a retrospective review," *Taiwanese Journal of Obstetrics and Gynecology*, vol. 49, no. 2, pp. 156–159, 2010.

[20] A. Goel, B. Ramakrishna, U. Zachariah et al., "How accurate are the Swansea criteria to diagnose acute fatty liver of pregnancy in predicting hepatic microvesicular steatosis?" *Gut*, vol. 60, no. 1, pp. 138-139, 2011.

[21] S. Wang, S.-L. Li, Y.-X. Cao, Y.-P. Li, J.-L. Meng, and X.-T. Wang, "Noninvasive Swansea criteria are valuable alternatives for diagnosing acute fatty liver of pregnancy in a Chinese population," *The Journal of Maternal-Fetal & Neonatal Medicine*, vol. 30, no. 24, pp. 2951–2955, 2017.

[22] H. H. Ko and E. Yoshida, "Acute fatty liver of pregnancy," *Canadian Journal of Gastroenterology*, vol. 20, no. 1, pp. 25–30, 2006.

[23] P. Vigil-De Gracia and J. A. Lavergne, "Acute fatty liver of pregnancy," *International Journal of Gynecology & Obstetrics*, vol. 72, no. 2, pp. 193–195, 2001.

[24] S. A. Geller, "Autoimmune hepatitis: histopathology," *Clinical Liver Disease*, vol. 3, no. 2, pp. 19–23, 2014.

[25] P. Bedossa, D. Dargère, and V. Paradis, "Sampling variability of liver fibrosis in chronic hepatitis C," *Hepatology*, vol. 38, no. 6, pp. 1449–1457, 2003.

[26] M.-C. Rousselet, S. Michalak, F. Dupré et al., "Sources of variability in histological scoring of chronic viral hepatitis," *Hepatology*, vol. 41, no. 2, pp. 257–264, 2005.

[27] J. N. Martin Jr, C. M. Briery, C. H. Rose, M. T. Owens, J. A. Bofill, and J. C. Files, "Postpartum plasma exchange as adjunctive therapy for severe acute fatty liver of pregnancy," *Journal of Clinical Apheresis*, vol. 23, no. 4, pp. 138–143, 2008.
[28] F. Jin, M. Cao, Y. Bai, Y Zhang, Y Yang, and B Zhang, "Therapeutic effects of plasma exchange for the treatment of 39 patients with acute fatty liver of pregnancy," *Discovery Medicine*, vol. 13, no. 72, pp. 369–373, 2012.
[29] M. R. Seyyed Majidi and J. Vafaeimanesh, "Plasmapheresis in acute Fatty liver of pregnancy: an effective treatment," *Case Reports in Obstetrics and Gynecolog*, vol. 2013, Article ID 615975, 23 pages, 2013.
[30] C.-B. Yu, J.-J. Chen, W.-B. Du et al., "Effects of plasma exchange combined with continuous renal replacement therapy on acute fatty liver of pregnancy," *Hepatobiliary & Pancreatic Diseases International*, vol. 13, no. 2, pp. 179–183, 2014.
[31] S. A. Ockner, E. M. Brunt, S. M. Cohn, E. S. Krul, D. W. Hanto, and M. G. Peters, "Fulminant hepatic failure caused by acute fatty liver of pregnancy treated by orthotopic liver transplantation," *Hepatology*, vol. 11, no. 1, pp. 59–64, 1990.
[32] J. Ringers, K. Bloemenkamp, N. Francisco, J. Blok, M. Arbous, and B. van Hoek, "Auxiliary or orthotopic liver transplantation for acute fatty liver of pregnancy: case series and review of the literature," *BJOG: An International Journal of Obstetrics & Gynaecology*, vol. 123, no. 8, pp. 1394–1398, 2016.
[33] T. Kushner, D. Tholey, J. Dodge, B Saberi, T Schiano, and N Terrault, "Outcomes of liver transplantation for acute fatty liver disease of pregnancy," *American Journal of Transplantation: Official Journal of the American Society of Transplantation and the American Society of Transplant Surgeons*, vol. 19, no. 7, pp. 2101–2107, 2019.
[34] M. M. Kaplan, "Acute fatty liver of pregnancy," *New England Journal of Medicine*, vol. 313, no. 6, pp. 367–370, 1985.
[35] A. G. Rajasri, R. Srestha, and J. Mitchell, "Acute fatty liver of pregnancy (AFLP) - an overview," *Journal of Obstetrics and Gynaecology*, vol. 27, no. 3, pp. 237–240, 2007.
[36] M. Varner and N. K. Rinderknecht, "Acute fatty metamorphosis of pregnancy. A maternal mortality and literature review," *The Journal of Reproductive Medicine*, vol. 24, no. 4, pp. 177–180, 1980.
[37] J. Liu, T. T. Ghaziani, and J. L. Wolf, "Acute fatty liver disease of pregnancy: updates in pathogenesis, diagnosis, and management," *American Journal of Gastroenterology*, vol. 112, no. 6, pp. 838–846, 2017.
[38] S. Tandra, M. M. Yeh, E. M. Brunt et al., "Presence and significance of microvesicular steatosis in nonalcoholic fatty liver disease," *Journal of Hepatology*, vol. 55, no. 3, pp. 654–659, 2011.
[39] R. Vuppalanchi, R. J. Gould, R. J. Gould et al., "Clinical significance of serum autoantibodies in patients with NAFLD: results from the nonalcoholic steatohepatitis clinical research network," *Hepatology International*, vol. 6, no. 1, pp. 379–385, 2012.
[40] H. Minakami, M. Morikawa, T. Yamada, T. Yamada, R. Akaishi, and R. Nishida, "Differentiation of acute fatty liver of pregnancy from syndrome of hemolysis, elevated liver enzymes and low platelet counts," *Journal of Obstetrics and Gynaecology Research*, vol. 40, no. 3, pp. 641–649, 2014.
[41] H. Reyes, L. Sandoval, A. Wainstein et al., "Acute fatty liver of pregnancy: a clinical study of 12 episodes in 11 patients," *Gut*, vol. 35, no. 1, pp. 101–106, 1994.
[42] H. Chen, L. Yuan, J. Tan, Y. Liu, and J. Zhang, "Severe liver disease in pregnancy," *International Journal of Gynecology & Obstetrics*, vol. 101, no. 3, pp. 277–280, 2008.
[43] M. M. Mellouli, F. B. Amara, H. Maghrebi, M. Bouchnack, N. Khaled, and H. Reziga, "Acute fatty liver of pregnancy over a 10-year period at a Tunisian tertiary care center," *International Journal of Gynecology & Obstetrics*, vol. 117, no. 1, pp. 88-89, 2012.
[44] A. Morton and J. Laurie, "Physiological changes of pregnancy and the Swansea criteria in diagnosing acute fatty liver of pregnancy," *Obstetric Medicine*, vol. 11, no. 3, pp. 126–131, 2018.

De Novo Autoimmune Hepatitis after COVID-19 Infection in an Unvaccinated Patient

Francisco A. Durazo,[1,2] Kelly Kristbaum,[1] James Miller,[3] Kia Saeian,[2] Motaz Selim,[1] and Johnny C. Hong[4]

[1]*Division of Transplant Surgery, Department of Surgery, Medical College of Wisconsin, Milwaukee, WI, USA*
[2]*Division of Gastroenterology and Hepatology, Department of Medicine, Medical College of Wisconsin, Milwaukee, WI, USA*
[3]*Department of Pathology and Laboratory Medicine, Medical College of Wisconsin, Milwaukee, WI, USA*
[4]*Division of Transplantation, Pennsylvania State University, College of Medicine Penn State Health Milton S. Hershey Medical Center Hershey, Pennsylvania, USA*

Correspondence should be addressed to Francisco A. Durazo; fdurazo@mcw.edu

Academic Editor: Mauro Vigano

Liver test abnormalities have been described during severe acute respiratory syndrome coronavirus (SARS-CoV)-2 infection causing coronavirus disease 2019. Most of them consist of elevation of the aminotransferases that resolve once the infection subsides. There are several reports of autoimmune hepatitis developing after vaccination against COVID-19 and one case of autoimmune hepatitis following COVID-19 infection. We present a patient that was not vaccinated against COVID-19 and developed resistant de novo autoimmune hepatitis following COVID-19 infection requiring aggressive immunosuppression.

1. Introduction

Severe acute respiratory syndrome coronavirus (SARS-CoV)-2 was first identified in December of 2019 in Wuhan City, China, and was declared a global pandemic by the World Health Organization (WHO) on March 11th, 2020. The disease is termed coronavirus disease 2019 (COVID-19). COVID-19 is typically characterized by fever, fatigue, dry cough, anosmia, and headache, which may evolve to respiratory failure [1]. COVID-19 infection has been associated with the development of autoimmune processes [2–5]. It seems as though the shared pathogenetic mechanisms and the clinical aspects between the hyper-inflammatory diseases and COVID-19 may suggest that SARS-CoV-2 could act as a triggering factor for the development of a rapid autoimmune and/or autoinflammatory dysregulation in genetically predisposed individuals [6]. There are several reports of autoimmune hepatitis that developed after COVID-19 vaccine [7–14] and one case report on a patient that developed autoimmune hepatitis during COVID-19 infection [15]. Molecular mimicry has been suggested as a potential mechanism for these associations [5]. We report the case of a patient, unvaccinated against COVID-19, that developed de novo autoimmune hepatitis after COVID-19 infection.

2. Clinical Presentation and Diagnostic Tests

A forty-nine-year-old Hispanic woman was in her usual state of health until 10/11/2020 when she presented with fever, cough, and loss of smell and taste. She saw her primary care provider (PCP) and tested positive for SARS-CoV-2 (nucleic acid amplification test per anterior nasal swab) on 10/11/20 and again on 10/21/20. She stayed home and was instructed to drink adequate liquids and to call back if shortness of breath would ensue. She recovered from her respiratory symptoms. Three weeks later she noted decreased appetite. In the beginning of December 2020, she called her primary care doctor with complaints of intermittent right upper quadrant abdominal pain, dark urine, and yellowing of the eyes. Laboratory studies revealed total bilirubin of 8.93 mg/dL, alanine aminotransferase (ALT) of 851 U/L [0–33], aspartate aminotransferase (AST) of 614 U/L [0–32], and alkaline phosphatase of 70 U/L [30–115]; therefore, she was instructed to go to the emergency department (ED).

Repeat laboratory studies in the ED revealed a total bilirubin of 10.82 mg/dL, ALT of 781 U/L, AST of 671 U/L, and alkaline phosphatase of 71 U/L. Urinalysis revealed urobilinogen of 2.0 mg/dL and a moderate amount of blood. Amylase was 67 U/L, and lipase was 101 U/L. The complete blood count showed white blood cell count of 6.1×10^3, hemoglobin of 13.1 g/dL, hematocrit of 41%, and a platelet count of 258×10^3. Troponin was negative. C-reactive protein was 13.68 mg/L. SARS-CoV-2 was not detected.

An ultrasound of the abdomen showed a markedly enlarged liver with normal echotexture, no intrahepatic biliary dilatation, and normal portal venous flow. The common bile duct (CBD) was dilated to eight millimeters (mm) with diffuse gallbladder wall thickening and edema but no stones.

Magnetic resonance cholangiopancreatography (MRCP) was obtained confirming diffuse gallbladder wall thickening without cholelithiasis, porta hepatis, and peripancreatic lymphadenopathy with reference to a porta hepatis lymph node measuring 4.5 by 2.5 centimeters (cm) without choledocholithiasis.

The surgical team was consulted and performed robotic assisted laparoscopic cholecystectomy with intraoperative cholangiogram and liver biopsy without complication. Liver pathology revealed variable, mild to moderate portal mononuclear cell inflammation with mixed plasma cells and eosinophils. There was no fibrosis, no iron deposition, and no bile duct injury. Further laboratory studies revealed non-reactive hepatitis A, B, and C serologies. She recovered favorably from the surgery and was discharged home.

She was referred to the Hepatology Clinic at our institution after her liver function tests did not improve post-cholecystectomy: total bilirubin increased to 11.41 mg/dL, ALT at 789 U/L, AST at 568 U/L, alkaline phosphatase at 66 U/L.

In clinic, she denied any previous problems with her liver or previous hospitalizations, and the available liver tests prior to her recent hospitalization were within normal limits. Her past medical history was significant for motion sickness. In addition to the recent laparoscopic cholecystectomy, her past surgical history was significant for a tonsillectomy, removal of a benign neck lymph node, and two benign breast mass excisions four years apart. Family history was negative for any autoimmune disorders or liver disease. She denied any herbal supplements or over-the-counter medications. She did report taking dextromethorphan/guaifenesin when experiencing flu-like symptoms after being diagnosed with COVID-19 four months prior. She reported not feeling well ever since being diagnosed with COVID-19.

She denied any recent travel, sick contacts, and blood transfusions. She had prior tattoos but none recently.

On physical examination, her vital signs were unremarkable. Physical assessment revealed an overweight female who was visibly jaundiced with no vascular angiomas and no lymphadenopathy. Lungs were clear to auscultation, and respiratory effort was normal. Heart auscultation showed a regular rate and rhythm without murmur, gallop, or rub. Her abdomen was soft, rounded, non-tender, and non-distended, with no organomegaly or masses. There was no peripheral edema. Neurological exam showed that she was alert and oriented without asterixis.

A complete serologic workup including hepatitis A IgM, hepatitis B core total and IgM, hepatitis C antibody and RNA, nuclear antibody, smooth muscle antibody, mitochondrial antibody, hepatitis E IgM, cytomegalovirus DNA, adenovirus, and Epstein–Barr DNA were all negative. Her immunoglobulin G (IgG) was 2093, alpha-1 antitrypsin was 204 mg/dL with M1M1 phenotype, and ceruloplasmin was 19 mg/dL. Iron panel showed a total iron binding capacity of 543 ug/dL, serum ferritin of 413 ng/mL, and a serum iron of 218 ug/dL. Lactate dehydrogenase (LDH) was 258 unit/L, creatinine phosphokinase (CPK) was 73 unit/L, and alpha-fetoprotein (AFP) was 7.0 ng/mL. Repeated SARS-CoV-2 (nucleic acid amplification test per anterior nasal swab) was negative.

According to the Revised Scoring System of the International Autoimmune Hepatitis Group, this patient had a score of 18 points, which is definite for the diagnosis of autoimmune hepatitis [16]. She was started on prednisone 40 milligrams (mg) daily for autoimmune hepatitis. Repeat blood work showed improvement with a total bilirubin of 3.6 mg/dL, ALT at 312 U/L, AST at 147 U/L, and alkaline phosphatase at 48 U/L. She was continued on corticosteroid therapy to which the total bilirubin responded favorably as low as 2.65 mg/dL; however, her aminotransferases remained unchanged.

She was sent for percutaneous lymph node biopsy of the enlarged porta hepatis lymph node which was unable to be completed due to position of the lymph node. Endoscopic ultrasound guided biopsy with fine needle aspiration was also attempted and aborted due to proximity of the node to the bile duct and portal vein.

She began a steroid taper that lasted four weeks. MRCP was repeated and unremarkable. Meanwhile, her total bilirubin increased to 4.51 mg/dL, ALT at 545 U/L, AST at 343 U/L, and alkaline phosphatase 63 U/L. Her prednisone was again increased to 40 mg. Her laboratory studies continued to worsen, and she complained of nausea and diarrhea. The INR slowly up trended to 2.0, and she complained of rectal bleeding. Colonoscopy was performed which revealed internal and external hemorrhoids—likely the source of rectal bleeding—as well as minimal diverticulosis.

Vitamin K was given for three days with no improvement of PT/INR. A second liver biopsy was taken showing severe cholestatic hepatitis with an atypical lymphocytic portal and sinusoidal infiltrate, with easily identifiable plasma cells and interface activity. Viral stains were negative (Figures 1–3).

Her Model for End-Stage Liver Disease (MELD) score had increased to 25, Na-MELD of 27, therefore she was referred for liver transplant due for concern for continued decompensation. Unfortunately, during this time she started

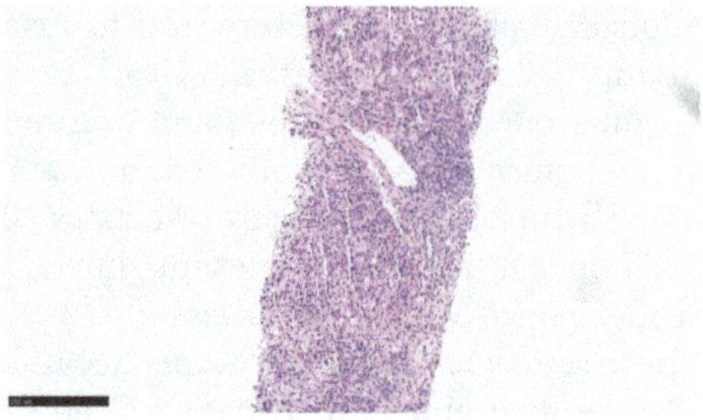

Figure 1: This low-power (100x) image of the second liver biopsy shows a moderate portal lymphoplasmacytic infiltrate with interface activity.

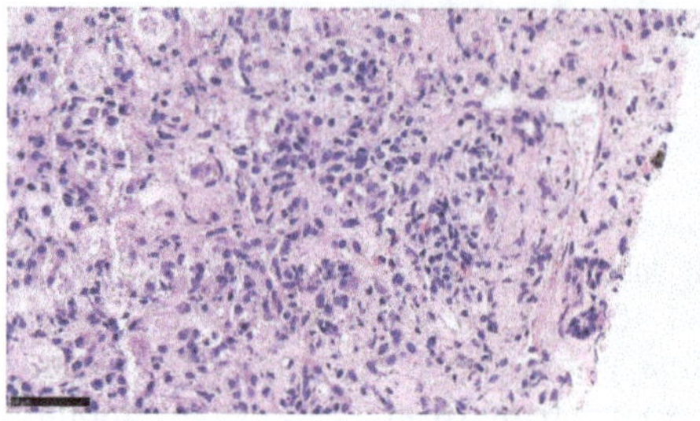

Figure 2: At 400x, plasma cells and eosinophils are easily identifiable as is surrounding interface activity.

to complain of abdominal pain, presented to the ED, and was admitted under the transplant surgery service for medical management. Computerized tomography (CT) of the abdomen and pelvis demonstrated extrahepatic mild biliary ductal dilatation measuring up to 9 mm and mild perihepatic ascites and portacaval lymphadenopathy. She improved with conservative management and was discharged home. Laboratory studies at time of discharge were total bilirubin 24.8 mg/dL, ALT 284 U/L, AST 442 U/L.

She returned to the ED three days later with right upper quadrant pain. T bilirubin increased to 30 mg/dL, ALT 289 U/L, AST 425 U/L, lipase 81. Liver doppler ultrasound demonstrated normal liver morphology and hemodynamics. MRCP demonstrated mild dilatation of bile ducts with CBD measuring up to 10 mm with decreased T2 signal and diffusion restriction with associated wall thickening and enhancement. She underwent endoscopic retrograde cholangiopancreatography which showed biliary dilation without any definite stricture or filling defect. A plastic biliary stent was placed. Her total bilirubin decreased to 21.9 mg/dL, and she was discharged home when symptoms improved.

Follow-up laboratory studies revealed a total bilirubin of 23 mg/dL, ALT of 140 U/L, AST of 225 U/L, and alkaline phosphatase of 101 U/L. PT/INR increased to 2.8. She was prescribed vitamin K 10 mg daily for three days, mycophenolate 1000 mg twice daily, and prednisone 20 mg daily.

On weekly labs, her total bilirubin improved to 16, 9, 8, and 6 mg/dL, respectively, and continued to downtrend. Her INR improved to 2.4, 2.0, 1.8, and 1.9 and continued to downtrend. Her immunoglobulin G continued to remain elevated in a range of 1500–2700. Her IGG subset showed elevation in IGG1 at 2257 (Table 1).

Her CA19-9 also continued to be elevated with a high of 2149 which was attributed to cholestasis. LDH also remained elevated in the 217–246 range.

She continued with transplant evaluation despite clinical improvement on mycophenolate and prednisone therapy. Workup revealed a breast mass 10 by 13 mm on mammogram. Biopsy confirmed invasive ductal carcinoma: 90% estrogen receptor positive and 60% progesterone receptor positive. Her transplant episode was closed, and she was referred to hematology/oncology for further treatment. She was BRCA negative. She continues to require prednisone

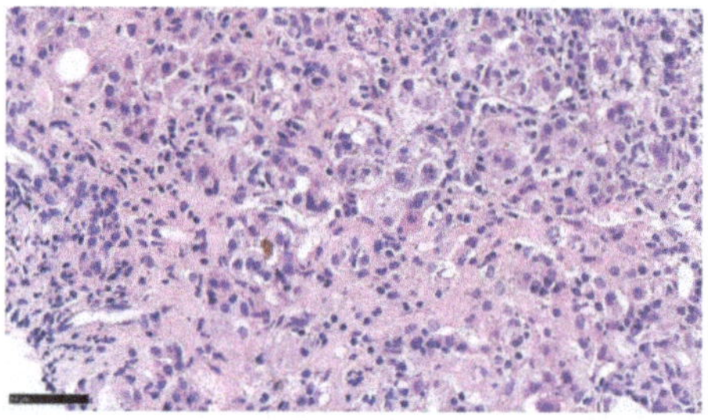

Figure 3: Another area shows canalicular cholestasis. Numerous background lymphocytes and plasma cells are also visible.

20 mg daily and mycophenolate 750 mg twice daily as maintenance therapy for autoimmune hepatitis.

3. Discussion

Liver test abnormalities have been identified as one of a growing list of findings in the spectrum of non-pulmonary manifestations described in COVID-19 infection. Different studies on COVID-19 have shown an incidence of liver injury ranging from 14.8% to 53%, mainly abnormal aminotransferases [17–21]. Currently, studies on the mechanisms of SARS-CoV-2-related liver injury are limited. It has been shown that SARS-CoV-2 uses ACE2 as its entry receptor. Both liver cells and bile duct cells express ACE2 [22]. However, the ACE2 expression of the bile duct cells is much higher than that of liver cells. Another study reported that the liver injury observed in COVID-19 patients might be caused by antivirals (lopinavir/litonavir) used for the treatment of SARS-CoV-2 infection [23].

COVID-19 infection has also been associated with the development of autoimmune processes [2–5]. Severe cases of COVID-19 infection are characterized by an autoinflammatory dysregulation that contributes to tissue damage [5]. The shared pathogenetic mechanisms and the clinical aspects between the hyper-inflammatory diseases and COVID-19 may suggest that SARS-CoV-2 could act as a triggering factor for the development of a rapid autoimmune and/or autoinflammatory dysregulation in genetically predisposed individuals [6]. There are several reports of autoimmune hepatitis that developed after COVID-19 vaccine [7–14] and one case report on a patient that developed autoimmune hepatitis during COVID-19 infection [15].

Table 1 Evolution of liver tests after COVID-19 infection.

Date	ALT	Bilirubin	IgG	INR	Alt/10	Alt/100
2/19/2021	851	8.9	2000	1.2	0.851	8.51
2/23/2021	469	6.7	2000	1.2	0.469	4.69
3/3/2021	789	11	2093	1.1	0.789	7.89
3/5/2021	781	11	2093	1.2	0.781	7.81
3/11/2021	736	9.4	1798	1.2	0.736	7.36
3/22/2021	312	3.6	1502	1.1	0.312	3.12
4/1/2021	637	2.6	1668	1.1	0.637	6.37
4/16/2021	693	4	1668	1.1	0.693	6.93
4/29/2021	538	3.7	1862	1	0.538	5.38
5/21/2021	545	4.5	1855	1.3	0.545	5.45
6/17/2021	552	17	1850	1.4	0.552	5.52
6/25/2021	496	17	1970	1.4	0.496	4.96
7/13/2021	393	22	1964	1.8	0.393	3.93
7/19/2021	262	20	2354	2.1	0.262	2.62
7/24/2021	289	31	2354	2.3	0.289	2.89
8/12/2021	129	16	2557	2.4	0.129	1.29
8/23/2021	114	9.4	2557	1.8	0.114	1.14
9/3/2021	81	6.6	1885	1.7	0.081	0.81
9/18/2021	60	4	1885	1.4	0.06	0.6
10/8/2021	56	2.2	1565	1.3	0.056	0.56
11/19/2021	42	0.8	1565	1.2	0.042	0.42
12/20/2021	38	1	1560	1.2	0.038	0.38
1/28/2022	128	1.1	1560	1.4	0.128	1.28
2/15/2022	84	1	1502	1.3	0.084	0.84
3/24/2022	45	0.6	1502	1.2	0.045	0.45
4/21/2022	30	0.6	1502	1.1	0.03	0.3

We report a case of a forty-nine-year-old unvaccinated female patient that developed new-onset autoimmune hepatitis after COVID-19 infection. She never recovered fully from her initial infection and complained of decreased appetite three weeks later and presented with jaundice approximately seven weeks later. She underwent a cholecystectomy with worsening of her liver tests and an intraoperative biopsy that showed portal mononuclear cell inflammation with mixed plasma cells and eosinophils and mild macrovesicular steatosis. Her serologic workup for viral infections, autoimmune, and metabolic diseases was non-contributory. She was not taking any hepatotoxic medications or supplements. She was started on prednisone, as a therapeutic trial for autoimmune hepatitis, without improvement of her liver tests. Prednisone was tapered. Her liver tests continued to worsen, and another therapeutic trial was attempted without much success. Due to her deterioration (total bilirubin 30 mg/dL, PT INR 2.8), she was evaluated for a liver transplant. She was then started on prednisone and mycophenolate. Her liver tests finally started to improve. Attempts were made to taper down prednisone but were unsuccessful. She still remains on dual therapy with prednisone and mycophenolate.

We suspect that COVID-19 infection may have triggered her autoimmune hepatitis. She had no history of liver disease in the past, and there was a temporal relation between COVID-19 infection and the onset of her symptoms. Her liver biopsy showed no fibrosis, suggesting absence of previous disease. She was unvaccinated against COVID-19.

The eventual dramatic response to prednisone and mycophenolate also supports the diagnosis of autoimmune hepatitis. In addition, the necessity of dual therapy to control the aminotransferases points toward a resistant autoimmune hepatitis. Further attempts at tapering the dose of prednisone have been futile.

4. Conclusion

We report a case of new-onset autoimmune hepatitis after COVID-19 infection in an unvaccinated patient. She presented three weeks after her diagnosis of COVID-19 infection with an aggressive steroid-resistant autoimmune hepatitis requiring prednisone and mycophenolate as dual maintenance therapy to control and prevent further progression of her disease.

References

[1] Z. Xu, L. Shi, Y. Wang et al., "Pathological findings of COVID-19 associated with acute respiratory distress syndrome," *The Lancet Respiratory Medicine*, vol. 8, no. 4, pp. 420–422, 2020.

[2] G. Toscano, F. Palmerini, S. Ravaglia et al., "Guillain-barre syndrome associated with SARS-CoV-2," *New England Journal of Medicine*, vol. 382, no. 26, pp. 2574–2576, 2020.

[3] A. A. Zulfiqar, N. Lorenzo-Villalba, P. Hassler, and E. Andres, "Immune thrombocytopenic purpura in a patient with covid-19," *New England Journal of Medicine*, vol. 382, no. 18, p. e43, 2020.

[4] L. Bowles, S. Platton, N. Yartey et al., "Lupus anticoagulant and abnormal coagulation tests in patients with covid-19," *New England Journal of Medicine*, vol. 383, no. 3, pp. 288–290, 2020.

[5] M. Ehrenfeld, A. Tincani, L. Andreoli et al., "COVID-19 and autoimmunity," *Autoimmunity Reviews*, vol. 19, no. 8, Article ID 102597, 2020.

[6] F. Caso, L. Costa, P. Ruscitti et al., "Could Sars-coronavirus-2 trigger autoimmune and/or autoinflammatory mechanisms in genetically predisposed subjects?" *Autoimmunity Reviews*, vol. 19, no. 5, Article ID 102524, 2020.

[7] F. Bril, "Autoimmune hepatitis developing after coronavirus disease 2019 (COVID-19) vaccine: one or even several swallows do not make a summer," *Journal of Hepatology*, vol. 75, no. 5, pp. 1256-1257, 2021.

[8] M. Ghielmetti, H. D. Schaufelberger, G. Mieli-Vergani et al., "Acute autoimmune-like hepatitis with atypical anti-mitochondrial antibody after mRNA COVID-19 vaccination: a novel clinical entity?" *Journal of Autoimmunity*, vol. 123, Article ID 102706, 2021.

[9] M. Rela, D. Jothimani, M. Vij, A. Rajakumar, and A. Rammohan, "Auto-immune hepatitis following COVID vaccination," *Journal of Autoimmunity*, vol. 123, Article ID 102688, 2021.

[10] A. Hines, J. G. Shen, C. Olazagasti, and S. Shams, "Immune thrombocytopenic purpura and acute liver injury after COVID-19 vaccine," *BMJ Case Reports*, vol. 14, no. 7, p. e242678, 2021.

[11] C. K. Tan, Y. J. Wong, L. M. Wang, T. L. Ang, and R. Kumar, "Autoimmune hepatitis following COVID-19 vaccination: true causality or mere association?" *Journal of Hepatology*, vol. 75, no. 5, pp. 1250–1252, 2021.

[12] P. Palla, C. Vergadis, S. Sakellariou, and T. Androutsakos, "Letter to the editor: autoimmune hepatitis after COVID-19 vaccination. A rare adverse effect?" *Hepatology*, vol. 75, no. 2, pp. 489-490, 2021.

[13] E. Vuille-Lessard, M. Montani, J. Bosch, and N. Semmo, "Autoimmune hepatitis triggered by SARS-CoV-2 vaccination," *Journal of Autoimmunity*, vol. 123, Article ID 102710, 2021.

[14] M. C. Londono, J. Gratacos-Gines, and J. Saez-Penataro, "Another case of autoimmune hepatitis after SARS-CoV-2 vaccination - still casualty?" *Journal of Hepatology*, vol. 75, no. 5, pp. 1248-1249, 2021.

[15] G. Rajendiran, B. Cowman, K. Erickson, T. Oliver, and W. Manatsathit, "Autoimmune hepatitis associated with COVID-19 infection - a diagnostic and therapeutic dilemma," *S D Med*, vol. 73, no. 11, pp. 528–532, 2020.

[16] A. J. Czaja, "Performance parameters of the diagnostic scoring systems for autoimmune hepatitis," *Hepatology*, vol. 48, no. 5, pp. 1540–1548, 2008.

[17] C. Huang, Y. Wang, X. Li et al., "Clinical features of patients infected with 2019 novel coronavirus in Wuhan, China," *The Lancet*, vol. 395, no. 10223, pp. 497–506, 2020.

[18] D. Wang, B. Hu, C. Hu et al., "Clinical characteristics of 138 hospitalized patients with 2019 novel coronavirus-infected pneumonia in wuhan, China," *JAMA*, vol. 323, no. 11, pp. 1061–1069, 2020.

[19] N. Chen, M. Zhou, X. Dong et al., "Epidemiological and clinical characteristics of 99 cases of 2019 novel coronavirus pneumonia in Wuhan, China: a descriptive study," *The Lancet*, vol. 395, no. 10223, pp. 507–513, 2020.

[20] Q. Cai, D. Huang, H. Yu et al., "COVID-19: abnormal liver function tests," *Journal of Hepatology*, vol. 73, no. 3, pp. 566–574, 2020.

[21] L. Xu, J. Liu, M. Lu, D. Yang, and X. Zheng, "Liver injury during highly pathogenic human coronavirus infections," *Liver International*, vol. 40, no. 5, pp. 998–1004, 2020.

[22] F. Qi, S. Qian, S. Zhang, and Z. Zhang, "Single cell RNA sequencing of 13 human tissues identify cell types and receptors of human coronaviruses," *Biochemical and Biophysical Research Communications*, vol. 526, no. 1, pp. 135–140, 2020.

[23] Z. Fan, L. Chen, J. Li et al., "Clinical features of COVID-19-related liver functional abnormality," *Clinical Gastroenterology and Hepatology*, vol. 18, no. 7, pp. 1561–1566, 2020.

27

A Case of Multiple Intratumoral Hemorrhage and Rupture of Hepatocellular Carcinoma after Starting Lenvatinib

Katsutoshi Ishihara

Department of Radiology, Yuai Memorial Hospital, 707 Higashiushigaya, Koga, Ibaraki, Japan

Correspondence should be addressed to Katsutoshi Ishihara; kishihara@yuai-hosp-jp.org

Academic Editor: Fumio Imazeki

A man in his 80s was administered lenvatinib to treat multiple hepatocellular carcinomas. After starting lenvatinib, he was admitted to our hospital for fever and epigastric tenderness. Conjunctival icterus and conjunctival pallor were observed. Computed tomography showed high density areas in his tumors which were suggestive of intratumoral hemorrhage and tumor rupture. As a result, the patient underwent an emergent angiography and arterial embolization.

1. Introduction

Lenvatinib is a multityrosine kinase receptor inhibitor that inhibits vascular endothelial growth factor (VEGF) receptor [1]. Lenvatinib can be used to treat patients with unresectable hepatocellular carcinoma (HCC).

The most common treatment-related adverse events among patients who received lenvatinib included hypertension, diarrhea, decreased appetite, and weight loss [2]. In a phase II trial, one patient died of liver tumor rupture that occurred within 30 days after receiving the last dose of lenvatinib [3]. The present study describe the case of a patient with advanced HCC who experienced multiple intratumoral hemorrhage and concomitant tumor rupture after the onset of treatment with lenvatinib.

2. Case Presentation

A man in his 80s with liver cirrhosis due to hepatitis C virus referred to our hospital for further examination and treatment of multiple hepatic masses. Computed tomography (CT) revealed multiple HCCs in both lobes of the liver (Figures 1(a) and 1(b)). PIVKA-II was 1000.51 mAU/ml on admission. Lenvatinib was started at a dose of 8 mg/day because surgery and radiofrequency ablation was not feasible.

Six days after starting lenvatinib, the patient experienced some epigastric discomfort. However, no clinically significant findings in the gastrointestinal endoscopic examination were observed. Twelve days after starting lenvatinib, he was admitted to our hospital for fever and epigastric tenderness. Conjunctival icterus and conjunctival pallor were observed. Laboratory results on admission showed a hemoglobin value of 8.5 g/dL, white blood cell count of 16100/μl, total bilirubin of 1.9 mg/dL, elevated transaminase (aspartate aminotransferase (AST) of 119 U/L; alanine aminotransferase (ALT) of 87 U/L), lactate dehydrogenase (LDH) of 406 U/L, and C-reactive protein (CRP) of 12.07 mg/dL. Platelet count was within normal limits. CT examination showed high-attenuation areas in the multiple HCCs (Figure 2), and perilesional blood was also observed near the hepatic tumor in the right lobe of the liver (Figure 3). Therefore, multiple intratumoral hemorrhage and HCC rupture were considered. The patient underwent an emergency angiography and arterial embolization. Pooling of contrast medium concerning intratumoral hemorrhage was observed in some tumors on angiography and CT during hepatic arteriography (CTHA) (Figures 4 and 5). CTHA also demonstrated a decrease in vascularity of the hepatic tumors mainly in the right lobe of the liver which was suggestive of a decrease in the viability of the tumor (Figure 5). In the left lobe of the liver, tumor stains were observed in more tumors than in the

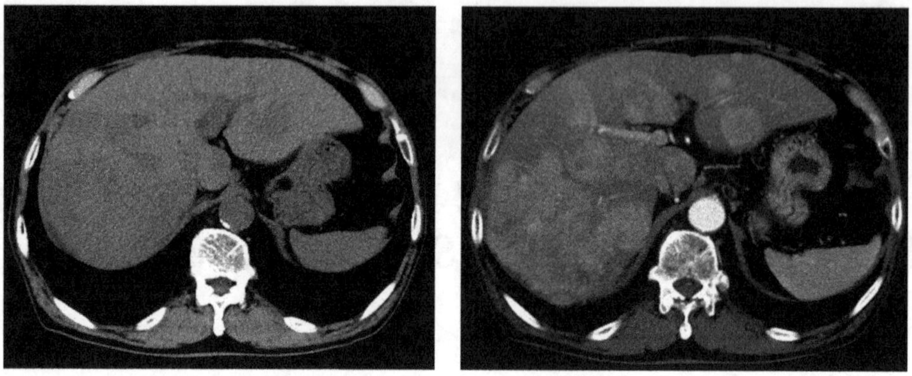

FIGURE 1: Nonenhanced computed tomography (a) and arterial phase of CT (b). Multiple liver tumors are depicted as low attenuation areas in nonenhanced CT and exhibited early enhancement in the arterial phase. These tumors were considered hepatocellular carcinomas.

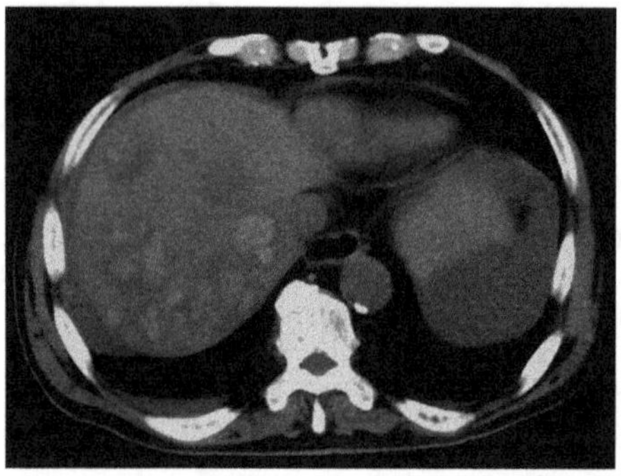

FIGURE 2: Nonenhanced computed tomography image. High-attenuation areas were observed in multiple HCCs considered to indicate multiple intratumoral hemorrhages.

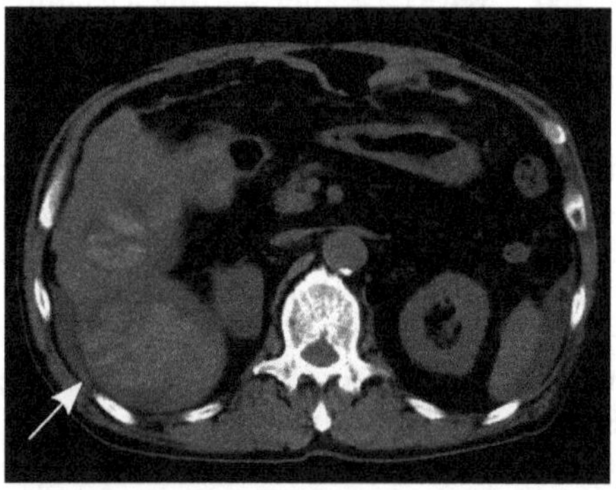

FIGURE 3: Nonenhanced computed tomography image. Perilesional blood was also observed near the hepatic tumor in the right lobe of the liver that was considered to indicate rupture of the HCC (arrow).

right lobe (Figure 6). Hepatic artery embolization was done with a gelatin sponge. Emulsion of lipiodol (2 ml) and epirubicin hydrochloride (20 mg) was also given before embolization to have an antitumor effect in the left lobe of the liver because tumor stains were observed in more tumors in the left lobe on CTHA than on the right lobe.

Eleven days after emergency embolotherapy, AST, ALT, and total bilirubin were recovered to normal levels. The hemoglobin level was recovered to 10.2 g/dl after embolization, and he was discharged from the hospital 18 days after embolotherapy. There was no fever or abdominal pain after discharge from the hospital. Administration of lenvatinib (4 mg/day) was resumed about two months after HCC rupture and intratumoral hemorrhage.

PIVKA-II was 1290.3 mAU/ml at three days after emergency angiography and 127.91 at two months after embolotherapy. Alpha-fetoprotein was within normal limits during the observation period.

3. Discussion

Lenvatinib is a multityrosine kinase inhibitor and inhibits tumor angiogenesis [1]. In the present case, some HCCs had decreased vascularity on CTHA. I believe that this decrease might be due to lenvatinib-induced inhibitions of tumor angiogenesis.

Sorafenib, like lenvatinib, is a multikinase inhibitor that inhibits VEGF. Rombolà et al. reported a case of HCC rupture and attributed the risk to sorafenib use [4]. Sorafenib inhibits VEGF signaling and is known to increase the risk of bleeding. VEGF is important for the survival of endothelial cells and for maintaining the architecture and integrity of the vasculature. Therefore, inhibition of the VEGF pathway may decrease the regeneration potential of damaged endothelial cells and may consequently increase the risk of hemorrhage [5]. The occurrence of hemorrhagic complications with lenvatinib use has been documented. In the REFLECT trial, cerebral hemorrhage was observed in 3 out of 462 patients [2]. In another phase II trial, one patient died because of a ruptured liver tumor within 30 days after receiving the last dose of lenvatinib [3]. Moreover, hemorrhagic events occurred in 35% of the patients treated with lenvatinib versus 18% of patients who received placebo against thyroid cancer [6]. In the present study, intratumoral hemorrhage and concomitant HCC rupture were observed. These phenomena may be attributable to the effect of lenvatinib as a VEGF inhibitor. Rupture of HCC may occur with the use of both lenvatinib and sorafenib.

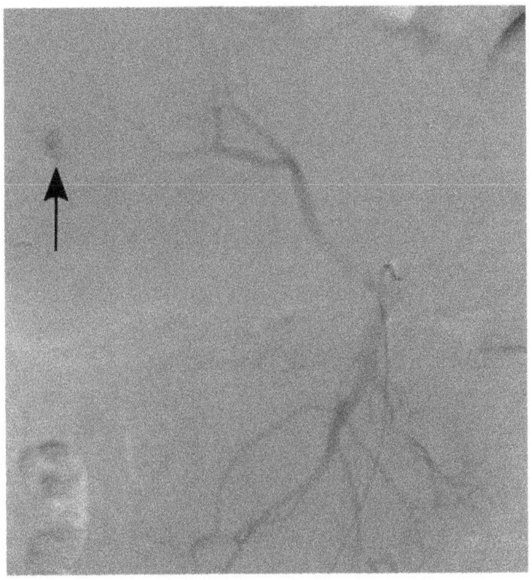

Figure 4: Pooling of contrast medium was observed on angiography (arrow). Right hepatic artery was replaced on the superior mesenteric artery.

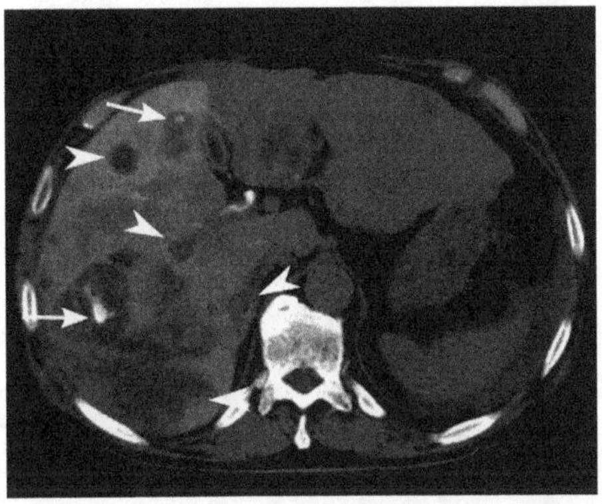

Figure 5: Arterial phase of computed tomography during right hepatic arteriography. Pooling of contrast medium was observed (arrows). Contrast effect of tumors was low (arrowheads) and it was considered to indicate decrease in vascularity of hepatocellular carcinomas.

High attenuation areas were seen in the multiple HCCs, and perilesional blood was observed near the hepatic tumor in the right lobe of the liver by CT examination in the present case. Therefore, multiple intratumoral hemorrhage and HCC rupture were considered. The pooling of contrast medium for intratumoral hemorrhage was observed in some tumors on angiography and CTHA. Uchida-Kobayashi et al. described that five of 68 cases treated with lenvatinib developed intraperitoneal or intratumoral hemorrhage, and they also observed pooling of contrast medium on angiography after intratumoral hemorrhage [7]. As they have pointed out, we also thought that pooling of contrast medium during angiography was similar to vascular lake phenomenon that was observed during TACE with drug-eluting beads (DEB-TACE). The etiology of the vascular lake phenomenon during DEB-TACE is not yet well understood. Seki et al. hypothesized that vascular lake phenomenon emerging during DEB-TACE could arise through the

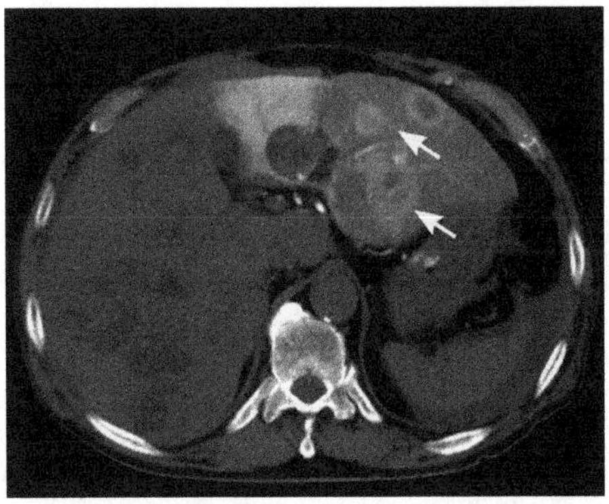

Figure 6: Arterial phase of computed tomography during left hepatic arteriography. In the left lobe of the liver, tumor stains were observed in more tumors than in the right lobe (arrowhead).

rupture of some of the vulnerable tumor microvasculature formed by tumor angiogenesis [8]. In our case, we thought that lenvatinib inhibited tumor angiogenesis and the remaining poorly developed tumor microvasculature tended to collapse. Therefore, pooling of contrast medium might be occurred and it suggested intratumoral hemorrhage.

The mechanism of spontaneous HCC rupture has not been understood. Several hypotheses have been proposed to explain the HCC rupture. It is said that tumor location is associated with spontaneous rupture of HCC [9]. Caudate lobe HCC or HCC which is subcapsular in location tends to rupture compared to a centrally located HCC because normal hepatic parenchyma surrounding the HCC can protect the tumor from rupture. Li et al. reported that most ruptured HCCs were localized to the left lateral segment (seg II and seg III) and right posterior-inferior segment (seg VI) [9]. These segments have relatively small room for a space occupying lesion compared to the other segments. Therefore, when the tumor grows beyond its capacity, the inner pressure splits open the surrounding parenchyma and tears the capsule leading to rupture. In the present case, ruptured HCC was localized to the subcapsular region in posterior-inferior segment. It might had been more prone to rupture because of the location of HCC and use of VEGF inhibitor.

There may not be a correlation between the dose of lenvatinib and hemorrhage because this report described that initiation doses of lenvatinib among the patients with hemorrhage were 12, 8, and 4 mg/day [7]. This report also described that the patients with hemorrhage had larger tumor than the patients without hemorrhage. So TACE prior to administration of lenvatinib for large HCC may be an option for precaution of HCC rupture.

This report describes multiple intratumoral hemorrhage and HCC rupture caused by lenvatinib administration in a patient with multiple HCC. It is important to know that HCC may be prone to rupture depending on the location of HCC and the use of lenvatinib.

Acknowledgments

The author would like to thank Shoichi Kato and Yuji Kumashiro for collecting data. The author would also like to thank Editage (http://www.editage.com) for English language editing.

References

[1] K. Suyama and H. Iwase, "Lenvatinib: a promising molecular targeted agent for multiple cancers," *Cancer Control*, vol. 25, pp. 1–5, 2018.

[2] M. Kudo, R. S. Finn, S. Qin et al., "Lenvatinib versus sorafenib in first-line treatment of patients with unresectable hepatocellular carcinoma: a randomised phase 3 non-inferiority trial," *The Lancet*, vol. 391, no. 10126, pp. 1163–1173, 2018.

[3] K. Ikeda, M. Kudo, S. Kawazoe et al., "Phase 2 study of lenvatinib in patients with advanced hepatocellular carcinoma," *Journal of Gastroenterology*, vol. 52, no. 4, pp. 512–519, 2017.

[4] A. Nair, S. J. Lemery, J. Yang et al., "FDA approval summary: lenvatinib for progressive, radio-iodine-refractory differentiated thyroid cancer," *Clinical Cancer Research*, vol. 21, no. 23, pp. 5205–5208, 2015.

[5] R. N. Cavalcante, F. Nasser, J. M. Motta-Leal-Filho et al., "Occurrence of vascular lake phenomenon as a predictor of improved tumor response in HCC patients that underwent DEB-TACE," *CardioVascular and Interventional Radiology*, vol. 40, no. 7, pp. 1044–1051, 2017.

[6] A. Seki, S. Hori, and C. Shimono, "Management of vascular lake phenomenon on angiography during chemoembolization with superabsorbent polymer microspheres," *Japanese Journal of Radiology*, vol. 33, no. 12, pp. 741–748, 2015.

[7] S. Uchida, K. Kageyama, A. Yamamoto et al., "Lenvatinib-induced tumor-related hemorrhages in patients with large hepatocellular carcinomas," *Oncology*, pp. 1–6, 2020.

[8] A. Seki, S. Hori, and C. Shimono, "Management of vascular lake phenomenon on angiography during chemoembolization with superabsorbent polymer microspheres," *Japanese Journal of Radiology*, vol. 33, no. 12, pp. 741–748, 2015.

[9] J. Li, L. Huang, C. F. Liu et al., "Risk factors and surgical outcomes for spontaneous rupture of BCLC stages A and B hepatocellular carcinoma: a case-control study," *World Journal of Gastroenterology*, vol. 2, no. 27, pp. 9121–9127, 2014.

Rare Histological Variants of Liver Cancer and their Management: A Single-Institution Experience

Brandon Swed[1] **Omar Gandarilla,**[1] **Kenrry Chiu,**[2] **Karim H. Halazun,**[3] **Benjamin Samstein,**[3] **Rhonda Yantiss,**[2] **and Gagandeep Brar**[1]

[1]*Division of Hematology and Medical Oncology, Department of Medicine, Weill Cornell Medicine/New-York Presbyterian, New York, New York, USA*
[2]*Department of Pathology and Laboratory Medicine, Weill Cornell Medicine/New-York Presbyterian, New York, New York, USA*
[3]*Division of Liver Transplantation and Hepatobiliary Surgery, Department of Surgery, Weill Cornell Medicine/New-York Presbyterian, New York, New York, USA*

Correspondence should be addressed to Gagandeep Brar; gab9046@med.cornell.edu

Academic Editor: Haruki Komatsu

Primary liver malignancies, including hepatocellular carcinoma (HCC) and cholangiocarcinoma, are a major cause of cancer-related morbidity and mortality worldwide. There are several histologically and biologically distinct subtypes of liver cancer that have previously been reported. However, literature regarding the nonsurgical management of these patients upon disease recurrence remains limited. These variants include combined HCC-cholangiocarcinoma (cHCC-CC), Epstein–Barr virus- (EBV-) associated carcinoma, undifferentiated carcinoma, and clear cell or thyroid-like variants of HCC. Here, we aim to highlight the pathologic features, clinical course, and outcomes of five patients with these unusual hepatic tumors and explain the rationale behind the choice of their systemic therapies upon disease recurrence. All patients underwent surgical resection as the standard of care for localized disease, and upon relapse, they were treated with either chemotherapy, targeted therapy, immunotherapy, or active surveillance based on the clinical context and tumor histology. These rare variants are important to recognize as they have prognostic and therapeutic implications, and there are currently insufficient data in the literature to guide further therapy.

1. Introduction

Primary liver cancers are a major cause of morbidity and mortality worldwide. Hepatocellular carcinoma (HCC), the most common type of liver cancer in adults, is ranked as the sixth most prevalent solid tumor malignancy and the third leading cause of cancer-related deaths globally [1]. Despite several recent advances in diagnostic and therapeutic modalities, prognosis generally remains poor, with a five-year relative survival rate of 18% observed in the United States [2]. Hepatic resection and liver transplantation are the standard of care for localized disease and are among the only treatment options with curative intent, as conventional chemotherapy and radiation therapy are generally ineffective [3]. Cholangiocarcinoma, the next most common primary liver cancer, is also associated with a high mortality that is generally attributed to advanced stage disease at the time of diagnosis. Several prognostic factors for liver cancers have been proposed, including tumor size, vascular invasion, elevated serum tumor markers (e.g., alpha-fetoprotein (AFP) and carbohydrate antigen 19-9 (CA 19-9)), resection margin status, and tumor histology [4].

Histologic analysis remains the gold standard for the diagnosis and classification of primary liver carcinomas, although the diagnosis of HCC can usually be made radiographically in the appropriate clinical context, and thus, many tumors are treated prior to histologic evaluation. However, there are some relatively rare variants that may be important to recognize because they either have prognostic and therapeutic implications or simulate features of other malignancies [5, 6]. These include combined HCC-cholangiocarcinoma (cHCC-CC), Epstein–Barr virus- (EBV-)

associated carcinoma, undifferentiated carcinoma, and clear cell or thyroid-like variants of HCC. Here, we report on the clinical course and outcomes of five patients with unusual hepatic tumors and describe their clinical and pathologic features.

2. Case Reports

2.1. Case 1: cHCC/CCA. A 67-year-old Caucasian male with a history of combined hepatitis C and alcoholic cirrhosis was found to have a small hepatic lesion in segment V on a screening ultrasound in November 2019. Follow-up abdominal MRI revealed a 1.5 cm Liver Imaging Reporting and Data System (LI-RADS) 4 lesion which was again confirmed on PET/CT (SUV 7.8) without evidence of distant metastases.

Given radiographic evidence of HCC and elevated AFP to 1017 ng/mL, he underwent a partial left hepatectomy the following month. The cirrhotic liver contained a 1.5 cm firm white tumor that showed morphologic and immunohistochemical features of a combined hepatocellular-cholangiocarcinoma (Figure 1). The adenocarcinomatous component showed CK7-positivity and was negative for arginase, whereas areas of hepatocellular differentiation were positive for arginase and negative for CK7. The tumor demonstrated extensive venous and lymphovascular invasion. Notably, his presurgical CA 19-9 was within normal limits.

Given pathology findings of positive margins and therefore high risk of recurrence, the decision was made to proceed with adjuvant stereotactic body radiation therapy (SBRT). His AFP declined to 9.8 ng/mL in the postoperative setting. He was started on systemic therapy with capecitabine in February 2020, with the intention of treating the more aggressive of the dual histologic subtypes, the cholangiocarcinoma. His AFP subsequently began to rise, and repeat imaging two months later unfortunately confirmed recurrence confined to the liver parenchyma. He had a repeat liver biopsy that demonstrated adenocarcinoma consistent with pancreaticobiliary origin. Further testing revealed PD-L1 positivity of 5% without targetable molecular alterations identified on next-generation Sequencing. He received local therapy with Y90 radioembolization and was started on nivolumab monotherapy which he is currently tolerating well. AFP has since downtrended.

2.2. Case 2: HCC/Undifferentiated Carcinoma. A 48-year-old Asian male was incidentally diagnosed with hepatitis B in June 2019 and started on antiviral therapy at that time. He developed focal right upper quadrant pain several months later prompting an abdominal ultrasound that revealed a region of heterogeneity in the right hepatic lobe, and follow-up abdominal MRI demonstrated a 14.7 × 10.1 cm LI-RADS TIV (tumor in vein) infiltrative hepatic mass consistent with HCC with extensive tumor thrombus. AFP level was elevated to 64.6 ng/mL, and staging CT scans and skeletal scintigraphy showed no evidence of distant metastatic disease.

The patient underwent a right hepatectomy in December 2019 with complete resection of a 14.2 cm heterogeneous tumor accompanied by satellite nodules with extensive venous invasion. The carcinoma showed hepatocellular differentiation as well as undifferentiated components (Figure 2). The latter consisted of broad trabeculae and sheets of high-grade tumor cells with extensive necrosis and readily apparent mitotic figures. These areas lacked convincing staining for Hepar-1 and arginase but had stronger, more diffuse CK7 staining. The tumor was negative for synaptophysin, chromogranin, and CK19.

He had a repeat MRI two months postresection in the setting of recurrent abdominal pain and rising AFP that demonstrated diffuse infiltrative tumor in the left hepatic lobe and suspected right lower lobe pulmonary metastases. He was started on palliative chemotherapy, and after one cycle, succumbed to his disease.

2.3. Case 3: HCC, Clear Cell Variant. A 59-year-old Asian male with a history of hepatitis B diagnosed in 2011 on antiviral therapy since that time was noted to have an elevated AFP to 21.8 ng/mL and liver mass on screening abdominal ultrasound in March 2019. Abdominal MRI, which was delayed due to lack of short-term follow-up, showed a dominant 5.5 cm segment V LI-RADS M (probably or definitely malignant, not necessarily HCC) hepatic mass. Notably, on staging PET/CT, there was no evidence of FDG-avid disease in the kidneys, gastrointestinal tract, or other sites where clear cell carcinoma is known to originate.

He underwent a right partial hepatectomy in October 2019 with complete resection of a 6.1 cm variegated tumor surrounded by multiple satellite nodules. Portal vein invasion was identified. Most (>80%) of the tumor cells contained abundant clear cytoplasm with some higher grade areas (Figure 3). The background liver showed chronic hepatitis with mild activity and thin septal fibrosis consistent with regressed cirrhosis.

Postoperatively, he was noted to have a rising AFP to 154 ng/mL and underwent SBRT to the resection cavity. Repeat imaging in April 2020 showed multifocal progressive liver lesions with suspected pulmonary and osseous metastatic disease, and AFP rapidly increased to 2728 ng/mL. He was subsequently started on palliative systemic therapy with lenvatinib, followed by second-line nivolumab for further disease progression.

2.4. Case 4: CCA, Thyroid-Like Variant. A 60-year-old Caucasian female with a history of Hashimoto's thyroiditis was incidentally noted to have a liver mass on CT imaging in 2009 performed as part of a workup for abdominal pain. Follow-up MRI demonstrated radiographic findings consistent with a hepatic adenoma. On surveillance imaging, this lesion was noted to be enlarging in size with associated hemorrhage, and she ultimately underwent a left hepatectomy ten years later in October 2019.

The resection specimen contained an 11.0 cm tan, variegated hemorrhagic tumor with cystic degeneration arising in a noncirrhotic liver. Resection margins were negative, and

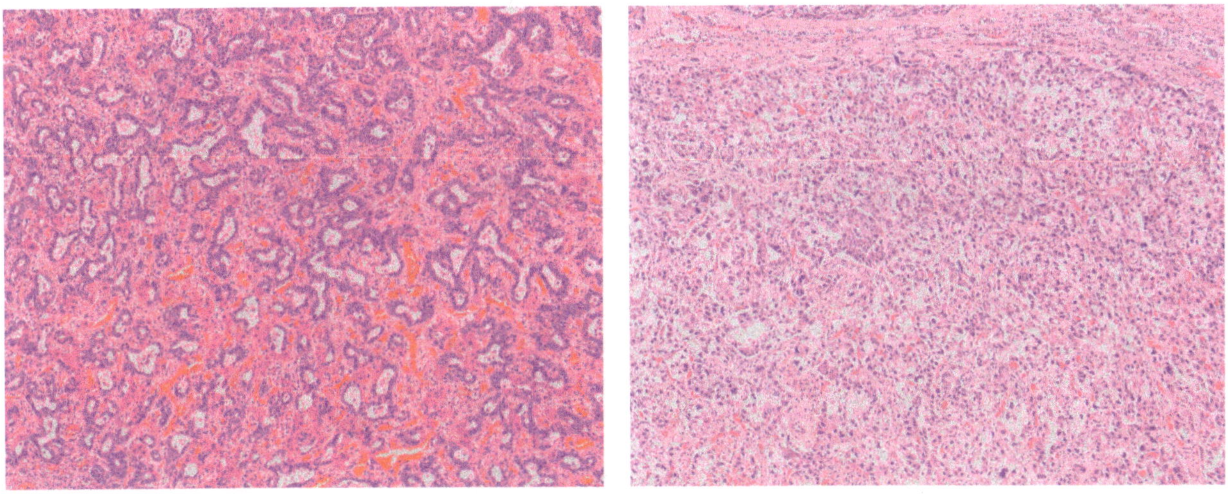

(a) (b)

FIGURE 1: The tumour showing mixed morphologic features with haphazardly arranged, irregularly shaped glands enmeshed in fibrotic stroma typical of cholangiocarcinoma (a) as well as sheet-like growth of solid cell nests and trabeculae showing morphologic and immunohistochemical evidence of hepatocellular differentiation (b).

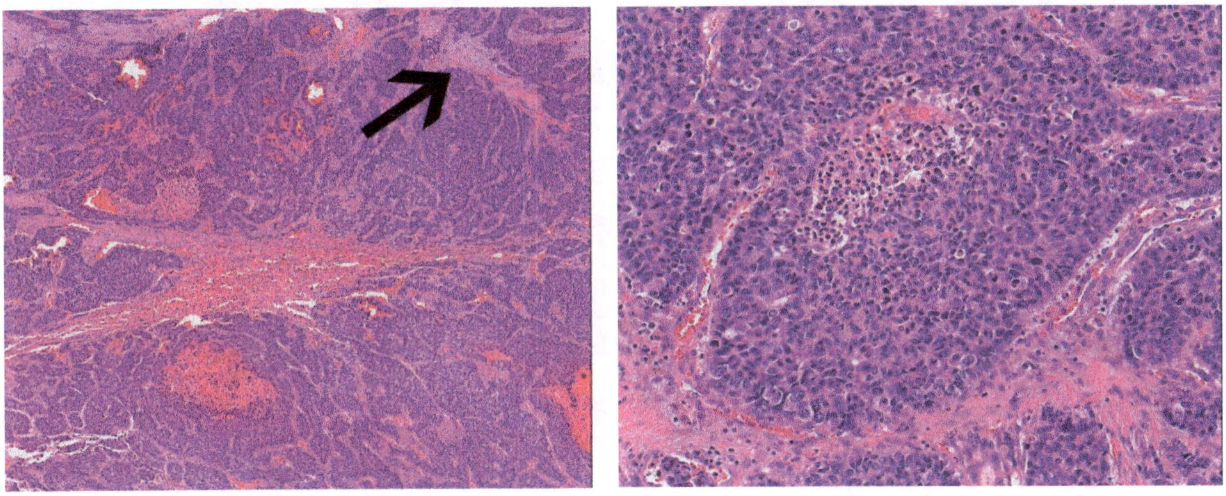

(a) (b)

FIGURE 2: The tumour composed of variably sized nests and trabeculae associated with desmoplasia (arrow) and hemorrhage. (a) High-grade tumour cells containing enlarged, hyperchromatic nuclei with relatively scant cytoplasm extensive necrosis. (b) The high-grade areas are positive for cytokeratin-7 and show patchy staining for arginase and Hepar-1.

no lymphovascular invasion was identified. Sheets of tumor cells were arranged in large, cystically dilated glands filled with eosinophilic material reminiscent of colloid seen in thyroid follicles (Figure 4). The entirety of the tumor demonstrated low-grade nuclear features without evidence of biliary dysplasia in the nonneoplastic parenchyma. The tumor cells were CK-7-positive and showed patchy synaptophysin staining, but were negative for arginase, TTF-1, and chromogranin. The tumor was classified as a thyroid-like variant of an intrahepatic cholangiocarcinoma.

A subsequent neck ultrasound showed no focal abnormalities to suggest metastatic disease from a primary thyroid malignancy. Given prior definitive surgical resection and the indolent nature of her neoplasm, the decision was made to defer adjuvant chemotherapy and instead pursue active radiographic surveillance. She has no evidence of recurrence nine months postresection.

2.5. Case 5: EBV-Associated CCA (Lymphoepithelioma-Like Carcinoma Variant of CCA). A 28-year-old Caucasian female with a history of ulcerative colitis and primary sclerosing cholangitis diagnosed at ages 16 and 23, respectively, was found to have a 6 cm mass adjacent to the caudate lobe on a screening abdominal MRI in October 2017. Tumor markers were notable for an elevated CA 19-9 to 2,733 U/

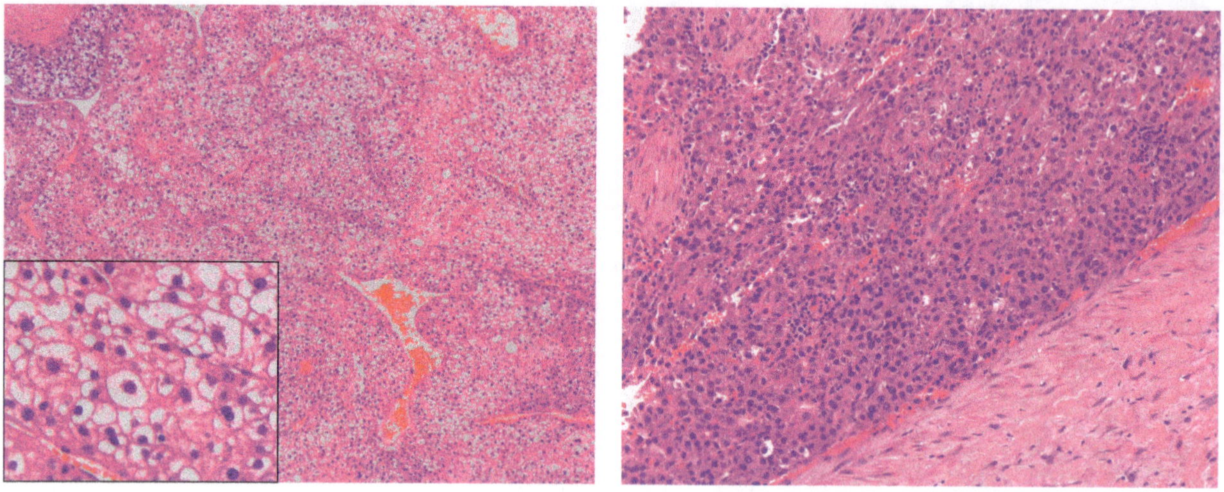

(a) (b)

FIGURE 3: This hepatocellular carcinoma containing broad trabaculae of tumour cells with abundant clear cytoplasm (a). Other high-grade areas resembling conventional hepatocellular carcinoma (b).

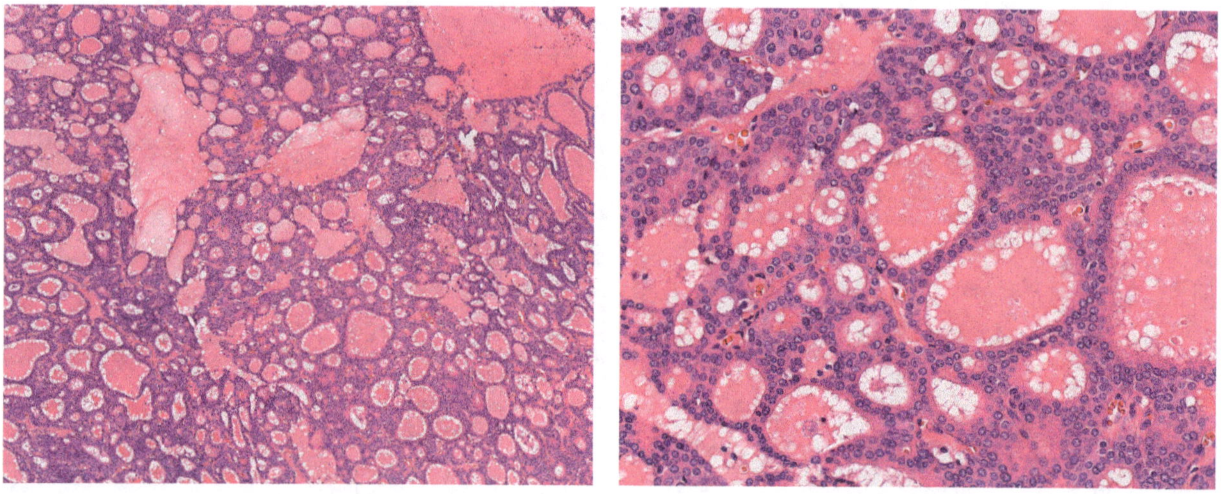

(a) (b)

FIGURE 4: Sheets of tumour cells arranged in cystically dilated glands (a) that contain brightly eosinophilic secretions reminiscent of colloid (b).

mL, while AFP and CEA were within normal limits. She underwent endoscopic biopsy of the subhepatic lesion, and fine needle aspiration (FNA) revealed adenocarcinoma, with a tumor profile that favored an upper gastrointestinal/pancreatobiliary primary. Staging PET/CT showed a peri-pancreatic/portacaval hypermetabolic mass likely representing the primary disease with suspected metastatic aortocaval lymphadenopathy but no evidence of distant metastatic disease. The following month, she had an excisional portal lymph node biopsy confirming metastatic adenocarcinoma.

She ultimately underwent a left hepatectomy with caudate lobectomy and hilar lymphadenectomy in March 2018. Surgical pathology revealed a 2.2 cm ill-defined, perihilar bile duct tumor centered at the confluence of the right and left hepatic ducts. The background liver showed features of primary sclerosing cholangitis with portal-based fibrosis. Microscopic examination of the tumor showed adenocarcinoma confined to the bile duct wall. The malignant glands were associated with a dense lymphoid infiltrate and tumor-infiltrating lymphocytes (Figure 5). In situ hybridization for EBV-encoded RNAs (EBER) demonstrated strong, diffuse labeling of tumor cells. One regional lymph node showed metastatic carcinoma. The findings were compatible with EBV-associated perihilar cholangiocarcinoma.

She experienced multiple postoperative complications including a hepatic abscess, severe gastroparesis, and

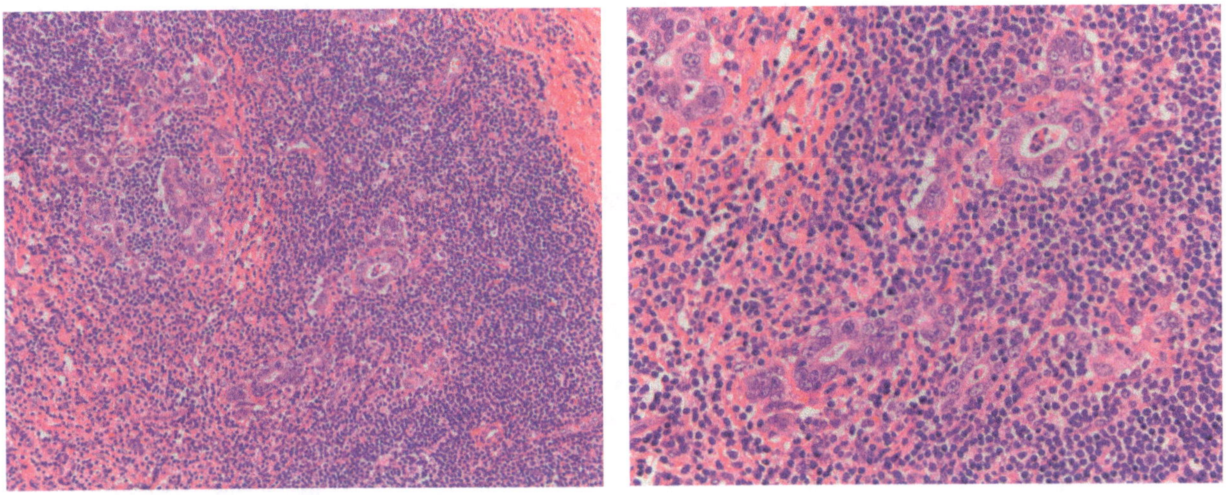

(a) (b)

FIGURE 5: Infiltrating malignant glands are intimately associated with a dense lymphoid infiltrate (a). Intraepithelial lymphocytes are also present (b) ([7–12]).

malnutrition that precluded adjuvant systemic therapy. Her CA 19-9 normalized in the postoperative period, and surveillance scans to date have shown no evidence of recurrent disease.

3. Discussion

Despite its overall high morbidity and mortality, primary liver cancer is a disease with a remarkably variable clinical course. A timely and accurate diagnosis is crucial for optimal management of these patients, as they generally have a poor response to systemic therapy [3]. This is, at least in part, explained by the several histologically and biologically distinct subtypes of liver cancer that have been reported.

Such heterogeneity of clinical findings, imaging characteristics, and histopathologic features can often obscure the precise diagnosis in these patients. [4] For example, cHCC/CCA described in case 1 displays phenotypic features suggestive of both hepatic and biliary differentiation, making the preoperative diagnosis exceptionally challenging. This is true of the other tumor subtypes as well. As described in case 3, it is important to distinguish the atypical clear cell variant of HCC from metastatic clear cell carcinomas that arise from various other primary sites, including the kidneys, ovaries, lungs, and other organs [13, 14]. Similarly, the thyroid-like variant of intrahepatic cholangiocarcinoma discussed in case 4 can be misconstrued as metastatic disease or ectopic normal thyroid tissue. However, the absence of a primary thyroid neoplasm and a lack of thyroid markers like TTF-1 in the liver tumor can be useful in distinguishing these two entities [15, 16].

The histologically distinct tumor features highlighted in this case series have important prognostic and therapeutic implications. However, literature regarding nonsurgical management in these rare subtypes is scarce and mainly limited to case reports, as outlined in Table 1. We report five patients with unique variants of liver cancer, all of whom underwent surgical resection as the standard of care for localized disease. These are among some of the first reports of using systemic therapy to treat these rare variants. Although data to support this is lacking, one of the five patients (case 1, cHCC/CCA) received adjuvant systemic therapy based on his anticipated poor clinical trajectory in the context of positive resection margins and high risk of recurrence. His treatment was targeted toward the more aggressive cholangiocarcinoma subtype. [6] This is in contrast to the patient in case 4, for instance, with a slow-growing thyroid variant that appears to behave more like a low-grade carcinoma. The exceedingly rare prior reports of this subtype suggest predominance in young females with a late presentation and large tumor burden, without apparent underlying liver parenchymal disease. Two of the patients (case 2 with undifferentiated carcinoma and case 3 with clear cell variant) received systemic therapy at the time of disease recurrence or metastases, and all three of the patients who received systemic therapy had further progression of disease. Clear cell carcinoma of the liver has traditionally been associated with a more favorable outcome than conventional HCC. However, the patient presented in case 3 had an unusually aggressive course, possibly attributed to a subpopulation of cells with higher grade cytology.

As we learn more about the subtleties of these uncommon liver cancers, diagnostic and therapeutic dilemmas remain. Treatment for these patients has generally been directed toward their dominant histologic subtype, as there are insufficient data in the literature to guide further therapy. This case series highlights the need for a deeper understanding of the biology of these tumors in order to select the most appropriate treatment options to improve patient outcomes. Although no

Table 1: Summary of selected prior case reports of liver cancer with rare histological features.

Reference	Patient demographics	Histological variant	HBV/ HCV status	Tumor size (cm)	Solitary or multiple	Treatment	Vital status
Sakhuja et al. [13]	32, F	Clear cell	−/−	18	Solitary	Hepatic resection	Alive
Albores-Saavedra et al. [14]	63, M	Clear cell	−/−	0.9	Solitary	Hepatic resection	Alive
Albores-Saavedra et al. [14]	25, F	Clear cell	−/−	1.1	Solitary	Hepatic resection	Alive
Albores-Saavedra et al. [14]	64, M	Clear cell	−/−	6	Solitary	Hepatic resection	Alive
Pecorella et al. [17]	35, F	Clear cell	−/−	NR	NR	Total hepatectomy, liver transplantation	Alive
Toriyama et al. [18]	56, M	Clear cell	+/−	2.2	Solitary	Surgical resection, adjuvant chemotherapy	Alive
Kothadia et al. [19]	51, F	Clear cell	−/−	20.7	Multiple	Transarterial chemoembolization	Alive
Chable-Montero et al. [15]	26, F	Follicular thyroid-like	−/−	NR	Solitary	Hepatic resection, adjuvant chemotherapy	Dead
Fornelli et al. [16]	52, M	Follicular thyroid-like	−/−	18	Solitary	None	Alive
Mittal et al. [20]	23, F	Follicular thyroid-like	−/−	12.1	Solitary	Hepatic resection	Alive
Chen et al. [21]	59, F	Follicular thyroid-like	+/−	3	Solitary	Hepatic resection	Alive
Hiraki et al. [22]	45, M	Undifferentiated	+/−	11.5	Solitary	Hepatic resection	Alive
Maeda et al. [23]	56, M	Undifferentiated	−/−	Very small	Multiple	None	Dead

HBV = hepatitis B virus; HCV = hepatitis C virus; M = male; F = female; NR = not reported. EBV = Epstein–Barr virus; cHCC/CCA = combined hepatocellular-cholangiocarcinoma.

clinically useful genomic alterations were detected by next-generation sequencing assays performed for each of the patients described, it is important to recognize that correlation of histology with molecular data remains a powerful tool in the understanding of the pathogenesis and behavior of liver cancers. More studies are needed to explore this, as greater awareness of these distinct entities can lead to improved treatment strategies and patient outcomes.

References

[1] A. Forner, M. Reig, and J. Bruix, "Hepatocellular carcinoma," *The Lancet*, vol. 391, no. 10127, pp. 1301–1314, 2018.

[2] American Cancer Society, *Cancer Facts & Figures 2020*, American Cancer Society, Atlanta, GA, USA, 2020.

[3] M. M. Kirstein and T. C. Wirth, "Multimodale therapie des hepatozellulären karzinoms," *Der Internist*, vol. 61, no. 2, pp. 164–169, 2020.

[4] A. Zimmerman, *Tumors and Tumor-like Lesions of the Hepatobiliary Tract: General and Surgical Pathology*, pp. 151–156, Springer International Publishing, Geneva, Switzerland, 1st edition, 2017.

[5] C. Stavraka, H. Rush, and P. Ross, "Combined hepatocellular cholangiocarcinoma (cHCC-CC): an update of genetics, molecular biology, and therapeutic interventions," *Journal of Hepatocellular Carcinoma*, vol. 6, pp. 11–21, 2018.

[6] K. O'Connor, J. C. Walsh, and D. F. Schaeffer, "Combined hepatocellular-cholangiocarcinoma (cHCC-CC): a distinct entity," *Annals of Hepatology*, vol. 13, no. 3, pp. 317–322, 2014.

[7] H. Nakasuka, S. Okada, T. Okusaka et al., "Undifferentiated carcinoma of the liver with neuroendocrine features: a case report," *Japanese Journal of Clinical Oncology*, vol. 28, no. 6, pp. 401–404, 1998.

[8] A. W. H. Chan, J. H. M. Tong, M. Y. M. Sung, P. B. S. Lai, and K.-F. To, "Epstein-Barr virus-associated lymphoepithelioma-like cholangiocarcinoma: a rare variant of intrahepatic cholangiocarcinoma with favourable outcome," *Histopathology*, vol. 65, no. 5, pp. 674–683, 2014.

[9] M. W. Si, J. A. Thorson, G. Y. Lauwers, P. Dalcin, and J. Furman, "Hepatocellular lymphoepithelioma-like carcinoma associated with Epstein barr virus," *Diagnostic Molecular Pathology*, vol. 13, no. 3, pp. 183–189, 2004.

[10] T.-C. Liao, C. A. Liu, N. C. Chiu, Y. C. Yeh, and Y. Y. Chiou, "Lymphoepithelioma-like cholangiocarcinoma: a mimic of hepatocellular carcinoma on imaging features," *World Journal of Gastroenterology*, vol. 21, no. 13, pp. 4089–4095, 2015.

[11] Y. Futsukaichi, K. Tajiri, S. Kobayashi et al., "Combined hepatocellular-cholangiocarcinoma successfully treated with sorafenib: case report and review of the literature," *Clinical Journal of Gastroenterology*, vol. 12, no. 2, pp. 128–134, 2019.

[12] S. Singh, S. Chakraborty, N. Bonthu, S. Radio, S. M. Hussain, and A. Sasson, "Combined hepatocellular cholangiocarcinoma: a case report and review of literature," *Digestive Diseases and Sciences*, vol. 58, no. 7, pp. 2114–2123, 2013.

[13] P. Sakhuja, P. K. Mishra, R. Rajesh, A. K. Sharma, R. Gondal, and M. Singh, "Clear cell hepatocellular carcinoma: back to the basics for diagnosis," *Journal of Cancer Research and Therapeutics*, vol. 11, no. 3, p. 656, 2015.

[14] J. Albores-Saavedra, M. P. Hoang, L. A. Murakata, P. Sinkre, and H. Yaziji, "Atypical bile duct adenoma, clear cell type,"

The American Journal of Surgical Pathology, vol. 25, no. 7, pp. 956–960, 2001.
[15] F. Chablé-Montero, A. Shah BS, D. Montante-Montes de Oca, A. Ángeles-Ángeles, D. E. Henson, and J. Albores-Saavedra, "Thyroid-like cholangiocarcinoma of the liver: an unusual morphologic variant with follicular, trabecular and insular patterns," *Annals of Hepatology*, vol. 11, no. 6, pp. 961–965, 2012.
[16] A. Fornelli, A. Bondi, E. Jovine, and V. Eusebi, "Intrahepatic cholangiocarcinoma resembling a thyroid follicular neoplasm," *Virchows Archiv*, vol. 456, no. 3, pp. 339–342, 2010.
[17] I. Pecorella, A. Ciardi, E. Aiello, M. R. Piras, C. Farci, and U. Di Tondo, "Clear cell hepatocellular carcinoma treated with liver transplantation," *Pathologica*, vol. 86, no. 3, pp. 307–310, 1994.
[18] E. Toriyama, A. Nanashina, H. Hayashi et al., "A case of intrahepatic clear cell cholangiocarcinoma," *World Journal of Gastroenterology*, vol. 16, no. 20, pp. 2571–2576, 2010.
[19] J. P. Kothadia, N. Kaur, R. Arju, M. Dakhel, and S. Giashuddin, "Primary clear cell carcinoma of the non-cirrhotic liver presenting as an acute abdomen: a case report and review of the literature," *Journal of Gastrointestinal Cancer*, vol. 48, no. 2, pp. 211–216, 2017.
[20] N. Mittal, M. Bal, M. Ramadwar, S. Patkar, and M. Goel, "Pathologic doppelgänger: thyroid? like intrahepatic cholangiocarcinoma with synchronous primary thyroid carcinoma in a young woman," *Annals of Hepato-Biliary-Pancreatic Surgery*, vol. 24, no. 2, pp. 182–187, 2020.
[21] S.-H. Chen, Z.-Y. Zheng, H. L. Wang et al., "Thyroid-like intrahepatic cholangiocarcinoma: report of a case and review of the literature," *International Journal of Surgical Pathology*, vol. 26, no. 7, pp. 649–654, 2018.
[22] M. Hiraki, K. Kitahara, A. Miyoshi et al., "A long-term survivor of undifferentiated carcinoma of the liver successfully treated with surgical treatments: a case report and literature review," *International Journal of Surgery Case Reports*, vol. 51, pp. 45–49, 2018.
[23] T. Maeda, H. Kayashima, and D. Imai, "Undifferentiated carcinoma of the liver: a case report with immunohistochemical analysis," *Surgical Case Reports*, vol. 3, no. 1, p. 12, 2017.

29

IgG4-Related Hepatic Pseudotumor Masquerading as a Klatskin Tumor

Jennifer Yoon[1], Steve Hu,[2] Daniel Phillips,[3] Amir Fathi,[4] and Adnan Ameer[2]

[1]*Department of Internal Medicine, University of California, Fresno, CA, USA*
[2]*Department of Gastroenterology and Hepatology, University of California, Fresno, CA, USA*
[3]*Department of Pathology, Community Regional Medical Center, Fresno, CA, USA*
[4]*Department of Surgery, University of California, Fresno, CA, USA*

Correspondence should be addressed to Jennifer Yoon; jennifer.yoon@ucsf.edu

Academic Editor: Zu-Yau Lin

Immunoglobulin G subclass 4 (IgG-4)-related disease (IgG4-RD) is an uncommon immune-mediated, fibro-inflammatory disease which has garnered recognition as a systemic condition. One manifestation of the disease in the hepatobiliary system is the development of hepatic inflammatory pseudotumors. These benign tumors are often misdiagnosed as malignant tumors and undergo unnecessary hepatic resections. We present a case of IgG4-related hepatic inflammatory pseudotumor (IPT) mimicking a Klatskin tumor. A high degree of clinical suspicion and extensive workup is imperative in reaching the correct diagnosis. IgG4-related inflammatory pseudotumor is a rare entity, but an important consideration in evaluating hepatic tumors.

1. Introduction

Inflammatory pseudotumors are benign, mass-forming lesions that consist of inflammatory cells, fibrous tissue, and myofibroblasts and are often mistaken for malignant tumors [1, 2]. They are commonly misconstrued as pancreatic cancer, Klatskin tumors, and lymphomas [3]. Hepatic IPTs can be due to viral or bacterial infections, congenital disease, gallstones, chronic biliary inflammation, and IgG4- related disease (IgG4-RD) [4]. IgG4-related hepatic IPTs are uncommon; differentiation from malignant tumors is crucial for management and avoiding unnecessary resection. Here, we describe a case of an IgG4-related hepatic IPT mimicking a Klatskin tumor.

2. Case Description

A 59-year-old incarcerated male with human immunodeficiency virus on highly active antiretroviral therapy presented with abdominal pain and jaundice. His liver panel was notably abnormal, with alkaline phosphatase 344 U/L (25–100 U/L), ALT 61 U/L (10–40 U/L), AST 44 U/L (8–40 U/L), total bilirubin 11.3 mg/dL (0.3–1.2 mg/dL), and direct bilirubin 7.2 mg/dL (0.0–0.4 mg/dL). An initial computed tomography (CT) scan revealed an amorphous-appearing pancreatic head mass with dilated intra- and extrahepatic bile ducts. A serum IgG4 level measured 354 mg/dL (4–86 mg/dL), and cancer antigen (CA) 19–9 was 97.9 U/ml (0–35.0 U/mL). Endoscopic ultrasound (EUS)-guided fine needle biopsy of the pancreatic head mass was performed. Pathology was consistent with type I autoimmune pancreatitis by immunohistochemistry, and no malignant cells were identified. Due to significant biliary obstruction, he underwent an endoscopic retrograde cholangiopancreatography (ERCP) with stenting of the distal inflammatory biliary stricture and initiated prednisone therapy with an extended taper, resulting in subsequent normalization of CT findings and liver labs.

Two years later, he again presented with similar symptoms. His liver enzymes were again elevated in a cholestatic pattern with a total bilirubin of 4.0 mg/dL, and his serum IgG4 was 458.9 mg/dL. The CT scan showed a mass-like mural thickening at the hepatic hilum concerning for a Klatskin tumor (Figure 1). EUS confirmed an irregular hypoechoic mass in the porta hepatis measuring 4.1×2.7 cm

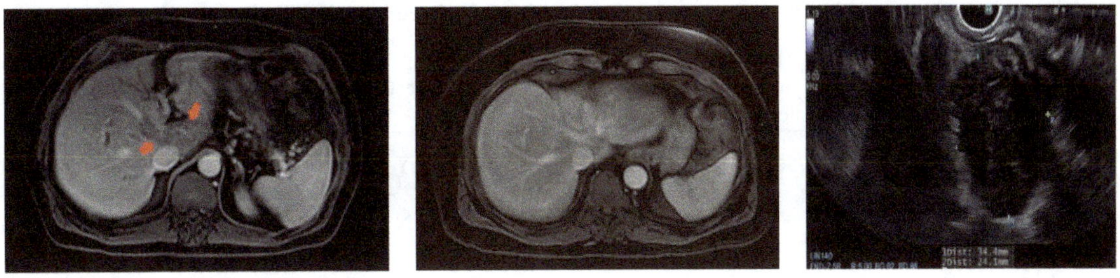

(a) (b) (c)

FIGURE 1: (a) Magnetic resonance imaging (MRI) of the abdomen demonstrating hepatic IPT prior to treatment with steroid taper. (b) MRI of the abdomen after treatment showing complete resolution of hepatic IPT. (c) Endoscopic ultrasound demonstrating a periportal mass.

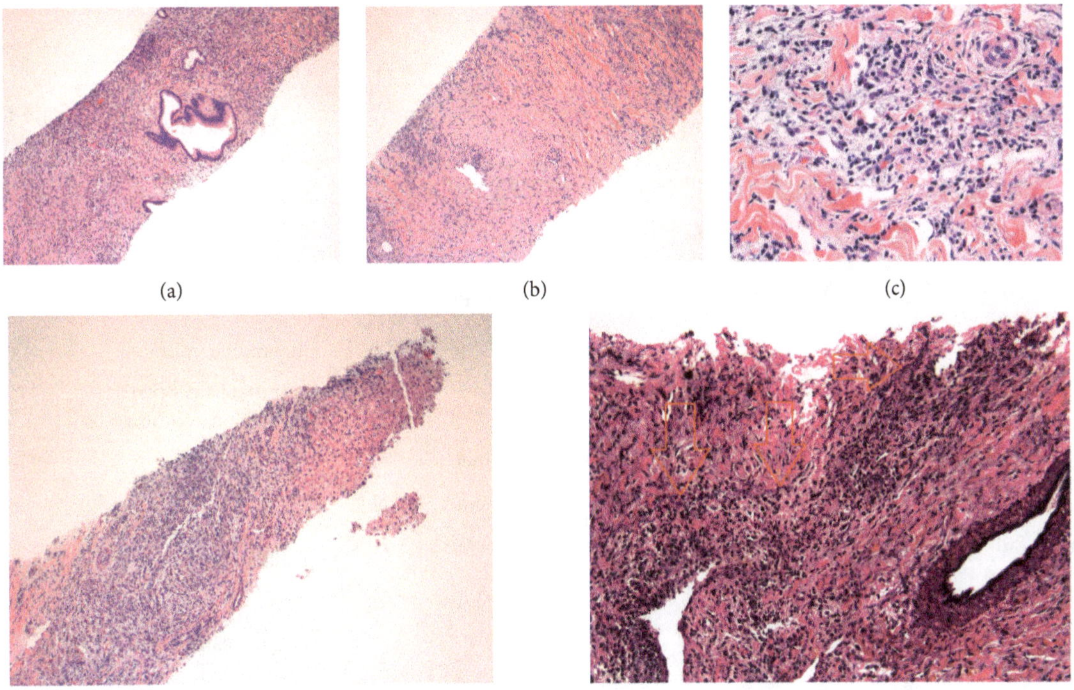

(a) (b) (c) (d) (e)

FIGURE 2: (a–d) Hepatocellular parenchyma with a mixed predominately mononuclear inflammatory infiltrate and reactive fibrosis, with residual bile duct elements present. (c) 400x total magnification; infiltrate is mainly comprised of lymphocytes and plasma cells. (d) The interface of the inflammatory process with background liver tissue. (e) Arrows highlight the residual elastic lamina.

(Figure 1). Histopathology showed dense lymphoplasmacytic infiltrating and a fibrosing process with residual bland pancreatic ducts and lobules. Immunohistochemistry demonstrated IgG4 plasma cell positivity (>10 per high-power field (HPF)). A subsequent CT-guided biopsy of the hilar mass also confirmed IgG4-positive plasma cells and obliterative phlebitis, consistent with IgG4 -associated hepatic IPT (Figure 2). He was again treated with a tapered course of prednisone with repeat imaging showing complete resolution of the pseudotumor.

3. Discussion

IgG4-RD is a chronic, immune-mediated, fibro-inflammatory disease that can involve multiple organ systems and often mimics malignancy, infection, or infiltrative disease. It is predominant in middle-aged to elderly men and commonly affects the pancreas, salivary glands, orbit, kidneys, and retroperitoneum [5, 6]. Diagnosis is based on a comprehensive workup of serology, imaging, histopathology, and response to steroids. While a histologic diagnosis was previously required, a clinical diagnosis can now be made using the 2019 American College of Rheumatology (ACR)/European League Against Rheumatism (EULAR) Executive Committee classification criteria [7]. Patients who meet the entry criteria in the absence of the exclusion criteria with a score of ≥20 are classified as having IgG4-RD, our patient scored a total of 38 points [7]. Histologically characteristic findings of IgG4-RD include a lymphoplasmacytic infiltrate, heavy IgG4-positive plasma cell infiltration, storiform fibrosis, and obliterative phlebitis [4, 7]. The most common manifestation of IgG4-RD in the hepatobiliary system is

Table 1: The literature review of reported IgG4-related hepatic IPTs to date.

Author	Year	Age	Sex	Tumor number/ location	Biopsy	Biopsy method	Resection	Initial diagnostic impression	Serum IgG4
Adachi K [14]	2017	60	M	1/Segment 3	N		Y	Hepatic cancer	Elevated
Adachi Y [15]	2020	80s	F	1	Y	Unspecified	N	Hepatic IPT	Elevated
Ahn KS [9]	2012	58	M	1			Y	Recurrence of Klatskin tumor	
		60	M	1			Y	Malignancy	
		76	M	2			N	Hepatic IPT	
		52	M	1			N	Hepatic IPT	
Buchter M [16]	2018	58	M		Y	Unspecified	N	Hodgkin's lymphoma	2528
Chia JS [17]	2020	53	M		N		Y		
Chung JW [18]	2019	67	M	1	Y	Percutaneous	Y	Abscess, cancer	2215
Fujisaki H [19]	2016	75	F	1/Segment 7	N		Y	Hepatic IPT	Serum normal, bx elevated
Hamano A [6]	2020	71	M	1/Segment 3	Y	Percutaneous	N	Hepatic cholangiocarcinoma	180
Hastir D [20]	2013	50	F	1/Segment 5	N		Y	Hepatocellular carcinoma	
Horiguchi S [21]	2012	76	M	1/Segment 2	Y	Laparoscopic	N		819
Itazaki Y [2]	2021	75	F	1			Y	Cholangiocarcinoma	
Kanno a [22]	2005	48	M		N		Y	Liver metastasis from cholangiocarcinoma	2150
Kataoka K [23]	2017	79	M		Y	Unspecified	N		Elevated
Kim F [24]	2011	58	M	1/Segment 4	Y	Percutaneous	N		1470
Lee YS [25]	2013	59	M	1/Segment 5	Y	Percutaneous	N	Inoperable gallbladder cancer	75
Legkiy O [26]	2019	60	M	2/Segment 2 & 6	Y	Percutaneous	Y		19.1
Matsuo Y [27]	2014	74	M	1/Segment 8	N		Y	Liver metastasis from GIST	
Miyajima S [28]	2017	50	F	1	Y	Unspecified	N	Cholangiocarcinoma	241
Mulki R [29]	2015	50	M	2	N		Y	Abscess with impending rupture	>182
Naitoh I [30]	2009	77	M	1/Segment 3	N		Y	Intrahepatic cholangitis	231
Patel H [10]	2018	48	M	1	Y	Unspecified	N		2228
Shibata M [4]	2016	72	M	1/Segment 7	Y	Percutaneous	N		137
Uchida K [31]	2007	54	M	1/Segment 4	Y	Unspecified	N	Pancreatic cancer with liver metastasis	213
Vadi S [32]	2018	54	M	1/ Gallbladder fossa	Y	Unspecified	N		356
Wang M [33]	2020	78	M	1/Segment 4	N		Y	Cholangiocarcinoma	
Yang L [34]	2015	60	M	1/Segment 3	Y	Unspecified	N		1590
Yueh HZ [35]	2021	47	M	Multiple	Y	Percutaneous	N	Metastatic cancer	1786

Zen Y(16 cases) [36]	1990–2005	Avg 67 (56–82)	11M 5F	N	Y	(All resected)	Hilar cholangiocarcinoma (8), intrahepatic cholangiocarcinoma (5), malignant hepatic tumor, undetermined origin (2), metastatic carcinoma (1)

cholangitis; rarely, hepatic IPTs can develop as a late-stage manifestation of the disease [8]. Due to the mass-forming nature of these lesions and nonspecific findings on imaging, these benign tumors are often mistaken for malignant tumors.

Traditionally, the first-line treatment has been systemic steroids, although some cases report spontaneous resolution [9,10]. Treatment is indicated for symptomatic patients or asymptomatic patients with progressive disease. Early recognition and prompt treatment are preferred due to concern for end-organ damage. Weight-based dosing of steroids, typically prednisone, is used to induce remission usually at a dose of 0.6 mg/kg/day for 2–4 weeks and gradually tapered off over the course of months depending on response to therapy [8, 11]. Use of systemic steroids may be limited due to side effects including poor glycemic control, infection, and weight gain [4]. Immunosuppressive agents such as rituximab, azathioprine, or mycophenolate mofetil may be used as adjunct agents for patient's intolerant systemic steroids due to significant side effects, nonresponse, or relapsing disease [8, 11]. More recently, rituximab has emerged as the preferred treatment due to a better side-effect profile with comparable efficacy to systemic steroids [12, 13].

Misclassification of hepatic IPTs for malignant tumors has resulted in unnecessary hepatic resections. IgG4-related hepatic IPTs are predominant in middle-aged to elderly males, a demographic which is more likely to lead physicians to suspect underlying malignancy. Our literature review has shown a total of 46 (36 males and 10 females) reported cases of hepatic IPTs, excluding this case (Table 1). Of the reported cases, initial diagnostic impressions were widely variable. Approximately 67% of the reported cases perceived the pseudotumor to be an underlying malignancy resulting in resections in 81% of cases. Of the 46 reported cases, 16 cases underwent a biopsy. Despite a negative biopsy result, still 12.5% of these cases underwent unnecessary liver resections. Of the patients who underwent biopsy with confirmed histopathologic diagnosis, 87.5% were spared surgical resections.

IgG4-related hepatic IPTs are rare and pose a diagnostic challenge given their resemblance to malignant tumors. A high degree of clinical suspicion and thorough workup is imperative in preventing patient harm from unnecessary resections. An accurate diagnosis can be established through tissue sampling with biopsy, and subsequently, hepatic resections can be circumvented. Our case details the definitive diagnosis and treatment of IgG4-associated hepatic IPT with successful avoidance of surgery. In addition, as IgG4-RD is a chronic disease, the development of the hepatic IPT may have been avoidable if the patient had been diagnosed with IgG4-RD at his first presentation and was sustained on maintenance therapy.

References

[1] S. Ichikawa, U. Motosugi, T. Suzuki, T. Shimizu, and H. Onishi, "Imaging features of hepatic inflammatory pseudotumor: distinction from colorectal liver metastasis using gadoxetate disodium-enhanced magnetic resonance imaging," *Abdom Radiol*, vol. 45, no. 8, pp. 2400–2408, 2020.

[2] Y. Itazaki, T. Einama, F. Konno et al., "IgG4-related hepatic inflammatory pseudotumor mimicking cholangiolocellular carcinoma," *Clinical Journal of Gastroenterology*, vol. 14, no. 6, pp. 1733–1739, 2021.

[3] W. Zhou, T. Murray, L. Cartagena et al., "IgG-4-Related disease as mimicker of malignancy," *SN Comprehensive Clinical Medicine*, vol. 3, no. 9, pp. 1904–1913, 2021.

[4] M. Shibata, H. Matsubayashi, T. Aramaki et al., "A case of IgG4-related hepatic inflammatory pseudotumor replaced by an abscess after steroid treatment," *BMC Gastroenterology*, vol. 16, no. 1, p. 89, 2016.

[5] A. Chougule and A. Bal, "IgG4-related inflammatory pseudotumor: a systematic review of histopathological features of reported cases," *Modern Rheumatology*, vol. 27, no. 2, pp. 320–325, 2016.

[6] A. Hamano, R. Yamada, K. Kurata et al., "Difficulty in differentiating between IgG4-related hepatic inflammatory pseudotumor and intrahepatic cholangiocarcinoma," *Clinical Journal of Gastroenterology*, vol. 14, no. 1, pp. 263–268, 2021.

[7] Z. S. Wallace, R. P. Naden, S. Chari et al., "The 2019 American College of Rheumatology/European League against rheumatism classification criteria for IgG4-related disease," *Annals of the Rheumatic Diseases*, vol. 79, no. 1, pp. 77–87, 2020.

[8] J. M. Lohr, U. Beuers, M. Vujasinovic et al., "European guideline on IgG4-related digestive disease - UEG and SGF evidence-based recommendations," *United European Gastroenterology Journal*, vol. 8, no. 6, pp. 637–666, 2020.

[9] K. S. Ahn, K. J. Kang, Y. H. Kim et al., "Inflammatory pseudotumors mimicking intrahepatic cholangiocarcinoma of the liver; IgG4-positivity and its clinical significance," *Journal of Hepato-Biliary-Pancreatic Sciences*, vol. 19, no. 4, pp. 405–412, 2011.

[10] H. Patel, S. Nanavati, J. Ha, A. Shah, and W. Baddoura, "Spontaneous resolution of IgG4-related hepatic inflammatory pseudotumor mimicking malignancy," *Case Reports in Gastroenterology*, vol. 12, no. 2, pp. 311–316, 2018.

[11] T. Kamisawa and K. Okazaki, "Diagnosis and treatment of IgG4-related disease," *Current Topics in Microbiology and Immunology*, vol. 401, pp. 19–33, 2017.

[12] MN. Carruthers, MD. Topazian, A. Khosroshahi et al., "Rituximab for IgG4-related disease: a prospective, open-label trial," *Annals of the Rheumatic Diseases*, vol. 74, no. 6,

[13] CA. Perugino and J. H. Stone, "Treatment of IgG4-related disease," *Zeitschrift für Rheumatologie*, vol. 75, no. 7, pp. 681–686, 2016.

[14] K. Adachi, K. Hashimoto, R. Nonaka et al., "[A case of an IgG4-related inflammatory pseudotumor of the liver showing enlargement that was difficult to differentiate from hepatic cancer]," *Gan To Kagaku Ryoho*, vol. 44, no. 12, pp. 1922–1924, 2017.

[15] Y. Adachi, N. Iwata, Y. Adachi et al., "[Coexistence of IgG4-pseudotumors of the liver:a case report]," *Journal of the Japanese Society of Gastroenterology*, vol. 117, no. 6, pp. 532–541, 2020.

[16] M. Büchter, G. Gerken, and A. Kahraman, "IgG4-associated inflammatory pseudotumor with bilobar hepatic foci," *Dtsch Arztebl Int*, vol. 115, no. 11, p. 181, 2018.

[17] J. S. Chia, H. Y. Chen, C. M. Ho, Y. M. Jeng, and H. L. Chen, "Existence of follicular helper T cells in an isolated IgG4-related hepatic inflammatory pseudotumor," *Journal of Gastrointestinal and Liver Diseases*, vol. 29, no. 4, p. 499, 2020.

[18] J. W. Chung, Y. S. Bae, J. H. Lim, D. K. Lee, and J. S. Yu, "IgG-4 related hepatic inflammatory pseudotumor complicated by actinomycosis during steroid therapy," *Journal of the Korean Society of Radiology*, vol. 80, no. 2, p. 351, 2019.

[19] H. Fujisaki, N. Ito, E. Takahashi et al., "A case of inflammatory pseudotumor of the liver with tumor enlargement," *Nihon Gekakei Rengo Gakkaishi (Journal of Japanese College of Surgeons)*, vol. 41, no. 1, pp. 105–109, 2016.

[20] D. Hastir, L. Verset, V. Lucidi, and P Demetter, "IgG4 positive lymphoplasmacytic inflammatory pseudotumour mimicking hepatocellular carcinoma," *Liver International*, vol. 34, no. 6, p. 961, 2013.

[21] S. Horiguchi, F. Ikeda, H. Shiraha et al., "Diagnostic usefulness of precise examinations with intraductal ultrasonography, peroral cholangioscopy and laparoscopy of immunoglobulin G4-related sclerosing cholangitis," *Digestive Endoscopy*, vol. 24, no. 5, pp. 370–373, 2012.

[22] A. Kanno, K. Satoh, K. Kimura et al., "Autoimmune pancreatitis with hepatic inflammatory pseudotumor," *Pancreas*, vol. 31, no. 4, pp. 420–423, 2005.

[23] K. Kataoka and K. Achiwa, "[Autoimmune pancreatitis and IgG4-related hepatic inflammatory pseudotumor complicated by an impacted pancreatic stone at the major papilla during steroid treatment]," *Journal of the Japanese Society of Gastroenterology*, vol. 114, no. 12, pp. 2158–2166, 2017.

[24] F. Kim, K. Yamada, D. Inoue et al., "IgG4-related tubulointerstitial nephritis and hepatic inflammatory pseudotumor without hypocomplementemia," *Internal Medicine*, vol. 50, no. 11, pp. 1239–1244, 2011.

[25] Y. S. Lee, S. H. Lee, M. G. Lee et al., "Immunoglobulin G4-related disease mimicking unresectable gallbladder cancer," *Gut and Liver*, vol. 7, no. 5, pp. 616–620, 2013.

[26] O. Legkiy, J. Wajda, A. Cwierz, J. Wysocka, and A. L. Komorowski, "Hepatic inflammatory pseudotumor related with IgG4," *Gastroenterología y Hepatología*, vol. 42, no. 3, pp. 176-177, 2019.

[27] Y. Matsuo, M. Sato, T. Shibata et al., "Inflammatory pseudotumor of the liver diagnosed as metastatic liver tumor in a patient with a gastrointestinal stromal tumor of the rectum: report of a case," *World Journal of Surgical Oncology*, vol. 12, no. 1, p. 140, 2014.

[28] S. Miyajima, A. Okano, and M. OHana, "Immunoglobulin G4-related hepatic inflammatory pseudotumor invading the abdominal wall," *Clinical Journal of Gastroenterology*, vol. 10, no. 1, pp. 57–62, 2017.

[29] R. Mulki, S. Garg, W. Manatsathit, and R Miick, "IgG4-related inflammatory pseudotumour mimicking a hepatic abscess impending rupture," *BMJ Case Reports*, vol. 2015, Article ID bcr2015211893, 2015.

[30] I. Naitoh, T. Nakazawa, H. Ohara et al., "IgG4-related hepatic inflammatory pseudotumor with sclerosing cholangitis: a case report and review of the literature," *Cases Journal*, vol. 2, p. 7029, 2009.

[31] K. Uchida, S. Satoi, H. Miyoshi et al., "Inflammatory pseudotumors of the pancreas and liver with infiltration of IgG4-positive plasma cells," *Internal Medicine*, vol. 46, no. 17, pp. 1409–1412, 2007.

[32] S. K. Vadi, R. Kumar, B. R. Mittal et al., "18F-FDG PET/CT in an atypical case of relapsed IgG4-related disease presenting as inflammatory pseudotumor in gall bladder fossa with extensive disease involvement," *Clinical Nuclear Medicine*, vol. 43, no. 10, pp. e357–e359, 2018.

[33] M. Wang, S. Zhang, and Q. Yang, "IgG4-Related hepatic inflammatory pseudotumor misdiagnosed as cholangiocellular carcinoma of the liver," *Journal of Gastrointestinal Surgery*, vol. 25, no. 4, pp. 1065-1066, 2021.

[34] L. Yang, P. Jin, and J. Q. Sheng, "Immunoglobulin G4-related disease (IgG4-RD) affecting the esophagus, stomach, and liver," *Endoscopy*, vol. 47, no. S 01, pp. E96–E97, 2015.

[35] H. Z. Yueh, K. K. Tung, and C. Tung, "IgG4-Related pseudotumors mimicking metastases in liver and lungs," *Case Rep Gastroenterol*, vol. 15, no. 1, pp. 163–170, 2021.

[36] Y. Zen, T. Fujii, Y. Sato, S. Masuda, and Y. Nakanuma, "Pathological classification of hepatic inflammatory pseudotumor with respect to IgG4-related disease," *Modern Pathology*, vol. 20, no. 8, pp. 884–894, 2007.

30

A Severe Case of Drug-Induced Liver Injury after Gemcitabine Administration: A Highly Probable Causality Grading as Assessed by the Updated RUCAM Diagnostic Scoring System

Ilenia Mascherona ,[1] Caterina Maggioli,[2] Maira Biggiogero,[3] Oreste Mora,[4] and Lucia Marelli[4]

[1]*Ospedale La Carità, Medicina Interna, Locarno, Switzerland*
[2]*AUSL di Bologna, Ospedale di Budrio, Bologna, Italy*
[3]*Clinica Luganese Moncucco, Unità di Ricerca Clinica, Lugano, Switzerland*
[4]*Clinica Luganese Moncucco, Oncologia Medica, Lugano, Switzerland*

Correspondence should be addressed to Ilenia Mascherona; ilenia.mascherona@eoc.ch

Academic Editor: Julio M. F. Chebli

Gemcitabine is an antineoplastic drug used in several forms of advanced pancreatic, lung, breast, ovarian, and bladder cancer. Common side effects include bone marrow suppression, fatigue, diarrhea, nausea, gastrointestinal upset, rash, alopecia, and stomatitis. Transient serum enzyme elevations could be observed during therapy, but clinically significant acute liver injury has been rarely associated with its use. Few cases of acute liver injury have been reported in the literature. We reported the clinical case of a 73--year-old man who developed clinically significant acute hepatic injury after using gemcitabine. Possible causes, clinical presentation, and treatments are discussed. According to the updated RUCAM score, the case was rated 10 points and became a suspected drug-induced liver injury. Moreover, on the liver biopsy, there were histological findings of mild-to-moderate portal hepatitis, eosinophilia, bile duct injury, and mild perisinusoidal fibrosis, suggesting drug damage.

1. Introduction

Gemcitabine is a cytosine analog [1, 2] which is used as an antineoplastic drug in the therapy of several forms of advanced pancreatic, lung, breast, ovarian, and bladder cancer. Common side effects include bone marrow suppression, fatigue, flu-like symptoms, diarrhea, nausea, gastrointestinal upset, and stomatitis.

Gemcitabine could be associated with transient serum enzyme elevations during therapy, but it is rarely a cause of acute, clinically apparent liver injury [3, 4]. Elevations in serum aminotransferase levels occur in 30% to 90% of patients [5–7]. These elevations are generally mild to moderate [8], asymptomatic, and self-limited, frequently resolving without discontinuation of the therapy. Serum bilirubin and alkaline phosphatase elevations are less common, but typically transient and mild. Few cases of acute hepatic injury due to gemcitabine have been reported. The clinical features of gemcitabine hepatotoxicity are not well described. Gemcitabine modification or discontinuation is considered only in drug-induced liver injury (DILI) cases.

We describe the case of a 73-year-old man who developed a DILI after gemcitabine treatment. A few DILI cases due to gemcitabine administration have been reported, most of them in patients with underlying chronic liver disease or extensive hepatic metastases [9–11].

Patient demographic data, details of diagnosis and treatment, and laboratory and radiological investigations were collected by the DPI electronic database of Clinica Luganese Moncucco (CLM), Lugano. The patient gave his informed consent before any data were entered into the database.

2. Case Presentation

On 21st September 2018, a 73-year-old man was admitted in the Department of Oncology of CLM for jaundice, itching, acholic feces, and hyperchromic urine. He was recently diagnosed with an urothelial carcinoma and treated with neoadjuvant chemotherapy (carboplatin and gemcitabine). One week before the admission, the patient reported an episode of diarrhea after eating cooked fish. The patient denied alcohol consumption and psychotropic drugs and herbal product assumption. He took his usual drug therapy (described in the following) and no other drugs.

On physical examination, the patient was alert, oriented to person, time, and place. Vital signs were normal, and body temperature was normal. The cutaneous examination revealed jaundice. No jugular turgescence, peripheral edema, flapping tremor, or hepatosplenomegaly was found. The rest of the clinical examination was without any particularities.

The patient's medical history reported benign prostatic hyperplasia, chronic gastritis, diverticulosis, right glaucoma, and iodinated contrast urticaria. His usual therapy was pantoprazole (40 mg/d), tamsulosin (400 mcg/d), and timolol (1 drop 2 times a day). On July 2018, a papillary urothelial carcinoma was diagnosed. This cancer infiltrated the bladder muscolaris propria, caused a perineural invasion, and was poorly differentiated (stage pT2N0M0, G3).

On 10th of August 2018, oncologists indicated neoadjuvant chemotherapy with carboplatin 5 AUC d1 and gemcitabine 1000 mg/sqm d1 and d8 every 21 days. Carboplatin was administered on the 10th and 31st of August, and gemcitabine was administered on the 10th, 17th, and 31st of August.

At admission, laboratory findings showed normocytic normochromic anemia (113 g/l); white blood cells and platelets were within normal limits. High hyperbilirubinemia (6.37 mg/dl) with a prevalence of conjugated bilirubin (5.96 mg/dl) and hypertransaminasemia (AST 82 U/l and ALT 158 U/l) were observed/found. Cholestasis enzymes were increased (ALP 407 U/l and GGT 186 U/l), and the ammonia level was high (134.54 ug/dl). Albumin level was within normal limits. No coagulation, renal, or electrolyte abnormalities were found (see Table 1).

A differential diagnosis of hepatitis was quickly started. Viral (HAV, HBV, HCV, HDV, HEV, CMV, and EBV) and autoimmune (ANA, ENA, ANCA, ASMA, AMA, anti-SLA/LP, anti-LC1, and anti-LKM immunoglobulins) hepatitis serology was performed with negative results. The celiac disease profile was negative. Alpha-1-antitrypsin, ceruloplasmin, carbohydrate-deficient transferrin (CDT), IgA, and alpha-fetoprotein (AFP) were normal. An abdominal CT scan and a magnetic resonance cholangiopancreatography (MRCP) were performed showing only an hepatic hemangioma of the VIII segment.

During the hospitalization, a symptomatic therapy with levocetirizine and dexamethasone was successfully carried out. On 24th September 2018, the patient was discharged with mild symptoms and improved laboratory findings (see Table 1).

No etiology was found, and an adverse drug reaction (ADR) was supposed. Hepatology consultation was performed, and chemotherapy (especially gemcitabine) was taken into account as a hepatitis cause. Gemcitabine was interrupted, and the patient underwent a liver biopsy. It suggested a drug injury, characterized by mild-to-moderate portal hepatitis, eosinophilia, bile duct injury, and mild perisinusoidal fibrosis (see Figure 1).

One month later, the patient was re-evaluated on an oncological check-up and showed a good health condition. There was no jaundice; urine and stools were normalized, and pruritus was resolved. Liver values were completely normalized, and an abdomen CT scan confirmed the absence of abnormalities.

3. Discussion

Drug-induced liver injury (DILI) is a common liver disease which generally occurs between several days and few months after drug ingestion [12]. It is a common side effect that often leads pharmaceutical companies to withdraw the responsible drug from the market [13]. Its prevalence is between 1 and 20 in 100,000 or less in developed countries [14]. Several risk factors are associated with the development of DILI [15]. For instance, it has been shown that adults are more at risk than children and women who seem to be more susceptible than men. Potentially, all drugs can be involved in DILI development, but it is more commonly experienced with acetaminophen [16, 17], antibiotics [18], NSAIDS, statins, antiplatelets, and immunosuppressant administration.

The clinical manifestations of DILI are usually nonspecific. The majority of patients manifests liver biochemical index abnormalities. Some patients might express unspecific symptoms such as fatigue, low-grade fever, anorexia, nausea, vomiting, liver pain, and epigastric discomfort. Besides, the patient with obvious cholestasis could manifest jaundice, itching, acholic stools, and hyperchromic urine. Rarely, the patient can experience hepatic failure. Hepatomegaly may be present on physical examination. In severe cases, coagulopathy and hepatic encephalopathy may develop, indicating acute liver failure. In acute DILI, the liver indexes are impaired for less than three months. In chronic DILI, instead, liver values remain altered for more than three months [19]. Chronic DILI may lead to fibrosis or cirrhosis and could have signs and symptoms associated with cirrhosis or hepatic decompensation [20–23]. The presence of jaundice, a double value of bilirubinemia, and an increase in transaminases are associated with a worse prognosis [24].

According to the pathogenesis, DILI can be classified into 2 types: intrinsic and idiosyncratic. The latter is more frequent, is not related to drug dosage, and has variable latency periods. The hypothesized mechanisms underlying hepatotoxicity include cell membrane destruction and cell death, development of an immunological reaction, inhibition of cellular metabolism pathways, abnormal bile flow, apoptosis, and inhibition of mitochondrial function.

According to the pattern of observed liver tests, there are 3 types of DILI: hepatocellular (hepatitis damage), cholestatic (biliary tract damage), and mixed, which was proposed

Table 1: Patient liver values from hospitalization up to the follow-up.

	23.10.18	11.10.18	03.10.18	28.09.18	24.09.18	23.09.18	22.09.18	21.09.18
Total bilirubin (<1.23 mg/dl)	1.12	2.02	3.64	7.49	6.67	6.08	6.37	6.78
Direct bilirubin (<0.29 mg/dl)	—	1.74	3.12	6.55	5.96	5.64	5.96	5.77
Aspartate aminotransferase (10–50 U/L)	24	61	100	154	94	88	82	76
Alanine transaminase (10–50 U/L)	46	158	329	325	182	167	158	161
Alkaline phosphatase (40–129 U/L)	108	199	292	347	381	385	407	444
Albumin (35–52 g/L)	40	36	36	36	34	—	—	37

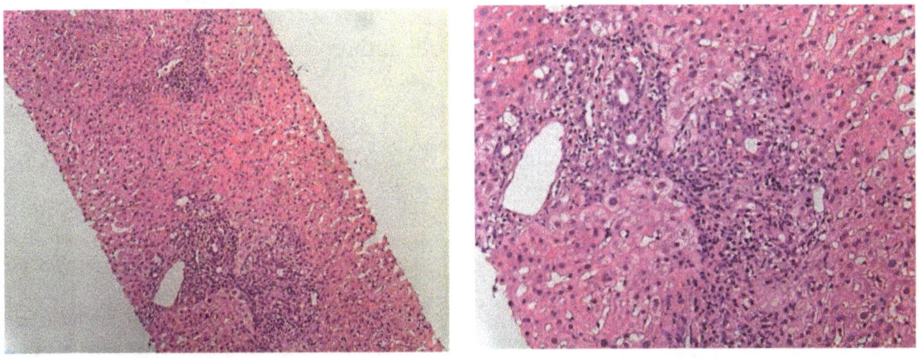

(a) (b)

Figure 1: (a) Performed liver biopsy which showed mild-to-moderate portal hepatitis with interface component, minimal lobular component, eosinophilia, bile duct injury, and mild perisinusoidal fibrosis. (b) Magnification.

by the Roussel Uclaf Causality Assessment Method (RUCAM) [12, 25]. DILI cholestasis is defined as an alanine aminotransferase (ALT) to alkaline phosphatase (ALP) ratio of less than 2. Injury is considered to be mixed if the ALT/ALP ratio is greater than 2 but less than 5 and hepatocellular if this ratio is >5.

Since there are no diagnostic tests or specific biomarkers for DILI, its diagnosis is made by exclusion of other causes of liver disease, including viral and autoimmune hepatitis, bile duct obstruction, hepatic ischemia, sepsis, and metabolic disorders. The updated RUCAM diagnostic criteria [12, 25] are also helpful: it stratifies the causal correlation between drugs and liver injury into 4 levels, high probable: score > 8, probable: $6 \leq$ score ≤ 8, possible: $3 \leq$ score $\leq$, and unlikely: $1 \leq$ score ≤ 2. Combined with these criteria, the diagnosis of DILI must rely on medical anamnesis and all clinical data. When necessary, DILI could be confirmed by liver biopsy.

If DILI is suspected, the primary treatment is the withdrawal of the offending drug. Thereafter, the patient should be treated on a symptomatic level. After the drug removal, the majority of patients clearly improved. 5 to 10% of cholestatic/mixed types of DILI, instead, progress to chronic disease [26].

DILI patients should be followed up with serial biochemical measurements until complete liver test resolution. Hepatology consultation should be considered in front of acute liver failure.

In our case report, the patient was a 73-year-old man who developed hepatitis with jaundice. He was treated with gemcitabine 21 days before his admission to CLM. Viral and autoimmune hepatitis and other hepatitis etiologies were excluded. The updated RUCAM scoring [12, 20, 25] was done, the patient was rated 10 points, and for this reason, our case had a high probability of being a DILI, a mixed-type DILI to be exact (ALT/ALP ratio of 2.75). The liver biopsy and the improvement in symptoms and liver values after gemcitabine discontinuation confirm the drug-induced liver injury.

Our case report evaluates gemcitabine inducing liver toxicity. Gemcitabine (2′,2′-difluoro-2′-deoxycytidine (dFdC)) is a deoxycytidine analog with multiple modes of action inside the cell. It is phosphorylated by deoxycytidine kinase to the active compounds gemcitabine di- and triphosphate. Gemcitabine diphosphate can be toxic if the pool of cellular ATP decreases. Its principal pharmacological activity is incorporated into DNA during replication in the S phase of the cell cycle, following the inactivation of DNA polymerases and the inhibition of DNA synthesis. Gemcitabine activity primarily consists of inducing cell cycle arrest and cell death. The induction of apoptosis through caspase signaling is also another important mechanism of action [27]. The precise molecular mechanisms determining tumor cell responses to gemcitabine and the impact of mechanistic interactions with other chemotherapeutic agents remain unelucidated [28]. Moreover, gemcitabine hepatic metabolism has its cornerstone into cytidine deaminase (CDA), encoded by the CDA gene located in locus 1p36.2–35 [29]. Several studies demonstrated that single-nucleotide polymorphism of CDA, resulting in decreased serum CDA concentration, may lead to severe toxicity induced by gemcitabine [30–32]. Usually, gemcitabine is well tolerated, with common side effects including nausea and vomiting, rash, fever, flu-like symptoms, and peripheral edema. Myelosuppression is the most common dose-limiting toxicity. Also, various pulmonary toxicities of gemcitabine have been reported [33]. Gemcitabine can cause a transient increase in liver indexes, whereas a more serious hepatic involvement up to fatal outcome is less frequent [7]. In our case report, in the absence of other causes, we believe that gemcitabine is the main cause of DILI. We do not consider carboplatin, concomitantly administered with gemcitabine [34, 35], as a DILI cause, due to very few cases of liver abnormalities in the literature, generally related to high dosages [36]. Discontinuation of gemcitabine, together with purely symptomatic therapy, lead us to a clinical resolution and normalization of laboratory indexes.

Moreover, comparing the case reports cited in [3, 4, 10, 11], our case report uses the RUCAM [12, 20, 25] diagnostic scoring system as a fundamental tool in the DILI diagnostic process.

4. Conclusion

In conclusion, clinicians should pay particular attention to the liver context, when starting a gemcitabine-based treatment regimen. A careful remote anamnesis and pharmacological history should be taken in order to identify risk factors that can contribute to the development of a drug-induced liver injury. Therefore, especially in follow-up care, clinicians should do thorough clinical and laboratory monitoring in order to promptly diagnose this rare adverse drug reaction.

Abbreviations

ADR: Adverse drug reaction
AFP: Alpha-fetoprotein
ALP: Alkaline phosphatase
ALT: Alanine aminotransferase
AMA: Antimitochondrial auto-antibodies
ANA: Antinuclear antibodies
ANCA: Antineutrophil cytoplasmic antibodies
Anti-LC1: Antiliver cytosolic antigen type 1
Anti-LKM: Liver/kidney microsomal antibodies
Anti-SLA/LP: Antisoluble liver antigen/liver-pancreas
ASMA: Anti-smooth muscle antibodies
AST: Aspartate aminotransferase
CDA: Cytidine deaminase
CDT: Carbohydrate-deficient transferrin
CLM: Clinica Luganese Moncucco
CMV: Cytomegalovirus
CT: Computed tomography
DILI: Drug-induced liver injury
EBV: Epstein–Barr virus
ENA: Extractable nuclear antigen
GGT: Gamma-glutamyl transferase
HAV: Hepatovirus A
HBV: Hepatovirus B
HCV: Hepatovirus C
HDV: Hepatovirus D
HEV: Hepatovirus E
MRCP: Magnetic resonance cholangiopancreatography
NSAIDS: Nonsteroidal anti-inflammatory drugs
RUCAM: Roussel Uclaf Causality Assessment Method.

Authors' Contributions

All authors contributed equally to this work.

References

[1] L. J. Ostruszka and D. S. Shewach, "The role of DNA synthesis inhibition in the cytotoxicity of 2′,2′-difluoro-2′-deoxycytidine," *Cancer Chemotherapy and Pharmacology*, vol. 52, no. 4, pp. 325–332, 2003.
[2] M. N. Kirstein and D. Yee, "Pharmacodynamic characterization of gemcitabine cytotoxicity in an in vitro cell culture bioreactor system," *Cancer Chemotherapy and Pharmacology*, vol. 61, no. 2, pp. 291–299, 2008.
[3] H. Tanaka, H. Takamori, S.-I. Eto et al., "Acute liver injury with hepatic encephalopathy associated with gemcitabine administration for adjuvant chemotherapy in an HBV carrier with pancreatic cancer," *Japanese Journal of Cancer and Chemotherapy*, vol. 37, pp. 1783–1786, 2010.
[4] D. C. Coeman, E. K. Verbeken, K. L. Nackaerts, M. G. Demedts, and J. F. Vansteenkiste, "A fatal case of cholestatic liver failure probably related to gemcitabine," *Annals of Oncology*, vol. 11, no. 11, pp. 1503-1504, 2000.
[5] M. Tonato and C. Martin, "Safety profile of gemcitabine," *Anticancer Drugs*, vol. 6, no. 6, pp. 27–32, 1995.
[6] https://livertox.nih.gov/Gemcitabine.htm.
[7] H. Anderson, B. Lund, F. Bach, N. Thatcher, J. Walling, and H. H. Hansen, "Single-agent activity of weekly gemcitabine in advanced non-small-cell lung cancer: a phase II study," *Journal of Clinical Oncology*, vol. 12, no. 9, pp. 1821–1826, 1994.
[8] N. Kaplowitz and L. D. DeLeve, Drug-nduced Liver Disease. Cancer Chemotherapy, pp. 541–567, Elsevier, Amsterdam, Netherlands, 3rd edition, 2013.
[9] M. Spielmann, A. Llombart-Cussac, S. Kalla et al., "Single-agent gemcitabine is active in previously treated metastatic breast cancer," *Oncology*, vol. 60, no. 4, pp. 303–307, 2001.
[10] M. Matsuda, G. Watanabe, S. Mine, and M. Hashimoto, "Fatal liver failure associated with gemcitabine hydrochloride therapy," *Japanese Journal of Cancer and Chemotherapy*, vol. 35, no. 1, pp. 157–159, 2008.
[11] K. Cheong, J. Li, and C. S. Karapetis, "Gemcitabine and reactivation of hepatitis B," *Medical Oncology*, vol. 20, no. 4, pp. 385–388, 2003.
[12] Li Xiao, X.-C. Liu, Y.-L. Song, R.-T. Hong, and H. Shi, "Suspected drug induced liver injury associated with iguratimod: a case report and review of the literature," *BMC Gastroenterology*, vol. 18, no. 1, p. 130, 2018.
[13] W. M. Lee, "Drug-induced hepatotoxicity," *New England Journal of Medicine*, vol. 349, no. 5, pp. 474–485, 2003.

[14] A. lIcata, M. G. Minissale, V. Calvaruso, and A. Craxì, "Focus on epidemiology of drug-induced liver injury: analysis of a prospective cohort," *European Review for Medical and Pharmacological Sciences*, vol. 21, no. 1, pp. 112–121, 2017.
[15] T. J. Davern, "Drug-induced liver disease," *Clinics in Liver Disease*, vol. 16, no. 2, pp. 231–245, 2012.
[16] G. Ostapowicz, R. J. Fontana, F. V. Schiødt et al., "Results of a prospective study of acute liver failure at 17 tertiary care centers in the United States," *Annals of Internal Medicine*, vol. 137, no. 12, pp. 947–954, 2002.
[17] A. M. Larson, J. Polson, R. J. Fontana et al., "Acetaminophen-induced acute liver failure: results of a United States multicenter, prospective study," *Hepatology*, vol. 42, no. 6, pp. 1364–1372, 2005.
[18] R. J. Andrade, M. I. Lucena, M. C. Fernández et al., "Drug-induced liver injury: an analysis of 461 incidences submitted to the Spanish registry over a 10-year period," *Gastroenterology*, vol. 129, no. 2, pp. 512–521, 2005.
[19] C. Bénichou, "Criteria of drug-induced liver disorders. Report of an international consensus meeting," *Journal of Hepatology*, vol. 11, no. 2, pp. 272–276, 1990.
[20] E. S. Bjornsson and J. G. Jonasson, "Drug-induced cholestasis," *Clinics in Liver Disease*, vol. 17, no. 2, pp. 191–209, 2013.
[21] M. V. Galan and S. C. Gordon, "The burden of acute non fulminant drug-induced hepatitis in a United States tertiary referral center," *Journal Of Clinical Gastroenterology*, vol. 129, no. 2, pp. 512–521, 2005.
[22] F. J. De Abajo, D. Montero, M. Madurga, and L. A. G. Rodriguez, "Acute and clinically relevant drug-induced liver injury: a population based case-control study," *British Journal of Clinical Pharmacology*, vol. 58, no. 1, pp. 71–80, 2004.
[23] M. W. Russo, J. A. Galanko, R. Shrestha, M. W. Fried, and P. Watkins, "Liver transplantation for acute liver failure from drug induced liver injury in the United States," *Liver Transplantation*, vol. 10, no. 8, pp. 1018–1023, 2004.
[24] E. Björnsson and R. Olsson, "Outcome and prognostic markers in severe drug-induced liver disease," *Hepatology*, vol. 42, no. 2, pp. 481–489, 2005.
[25] G. Danan and R. Teschke, "RUCAM in drug and herb induced liver injury: the update," *International Journal of Molecular Sciences*, vol. 17, no. 1, p. 14, 2016.
[26] R. J. Andrade, M. I. Lucena, N. Kaplowitz et al., "Outcome of acute idiosyncratic drug-induced liver injury: long-term follow-up in a hepatotoxicity registry," *Hepatology*, vol. 44, no. 6, pp. 1581–1588, 2006.
[27] S. Noble and K. L. Goa, "Gemcitabine," *Drugs*, vol. 54, no. 3, pp. 447–472, 1997.
[28] S. S. Hamed, R. M. Straubinger, and W. J. Jusko, "Pharmacodynamic modeling of cell cycle and apoptotic effects of gemcitabine on pancreatic adenocarcinoma cells," *Cancer Chemotherapy and Pharmacology*, vol. 72, no. 3, pp. 553–563, 2013.
[29] D. Micozzi, F. M. Carpi, S. Pucciarelli et al., "Human cytidine deaminase: a biochemical characterization of its naturally occurring variants," *International Journal of Biological Macromolecules*, vol. 63, pp. 64–74, 2014.
[30] M. Tanaka, M. Javle, X. Dong, C. Eng, J. L. Abbruzzese, and D. Li, "Gemcitabine metabolic and transporter gene polymorphisms are associated with drug toxicity and efficacy in patients with locally advanced pancreatic cancer," *Cancer*, vol. 116, no. 22, pp. 5325–5335, 2010.
[31] J. J. Farrell, K. Bae, J. Wong, C. Guha, A. P. Dicker, and H. Elsaleh, "Cytidine deaminase single-nucleotide polymorphism is predictive of toxicity from gemcitabine in patients with pancreatic cancer: RTOG 9704," *The Pharmacogenomics Journal*, vol. 12, no. 5, pp. 395–403, 2012.
[32] X. Ding, W. Chen, H. Fan, and B. Zhu, "Cytidine deaminase polymorphism predicts toxicity of gemcitabine-based chemotherapy," *Gene*, vol. 559, no. 1, pp. 31–37, 2015.
[33] M. W. Saif, "Pulmonary toxicity associated with gemcitabine," *Journal of the Pancreas*, vol. 11, no. 2, pp. 189-190, 2010.
[34] M. De Santis, J. Bellmunt, G. Mead et al., "Randomized phase II/III trial assessing gemcitabine/carboplatin and methotrexate/carboplatin/vinblastina in patients with advanced urothelial cancer who are unfit for cisplatin-based chemotherapy: EORTC study 30986," *Journal of Clinical Oncology*, vol. 30, no. 2, pp. 191–199, 2012.
[35] L. Dogliotti, G. Cartenì, S. Siena et al., "Gemcitabine plus cisplatin versus gemcitabine plus carboplatin as first-line chemotherapy in advanced transitional cell carcinoma of the urothelium: results of a randomized phase 2 trial," *European Urology*, vol. 52, no. 1, pp. 134–141, 2007.
[36] R. H. Hruban, S. S. Sternberg, P. Meyers, M. Fleisher, C. Menendez-Botet, and J. K. Boitnott, "Fatal thrombocytopenia and liver failure associated with carboplatin therapy," *Cancer Investigation*, vol. 9, no. 3, pp. 263–268, 1991.

Gas-Forming Liver Abscess versus Emphysematous Hepatitis: A Radiologic Diagnostic Dilemma—A Case Report and Review of the Literature

Youssef Ghosn,[1] Ali Abdallah,[2] Mohammed Hussein Kamareddine,[1] Amine Geahchan,[2] Ahmad Baghdadi,[1] Ziad El-Rassi,[3] Abbas Chamseddine,[2] and Raja Ashou[2]

[1] *Faculty of Medicine and Medical Sciences, University of Balamand, Achrafieh, Beirut, Lebanon*
[2] *Department of Diagnostic Radiology, Saint George Hospital University Medical Center, University of Balamand, Achrafieh, Beirut, Lebanon*
[3] *Department of General Surgery, Saint George Hospital University Medical Center, University of Balamand, Achrafieh, Beirut, Lebanon*

Correspondence should be addressed to Youssef Ghosn; youssef.ghosn994@gmail.com

Academic Editor: Haruki Komatsu

A 38-year-old diabetic woman, with history of cholecystectomy and ventral hernia repair, was hospitalized due to sudden-onset abdominal pain and fever. Computed tomography revealed a mixed collection containing necrotic debris and emphysematous change in the left lobe of the liver mainly in segments II and III. These radiological findings suggested emphysematous hepatitis (EH). The patient's condition deteriorated rapidly, and she was rushed to the operating room for urgent exploratory laparotomy where debridement was performed. Intraoperatively the patient was found to have an abscess with incomplete capsule concurrent with hepatic necrosis suggesting the co-occurrence of abscess and EH. The patient survived and was discharged after 13 days. Relevant literature was reviewed, and to the best of our knowledge, EH is an extremely rare entity with limited data regarding its pathogenesis, causative organisms, and management. EH is a rapidly invasive disease process that can be fatal if appropriate therapeutic intervention is delayed. Initial presentations are usually subtle, thus high clinical and radiological suspicion is required for early diagnosis and management to decrease associated mortality and morbidity. We hence report the first successfully treated case of EH with review of the literature.

1. Introduction

Intra-abdominal emphysematous parenchymal infections have been widely recognized involving a variety of abdominal organs, including the urinary tract, gallbladder, uterus, stomach, and pancreas. However, few reported cases have described similar emphysematous changes occurring in the liver [1, 2]. Although the spectrum of causes of hepatic gas detected with computed tomography (CT) is broad, emphysematous parenchymal involvement of the liver is extremely rare [3]. The first case of replacement of the liver parenchyma by air with no evidence of abscess was reported by Blachar et al. (2001) [4]. The diagnosis of this condition requires high clinical suspicion for a hepatobiliary pathology coupled with imaging and the ability of radiologists to identify the pathological process. Emphysematous hepatitis (EH) shares some radiological and clinical features with other entities caused by acute necrotizing, gas-forming infection such as emphysematous pyelonephritis [5]. However, EH is still poorly characterized and could be hard to differentiate from gas-forming pyogenic liver abscess (PLA). We herein report a case of EH in a diabetic, 38-year-old female, successfully treated with antibiotics and rapid surgical debridement. Unfortunately, all other reported cases with EH have led to fatality within one to three days of admission. A complete review of the literature is also presented.

2. Case Presentation

A 38-year-old woman was admitted to the Medical Intensive Care Unit (MICU) at Saint Georges University Hospital,

Beirut, because of a 2 day history of chills and fever (reaching 39.5 degrees Celsius), along with nausea and vomiting (2 episodes), and 1 day history of severe abdominal pain that was diffuse and did not respond to symptomatic treatment. Patient then noted abdominal fullness, so she presented to our emergency department. The patient had a past medical history remarkable for gestational diabetes mellitus and a past surgical history of two C-sections, cholecystectomy (4 years prior to presentation), and most recently surgical repair of a ventral hernia with a mesh placement (4 years prior to presentation).

On presentation, the patient was awake, alert, and oriented to time, place, and person. However, the patient was in severe pain and acutely ill in appearance. She was febrile 38.9 C, but the rest of her vitals were stable. Examination was remarkable for mild scleral icterus, right upper quadrant tenderness, abdominal rigidity, and guarding, but the liver and spleen were not palpable. Initial complete blood count showed leukocytosis of 54.9 x109/L with 88.3% neutrophils, anemia with hematocrit of 26.1 % and hemoglobin of 8.3 g/dL, and platelet count of 280 x103/mL. C-reactive protein (CRP) was remarkably elevated measuring 49.33 mg/L.

Blood urea nitrogen was 53 mg/dL and creatinine 0.66 mg/dL. Liver function tests showed aspartate aminotransferase (AST) of 434 u/L, alanine aminotransferase (ALT) of 296 u/L, alkaline phosphatase of 133 u/L, gamma-glutamyltransferase of 29 u/L, total bilirubin of 4.28 mg/dL, and direct bilirubin of 1.89 mg/dL. Coagulation studies showed a prolonged prothrombin time (PT) of 15.44 seconds, with International Normalized Ratio (INR) of 1.29, and partial thromboplastin time (PTT) of 39.49 seconds. The rest of the serum biochemistry panel showed normal pancreatic enzymes, increased serum glucose of 281 mM, decreased total protein of 6 g/dL, and albumin of 3.4 g/dL.

As for the imaging done, chest X-ray was unremarkable. However, abdominal CT scan with oral and IV contrast demonstrated a mixed collection containing air and debris measuring 8x7x5.5 cm limited laterally by the left portal vein and extending medially toward the lesser curvature of the stomach associated with moderate intra- and extrahepatic biliary dilation. Moreover, it is spreading at the posterior aspect of the left lobe of the liver mainly in segments II and III. Emphysematous alveolarization of the adjacent hepatic parenchyma was also noted (Figures 1 and 2). The absence of cluster signs, septal breakage, collections in favor of pus, fluid collections and the lack of capsular enhancement of an abscess capsule made EH more likely than PLA.

The patient underwent urgent exploratory laparotomy. Preoperative Amoxicillin-Clavulanic acid was given. A huge cavity in the hepatic parenchyma was noted involving segments II and III along with necrotic liver parenchyma which underwent debridement. Exploration of the abdomen was done, with no other collection or pathology found. Liver necrotic tissue was sent to pathology and fluid was sent for culture. Pathology results showed liver parenchyma with marked mixed inflammatory prominent necrosis and focal accumulation of pus, with no evidence of granulomas or malignancy. Fluid culture grew *Escherichia coli* and *Enterococcus faecium*, so the patient was started on tigecycline. The surgery was uneventful and the patient was transferred to the ICU for monitoring and further management. Patient was stable in the ICU and her lab results improved significantly, so she was transferred to the floor and discharged home 13 days after her presentation.

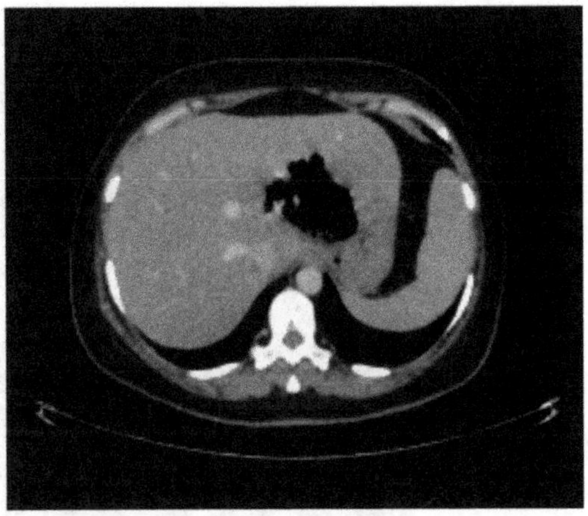

FIGURE 1: Axial abdominal CT scan with oral and IV contrast. Mixed collection containing air and debris spreading at the posterior aspect of the left lobe of the liver mainly in segments II and III, limited laterally by the left portal vein and extending medially towered the lesser curvature of the stomach associated with moderate intra- and extrahepatic biliary dilation. Sharply marginated left borders are noted.

3. Review of the Literature

3.1. Causes and Differential Diagnosis . EH seems to share similar risk factor with other manifestations of gas-producing infections which are related to anaerobic bacteria and usually associated with immunosuppressive pathologies such as diabetes mellitus (DM) and cancer. Interestingly, most of these patients had history of recent abdominal surgery.

DM appears to be highly associated with EH. Similar to our case, the first case reported by Blachar et al. (2001) was of a patient with DM. This 43-year-old woman had short gut syndrome with the most recent bowel resection preformed 6 weeks before presentation [4]. Another case by Chauhan U et al. (2012) describes fulminant EH in a diabetic patient with replacement of the entire liver parenchyma by air [6].

Other than diabetes, gastrointestinal cancers seem to be associated with EH. One case reported by Kim JH et al. (2012) Showed EH in an 80-year-old patient with hilar cholangiocarcinoma [1]. Similarly, Letourneau-Guillon et al. (2010) reported a case of EH in 53-year-old patient with cholangiocarcinoma three months after undergoing left hepatectomy with hepaticojejunostomy and left hepatic duct extension [7]. Another case by Nada KM el al. (2017) reported EH in a patient with a history of pancreatic cancer and liver metastasis who underwent Whipple procedure 8 month prior to presentation [2].

Because EH is commonly related to liver infarction and infection, the pathophysiology of EH is thought to be

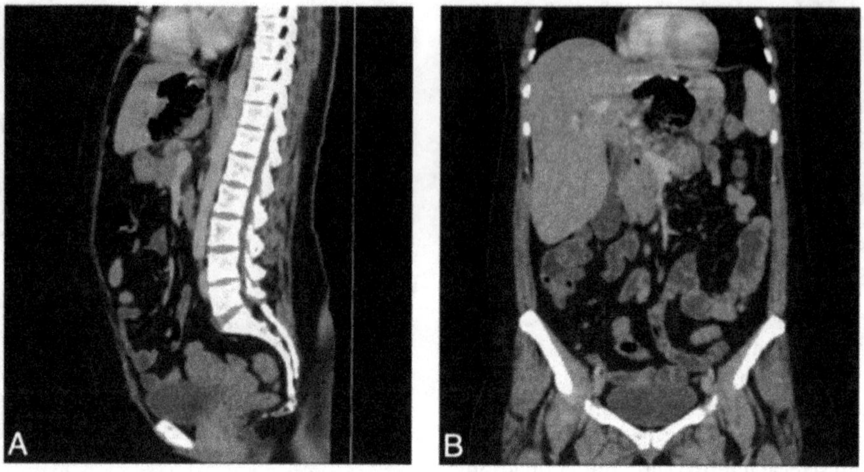

(a) (b)

FIGURE 2: Sagittal (a) and coronal (b) abdominal CT scan with oral and IV contrast. Mixed collection containing air and debris measuring 8x7x5.5 cm is present. The lesion is spreading at the posterior aspect of the left lobe at segments II and III. Emphysematous changes of the adjacent parenchyma are noted.

due to superinfection of infarcted liver parenchyma [3]. It is usually caused by bacterial pathogens associated with emphysematous infections such as *Streptococcus mutans*, *Enterococcus faecalis* [2], *E. coli*, *Klebsiella*[8], *Enterobacter*, *Pseudomonas*, and *Proteus* [9] causing acid fermentation from tissue necrosis that ultimately forms a mixture of gases that could not be transported out of the liver due to the necrotic tissue [5, 10].

The differential diagnosis for gas in the liver is broad. Emphysematous changes in the liver has typically been seen in clinical situations involving gas-forming bacteria [11] and bowel infarction or following invasive procedures or therapeutic interventions such as sphincterotomy [12], hepatic artery thrombosis after liver transplantation (caused by damage of hepatic circulation) [13], radiofrequency ablation, and percutaneous ethanol injection in hepatocellular carcinoma [14]. Gas gangrene in the liver, which necessitates compromise of both the portal and arterial supply, has been reported in the setting of liver transplantation and hepatic trauma [13].

3.2. Clinical Manifestation and Outcome. Initial clinical manifestations are usually subtle and progress rapidly in the absence of therapeutic interventions [2]. Symptoms and signs include sudden-onset right upper abdominal pain, hepatomegaly, icterus, and altered mental status fever with eventual progression to septic shock [1, 2]. Lab values generally show leukocytosis and elevated LFTs [1, 2, 4, 6].

This entity has significant poor outcome, since most patients with this severe infection do not improve despite application of aggressive management (antibiotic therapy with or without drainage) and progress rapidly. The clinical outcome of EH appears to be fatal, as seen in all other reports, with death between one to three days after presentation [1, 2, 4, 6, 7]. Therefore, a more aggressive therapeutic modality is emphasized and surgical intervention should not be delayed in patients with EH in order to avoid total emphysematous replacement of hepatic parenchyma leading to death.

3.3. Radiological Features. When emphysematous liver changes are noted, it is important to check whether the gas is located in the bile ducts, liver parenchyma, vascular structures, or the lymphatic system in order to determine the origin. When the gas is located in the liver parenchyma, we should think of an infectious process like a liver abscess due to septic emboli, ascending cholangitis, or EH. Once gas is present in the liver parenchyma, it can spread through the hepatic veins, bile ducts, or the lymphatic system [3].

Although these two entities can present similarly, it important to differentiate between PLA and EH; however, EH is a new characterized entity with limited cases to be able to form definitive radiological diagnostic criteria. The difference between EH and gas-forming pyogenic liver abscesses is that PLA usually has clustered or multiseptated lesion (cluster signs and septal breakage) generally with pus and fluid collections [1, 8]. Often there is a double target sign due to the enhancement of the abscess capsule and the surrounding edema in the liver parenchyma [3]. In few cases of gas-forming PLA, air-fluid level or air bubbles can be present. On the other hand, in EH, the affected liver is totally replaced by air with no fluid content [1].

Moreover, in EH the arterial and portal venous blood supply is impaired causing sharply marginated wedge shaped areas, corresponding to the liver segments without contrast enhancement. In these infarcted liver segments, the parenchyma is replaced by gas which can further spread through the hepatic veins, biliary tract, or the lymphatic system [3].

For now, it seems that the definitive diagnosis requires surgical exploration. Our example demonstrates radiological features of EH; however, upon surgical exploration both entities (abscess and EH) were present, suggesting that both could be co-manifested with the probability that PLA contributed to EH.

4. Conclusion

EH is rare clinical entity with poor characterization. It is important to distinguish between EH and gas-forming PLA, knowing that both entities might be co-manifested. Patients should be treated with urgent exploratory laparotomy with surgical debridement. Appropriate antibiotics should be administered. For now, this is the only successfully treated case of EH.

References

[1] J. H. Kim, E. S. Jung, S. H. Jeong et al., "A case of emphysematous hepatitis with spontaneous pneumoperitoneum in a patient with hilar cholangiocarcinoma," *Clinical and Molecular Hepatology*, vol. 18, no. 1, pp. 94–97, 2012.

[2] K. M. Nada, I. El Husseini, M. E. Abu Hishmeh, N. S. Shah, N. Ibragimova, and R. Basir, "A rare case of septic shock secondary to emphysematous hepatitis," *Case Reports in Critical Care*, vol. 2017, Article ID 3020845, 3 pages, 2017.

[3] W. Verwimp, O. de Beeck, A. Snoeckx et al., "Gas in the liver what radiologist needs to know," in *Poster presented at: European congress of radiology*, Vienna, Austria, 2013.

[4] A. Blachar, M. P. Federle, and G. Brancatelli, "Acute fulminant hepatic infection causing fatal 'emphysematous hepatitis': case report," *Abdominal Imaging*, vol. 27, no. 2, pp. 188–190, 2002.

[5] L. I. Schainuck, R. Fouty, and R. E. Cutler, "Emphysematous pyelonephritis. A new case and review of previous observations," *American Journal of Medicine*, vol. 44, no. 1, pp. 134–139, 1968.

[6] U. Chauhan, S. M. Prabhu, G. S. Shetty, R. S. Solanki, A. K. Udiya, and A. Singh, "Emphysematous hepatitis - a fatal infection in diabetic patients: case report," *Clinics and Research in Hepatology and Gastroenterology*, vol. 36, no. 6, pp. e114–e116, 2012.

[7] L. Létourneau-Guillon, P. Audet, M. Plasse, and L. Lepanto, "Answer to case of the month# 162: emphysematous infection of the liver parenchyma," *Canadian Association of Radiologists Journal*, vol. 61, no. 2, pp. 117–119, 2010.

[8] L. Yang-Sheng, W. Wei-Sheng, and C. Ming-Jen, "Emphysematous changes of the liver," *Clinical challenges and Images in GI*, pp. 213, 413–414, 2012.

[9] Y.-L. Wan, T.-Y. Lee, M. J. Bullard, and C.-C. Tsai, "Acute gas-producing bacterial renal infection: correlation between imaging findings and clinical outcome," *Radiology*, vol. 198, no. 2, pp. 433–438, 1996.

[10] J. Huang, K. Chen, and M. Ruaan, "Mixed acid fermentation of glucose as a mechanism of emphysematous urinary tract infection," *The Journal of Urology*, vol. 146, no. 1, pp. 148–151, 1991.

[11] T. Y. Lee, Y. L. Wan, and C. C. Tsai, "Gas-containing liver abscess: radiological findings and clinical significance," *Abdominal Imaging*, vol. 19, no. 1, pp. 47–52, 1994.

[12] D. E. Grayson, R. M. Abbott, A. D. Levy, and P. M. Sherman, "Emphysematous infections of the abdomen and pelvis: a pictorial review," *RadioGraphics*, vol. 22, no. 3, pp. 543–561, 2002.

[13] S. Doblecki-Lewis, E. Palaios, P. A. Bejarano, A. G. Tzakis, G. Selvaggi, and M. I. Morris, "Hepatic gas gangrene following orthotopic liver transplantation: three cases treated with re-transplantation and a review of the literature," *Transplant Infectious Disease*, vol. 10, no. 4, pp. 280–285, 2008.

[14] A. Solinas, G. S. Erbella, E. Distrutti et al., "Abscess formation in hepatocellular carcinoma: Complications of percutaneous ultrasound-guided ethanol injection," *Journal of Clinical Ultrasound*, vol. 21, no. 8, pp. 531–533, 1993.

32

Postliver Transplantation Rhino-Orbital Mucormycosis, an Unexpected Cause of a Downhill Course

Swapnali Sabhapandit,[1] Mithun Sharma,[2] Anuradha Sekaran,[3] Balachandran Menon,[4] Anand Kulkarni,[2] Soumya TR,[2] Padaki Nagaraja Rao,[2] and Duvurr Nageshwar Reddy[5]

[1]*Department of Ophthalmology, AIG Hospitals, Hyderabad, India*
[2]*Department of Hepatology and Liver Transplantation, Asian Institute of Gastroenterology, Hyderabad, India*
[3]*Department of Pathology, Asian Institute of Gastroenterology, Hyderabad, India*
[4]*Department of Liver Transplantation, Asian Institute of Gastroenterology, Hyderabad, India*
[5]*Department of Gastroenterology, Asian Institute of Gastroenterology, Hyderabad, India*

Correspondence should be addressed to Mithun Sharma; drmithunsharma@gmail.com

Academic Editor: Haruki Komatsu

The COVID-19 pandemic has impacted transplantation worldwide in a major way with infections and post-COVID-19 complications contributing to increased mortality and morbidity. We present a case of a 42-year-old lady who developed rhino-orbital mucormycosis in a postliver transplantation period. The initial presentation of the patient was very subtle. She never had overt COVID-19 infection before surgery and in the recovery period. Though cases of mucormycosis in the wound site have been reported, this would be one of the rare cases of rhino-orbital mucormycosis postliver transplantation. This infection leads to a rapid downhill course and the death of the patient. Atypical infections and presentations need to be monitored in postliver transplantation patients who are getting operated on during this pandemic, and a high level of clinical suspicion is required to pick up these cases at an early stage.

1. Introduction

Coronavirus disease-2019 (COVID-19) pandemic has affected liver transplantation programmes worldwide and has thrown new challenges in both the pre and post-transplantation periods. Though, currently, many guidelines are in place, yet in the initial phase of pandemic, weighing the risk-benefit ratio of transplantation versus adverse outcome due to SARS-CoV-2 infection was tough [1].

Postliver transplantation outcome has shown varied results during the pandemic. In a systematic review, 23% of posttransplantation patients were found to be infected with severe COVID-19 infection with 55.9% cases requiring modification of immunosuppression [2]. In addition, recent data from the West have shown "excess deaths" in all solid organ transplantations during the pandemic, with the number of deaths mirroring the COVID-19 incidence [3].

In India, during the second wave of the COVID-19 pandemic, rhino-orbital mucormycosis was increasingly reported in diabetic patients (81.2%) and patients with corticosteroid use (79.69%) requiring oxygen supplementation [4]. However, in the published case series, no case was reported in postliver transplantation patients, though they too had a common risk factor of use of corticosteroids. The worst prognosis has been noted in patients with involvement of the brain and those who had a SOFA score of greater than 2 at presentation [5].

We present a case of rhino-orbital mucormycosis in a postliver transplantation patient. The case brings to forefront the subtle onset of the disease and the need of high

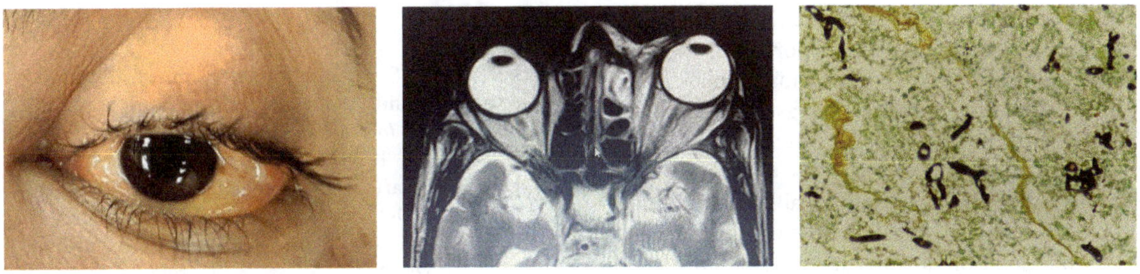

(a) (b) (c)

FIGURE 1: Picture showing lid edema and ptosis of left eye lid (a) with MRI showing mucormycosis deposits in the left paranasal sinuses and orbit (b). Staining with Grocott methenamine silver stain showing septate hyphae of mucormycosis (c).

index of clinical suspicion for diagnosis. Early diagnosis can save the life of many of these patients with good outcome [6].

2. Case Report

We present a case of a 42-year-old gentleman who underwent living donor liver transplantation on 25th May 2021 for alcohol use disorder-related decompensated chronic liver disease with MELD score 28. The ABO compatible donor was his wife who had no comorbidities except for hypothyroidism. Both the donor and the recipient were negative for severe acute respiratory syndrome virus 2 (SARS-CoV-2) on reverse transcriptase polymerase chain reaction (RT-PCR) done on two occasions with the last test done 24 hours before surgery. As per protocol of our institute, the COVID-19 antibodies were also tested and found to be negative 24 hours prior to liver transplantation. Neither the recipient nor the donor was vaccinated against SARS-CoV-2.

The postoperative recovery period was uneventful, and the patient was treated with steroids, tacrolimus, and mycophenolate mofetil as per protocol. The dose of prednisolone was tapered to 15 mg/day on the fifteenth day postsurgery. The patient did not have any fever or constitutional symptoms in the postoperative period. However, on posttransplantation day 20, he complained of sudden onset redness of the left periorbital area with pain in the left eye (Figure 1(a)). An immediate in-house ophthalmology consultation was sought. On examination, there was ptosis of the left upper eyelid and mild proptosis of the left eye along with conjunctival redness. Contrast-enhanced magnetic resonance imaging of the orbit, paranasal sinuses, and the brain showed thickening of the medial rectus and superior oblique muscles with fat stranding. In addition, contiguous areas of nonenhancing tissue were noted in the paranasal sinuses suggestive of angioinvasive fungal infection (Figure 1(b)). Qualitative PCR from swabs taken from the left nostril was positive for *Mucorales* deoxyribonucleic acid, which is a sensitive marker for invasive mucormycosis. His repeat test for SARS-CoV-2 RT-PCR and rapid antigen tests were negative. However, his immunoglobulin (Ig) G for COVID-19 was now positive, while IgM was negative. A computerized tomography of the chest showed no evidence of pulmonary COVID-19 infection or any pulmonary mucormycosis.

Nasal swab stain revealed hyphae of mucormycosis on Grocott methenamine silver stain (Figure 1(c)). Based on reports of nasal swab, positive DNA for *Mucorales* and radiographic features [7], a diagnosis of rhino-orbital mucormycosis was made. Systemic antifungals (intravenous liposomal-amphotericin *B*, 10 mg/kg/day, with oral posaconazole 300 mg twice daily on day 1 followed by 300 mg once daily) were initiated. Immunosuppressants tacrolimus and mycophenolate mofetil were stopped. However, even after five days of initiation of antifungals, the patient did not show any clinical signs of improvement. A repeat contrast enhanced MRI of the orbit and paranasal sinuses showed worsening of the lesions with invasion of the orbital bone. Orbital exenteration with the eyelid sparing technique was planned, but surgical consent was refused by the family. Despite continuing conservative management for next 3 days, the patient had a downhill course and succumbed to his infection.

Informed written consent was taken for publication of this case from the patient and also next of kin.

3. Discussion

Rhino-orbital mucormycosis is frequently caused by fungal infection due to *Rhizopus* spp., *Mucor* spp., and *Lichtheimia* spp. [8] During the COVID-19 pandemic, there has been an increase in the incidence of such cases [9]. The source of infection is usually from the paranasal sinuses, and majority of the patients presents with unilateral facial edema and proptosis [10]. The European Confederation of Medical Mycology (ECMM) has laid down specific guidelines for diagnosis and includes demonstration of fungal hyphae in microscopy and culture along with molecular methods for direct detection of fungal deoxyribonucleic acid [11].

Steroids use during the pandemic has been implicated as the most common predisposing factor for rhino-orbital mucormycosis [12]. Other coexisting diseases such as diabetes mellitus has been associated with majority of the cases [13]. Longer length of hospital stay in posttransplantation immunosuppressed patients may predispose them to multiple infections including mucormycosis [14]. A rare case report of rhino-orbital maxillary mucormycosis after solid organ transplantation has been reported in the non-pandemic era also [15].

One interesting finding is that despite the use of steroids in posttransplantation patients, the reported incidence of invasive mucormycosis is rare in the nonpandemic era, and therefore, questions have been raised as to whether the SARS-CoV-2 virus itself predisposes patients to mucormycosis.

After solid organ transplantation, abdominal mucormycosis has been reported, and the most common route of infection is contamination during surgery [16]. However, in our case, since the surgical wound was not involved, the chances of contacting the infection from the operation theatre during surgery were very remote. The possibility of SARS-CoV-2 RT-PCR-negative COVID-19 infection was assumed as IgG and IgM which was negative pre-transplantation changed to IgG positive posttransplantation. SARS-CoV-2 IgG positivity indicates asymptomatic COVID-19 during the recovery period, which may be masked by immunosuppressants.

Though COVID-19 is showing a downward trend, possibility of a fourth wave still looms large. This case would serve as an index case of rhino-orbital mucormycosis in postliver transplantation patients and make transplant physicians keep their index of suspicion high for any periorbital swelling or ocular pain after transplantation.

4. Conclusion

Despite extensive screening of patients in the pre-transplantation period, the risk of contracting asymptomatic COVID-19 in the posttransplantation period is possible. However, the exact source and predisposing factor in this rare case will remain an enigma. High index of suspicion is required for any atypical symptom that may occur in the posttransplantation period in this era of COVID-19 pandemic.

Abbreviations

SARS-CoV-2:	Severe acute respiratory syndrome coronavirus 2
IgG:	Immunoglobulin G
RT-PCR:	Reverse transcriptase polymerase chain reaction.

Authors' Contributions

SS, MS, and BM conceptualized and designed the study. AS analysed the pathology specimens, AVK, SS, and MS collected data. SS and MS did compilation. MS, SS, and PNR did the initial draft. SS, AS, and MS provided figures. DNR, PNR, SS, and MS edited and revised the article. All members approved the final draft.

References

[1] S. Gupta, S. Sudhindran, N. Saraf et al., "Liver transplant society of India guidelines for liver transplant during COVID-19 times," *Journal of Clinical and Experimental Hepatology*, vol. 12, no. 1, pp. 180–185, 2022.

[2] A. V. Kulkarni, H. V. Tevethia, M. Premkumar et al., "Impact of COVID-19 on liver transplant recipients-A systematic review and meta-analysis," *EClinicalMedicine*, vol. 38, Article ID 101025, 2021.

[3] A. B. Massie, W. A. Werbel, R. K. Avery, T. Po-Yu Chiang, J. J. Snyder, and D. L. Segev, "Quantifying excess deaths among solid organ transplant recipients in the COVID-19 era," *American Journal of Transplantation*, 2022.

[4] R. Patel, J. Jethva, P. R. Bhagat, V. Prajapati, H. Thakkar, and K. Prajapati, "Rhino-orbital-cerebral mucormycosis: an epidemiological study from a tertiary care referral center in Western India," *Indian Journal of Ophthalmology*, vol. 70, no. 4, pp. 1371–1375, 2022.

[5] H. R. Nehara, S. Kumawat, J. Gupta, G. Gupta, P. Sirohi, and B. Gupta, "Coronavirus disease, diabetes and glucocorticoid a terrible trio for invasive mucormycosis: an observational study from northwest Rajasthan," *Journal of the Association of Physicians of India*, vol. 69, no. 12, pp. 11-12, 2022.

[6] J. C. Deyo, N. Nicolsen, A. Lachiewicz, and T. Kozlowski, "Salvage treatment of mucormycosis post-liver transplant with Posaconazole during sirolimus maintenance immunosuppression," *Journal of Pharmacy Practice*, vol. 30, no. 2, pp. 261–265, 2017.

[7] S. Safder, J. S. Carpenter, T. D. Roberts, and N. Bailey, "The "Black Turbinate" sign: an early MR imaging finding of nasal mucormycosis," *American Journal of Neuroradiology*, vol. 31, no. 4, pp. 771–774, 2010.

[8] O. A. Cornely, A. Alastruey-Izquierdo, D. Arenz et al., "Global guideline for the diagnosis and management of mucormycosis: an initiative of the European confederation of medical Mycology in cooperation with the mycoses study group education and research consortium," *The Lancet Infectious Diseases*, vol. 19, no. 12, pp. e405–e421, 2019.

[9] K. Ahmadikia, S. J. Hashemi, S. Khodavaisy et al., "The double-edged sword of systemic corticosteroid therapy in viral pneumonia: a case report and comparative review of influenza-associated mucormycosis versus COVID-19 associated mucormycosis," *Mycoses*, vol. 64, no. 8, pp. 798–808, 2021.

[10] M. S. Bae, E. J. Kim, K. M. Lee, and W. S. Choi, "Rapidly progressive rhino-orbito-cerebral mucormycosis complicated with unilateral internal carotid artery occlusion: a case report," *Neurointervention*, vol. 7, no. 1, pp. 45–49, 2012.

[11] M. Chermetz, M. Gobbo, K. Rupel et al., "Combined orofacial aspergillosis and mucormycosis: fatal complication of a recurrent paediatric glioma-case report and review of literature," *Mycopathologia*, vol. 181, no. 9-10, pp. 723–733, 2016.

[12] M. Sen, S. G. Honavar, N. Sharma, and M. S. Sachdev, "COVID-19 and eye: a review of ophthalmic manifestations of COVID-19," *Indian Journal of Ophthalmology*, vol. 69, no. 3, pp. 488–509, 2021.

[13] J. A. Al-Tawfiq, S. Alhumaid, A. N. Alshukairi et al., "COVID-19 and mucormycosis superinfection: the perfect storm," *Infection*, vol. 49, pp. 1–21, 2021.

[14] M. Salehi, K. Ahmadikia, H. Badali, and S. Khodavaisy, "Opportunistic fungal infections in the epidemic area of COVID-19: a clinical and diagnostic perspective from Iran," *Mycopathologia*, vol. 185, no. 4, pp. 607–611, 2020.

[15] R. Farojov, O. Aydın, C. Yılmaz et al., "Rhino-orbita-maxillary mucormycosis after liver transplantation: a case report," *Transplantation Proceedings*, vol. 48, no. 9, pp. 3210–3213, 2016.

[16] M. Kueht, J. A. Villarreal, E. Reece et al., "Cutaneous mucormycosis in solid organ transplant recipients after hurricane harvey: short- and long-term management," *Plastic and Reconstructive Surgery—Global Open*, vol. 7, no. 1, Article ID e2041, 2019.

33

Rifampicin for Treatment of Cholestatic Pruritus Caused by Drug-Induced Acute Liver Injury as Assessed by the RUCAM Classification

Ali R. Ahmadi,[1,2] Maria Chicco,[3] and Marcel van den Berge[1,2]

[1]*Department of Internal Medicine, Erasmus MC, Rotterdam, Netherlands*
[2]*Department of Internal Medicine, Admiraal de Ruyter Ziekenhuis, Goes, Netherlands*
[3]*Department of General Surgery, Wexham Park Hospital, Frimley Health NHS Trust, Frimley, UK*

Correspondence should be addressed to Ali R. Ahmadi; a.ahmadi@erasmusmc.nl

Academic Editor: Sorabh Kapoor

A male bodybuilder of 39 years of age developed severe pruritus, nausea, and jaundice after injecting anabolic steroids purchased on the black market. The patient had no history of liver disease and no risk factors for viral hepatitis. Extensive laboratory testing, radiographic imaging, and liver biopsy excluded a majority of potential pathologies. The patient was diagnosed with drug-induced acute liver injury and secondary acute renal failure most likely caused by testosterone purchased on the black market. The pruritus caused insomnia and significant psychological distress. Treatment was initiated with cholestyramine and naltrexone for one week with no effect on the pruritus. Subsequently, all medications were stopped, and rifampicin was started. Pruritus resolved after starting rifampicin, and liver and kidney function improved rapidly and normalized within 5 months.

1. Background

Drug-induced liver injury (DILI) is the most common cause of acute liver failure in the Western world [1]. It is a rare disease with possible fatal outcome with limited treatment options. Cholestatic pruritus is a common symptom of DILI caused by increased levels of serum bilirubin. It is recognized as a troublesome symptom, which significantly affects patients' daily activities, including sleep and the ability to work or attend school [2]. The negative impact of pruritus on patients' quality of life has been demonstrated in numerous studies: chronic pruritus can lead to anxiety, depression, and even suicide. In this case report, our patient experienced extreme discomfort because of pruritus caused by DILI. He was unable to sleep, which had significant impact on his mood and overall mental status. We used the Roussel Uclaf Causality Assessment Method (RUCAM) to quantitatively assess causality in this suspected case of DILI [3]. RUCAM represents a structured, standardized, validated, and hepatotoxicity-specific diagnostic approach that attributes scores to individual key items, providing final quantitative gradings of causality for each suspect drug/herb in a case report. Based on this scoring system, DILI was likely to be the cause. After several unsuccessful attempts to alleviate pruritus, we resorted to the use of rifampicin with remarkable success. Rifampicin is most commonly used as an antibiotic for treatment of tuberculosis. An additional and not well-known off-label indication of rifampicin is to treat cholestatic pruritus.

2. Case Presentation

The patient saw his general practitioner because of malaise, nausea, and severe generalized pruritus. The patient was referred to the hospital the same day. He had no prior disease history. He had not recently traveled abroad and had no fever or weight loss. The patient mentioned he had loss of appetite, discoloured faeces, and dark "coca-cola-like" urine. He reported use of certain supplements, such as mesterolone, exemestane, and taladafil, which he had acquired from a pharmacy abroad. He also indicated that he had

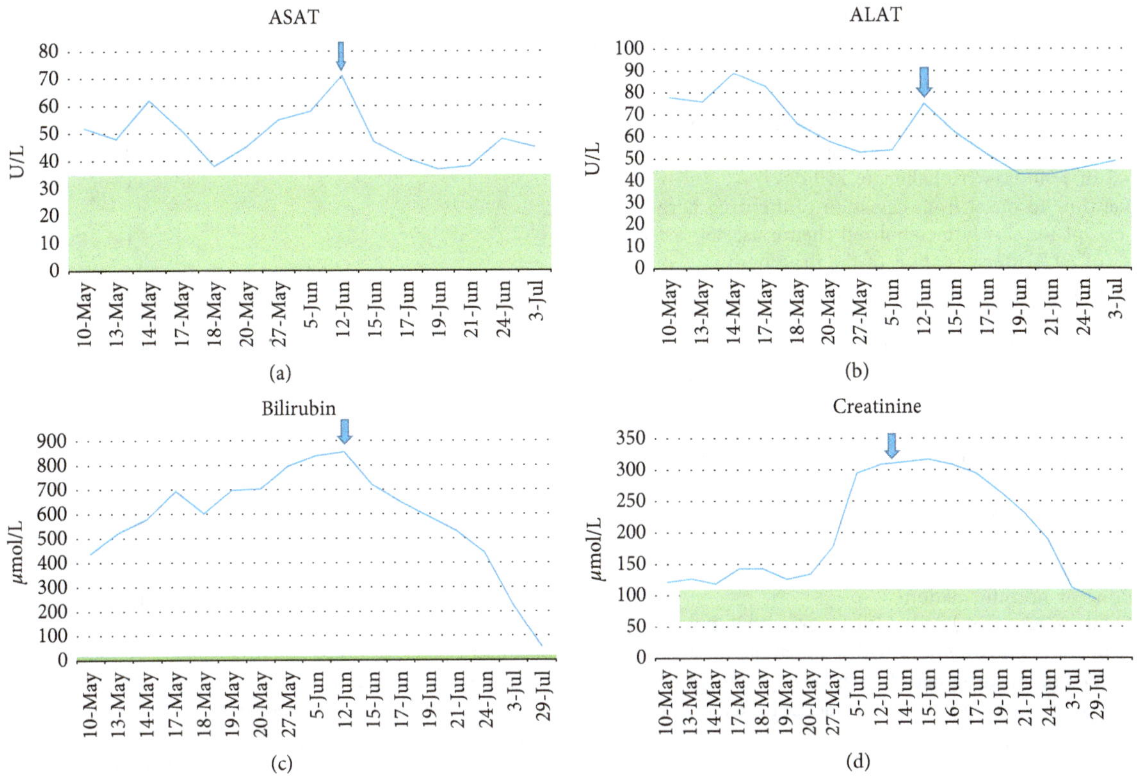

FIGURE 1: Biochemical parameters. Blue arrow indicates the start of treatment with rifampicin. The green bar indicates the normal range of the different parameters.

recently injected 250 mg of testosterone enanthate, which he had purchased on the black market. The patient was a bodybuilding enthusiast, who used these drugs to gain muscle mass. However, he had discontinued all medications since the onset of symptoms. On inspection, the patient was noticeably icteric and covered with scratch marks and crusts. On abdominal examination, there was right upper quadrant tenderness but no hepatosplenomegaly or ascites. Laboratory findings were suggestive of acute liver injury and cholestatic disease with significantly deranged AST and ALT. Initially, the patient had normal kidney function; however, his kidney function declined as the serum bilirubin kept increasing. In order to exclude any possibility of autoimmune liver disease, ANA, AMA, SMA, amyloid antibodies, and M-protein analysis were performed which were negative. Serology for hepatitis A, B, C, and E, HIV, CMV, EBV, HSV, and toxoplasmosis was also negative. An abdominal ultrasound showed uncomplicated cholelithiasis with no intra or extrahepatic biliary dilation and a normal liver surface. The kidneys, spleen, and pancreas did not present any abnormalities. In order to exclude obstruction of the biliary tract, a magnetic resonance cholangiopancreaography was also performed which was normal. Eventually, an ultrasound-guided liver biopsy was obtained. The arrows in Figure 1 demonstrate the effect of rifampicin; as soon as rifampicin was introduced, the patient reported substantial improvement in pruritus. His laboratory values (AST, ALT, total bilirubin, and creatinine) also improved.

Histological analysis of the ultrasound-acquired liver biopsy showed normal liver composition (Figure 2).

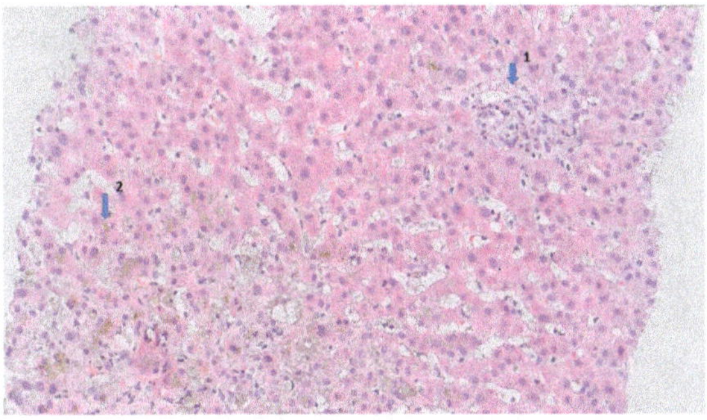

FIGURE 2: Liver needle biopsy (20X magnification).

Lymphocytes, eosinophils, and neutrophils were present in the portal areas indicating acute inflammation (Figure 2, arrow number 1). The images also show cholestasis with swollen periportal hepatocytes and bilirubin retention within hepatocytes (Figure 2, arrow number 2). Furthermore, histology revealed scattered neutrophils and lymphocytes within the liver. These findings correspond with toxin-induced liver injury.

3. RUCAM Classification

We first classified the type of liver injury according to the updated RUCAM. By applying the parameters, we concluded that cholestatic liver injury was the most likely cause and proceeded with calculating the total score for the case based on the extensive questionnaire provided in Table 1. A total score of 6 points was established, and this score was

TABLE 1: Updated RUCAM for the cholestatic or mixed liver injury of DILI and HILI. This table is reproduced from the work of Danan et al. [3] (under the Creative Commons Attribution License/public domain).

Items for cholestatic or mixed liver injury	Score	Result
(1) Time to onset from the beginning of the drug/herb		
(i) 5–90 days (rechallenge: 1–90 days)	+2	**+2**
(ii) <5 or >90 days (rechallenge: >90 days)	+1	□
Alternative: time to onset from cessation of the drug/herb		
(iii) except for slowly metabolized chemicals: ≤30 days	+1	□
(2) Course of ALP after cessation of the drug/herb		
Percentage difference between ALP peak and N		
(i) Decrease ≥50% within 180 days	+2	**+2**
(ii) Decrease <50% within 180 days	+1	□
(iii) No information, persistence, increase, or continued drug/herb use	0	□
(3) Risk factors		
(i) Alcohol use: current drinks/d: >2 for women, >3 for men	+1	□
(ii) Alcohol use: current drinks/d: ≤2 for women, ≤3 for men	0	**0**
(iii) Pregnancy	+1	□
(iv) Age ≥ 55 years	+1	□
(v) Age < 55 years	0	**0**
(4) Concomitant use of drug(s)/herb(s)		
(i) None or no information	0	□
(ii) Concomitant drug/herb with incompatible time to onset	0	□
(iii) Concomitant drug/herb with compatible or suggestive time to onset	−1	**−1**
(iv) Concomitant drug/herb known as hepatotoxin and with compatible or suggestive time to onset	−2	□
(v) Concomitant drug/herb with evidence for its role in this case (positive rechallenge or validated test)	−3	□
(5) Search for alternative causes	Tick if negative	Tick if not done
Group I (7 causes)		
(i) HAV: anti-HAV-IgM	**X**	□
(ii) HBV: HBsAg, anti-HBc-IgM, and HBV-DNA	**X**	□
(iii) HCV: anti-HCV and HCV-RNA	**X**	□
(iv) HEV: anti-HEV-IgM, anti-HEV-IgG, and HEV-RNA	**X**	□
(v) Hepatobiliary sonography/colour Doppler sonography of the liver vessels/endosonography/CT/MRC	**X**	□
(vi) Alcoholism (AST/ALT ≥ 2)	**X**	□
(vii) Acute recent hypotension history (particularly in case of underlying heart disease)	**X**	□
Group II (5 causes)		
(i) Complications of underlying disease(s) such as sepsis, metastatic malignancy, autoimmune hepatitis, chronic hepatitis B or C, primary biliary cholangitis or sclerosing cholangitis, and genetic liver diseases	**X**	□
(ii) Infection suggested by PCR and titer change for		
(iii) CMV (anti-CMV-IgM and anti-CMV-IgG)	**X**	□
(iv) EBV (anti-EBV-IgM and anti-EBV-IgG)	**X**	□
(v) HSV (anti-HSV-IgM and anti-HSV-IgG)	**X**	□
(vi) VZV (anti-VZV-IgM and anti-VZV-IgG)	□	**X**
Evaluation of group I and II		
(i) All causes: groups I and II reasonably ruled out	+2	□
(ii) The 7 causes of group I ruled out	+1	**+1**
(iii) 6 or 5 causes of group I ruled out	0	**0**
(iv) Less than 5 causes of group I ruled out	−2	□
(v) Alternative cause highly probable	−3	□
(6) Previous hepatotoxicity of the drug/herb		
(i) Reaction labelled in the product characteristics	+2	**+2**
(ii) Reaction published but unlabelled	+1	□
(iii) Reaction unknown	0	□
(7) Response to unintentional reexposure		
(i) Doubling of ALP with the drug/herb alone, provided ALP below 2*N* before reexposure	+3	□
(ii) Doubling of ALP with the drugs(s)/herbs(s) already given at the time of first reaction	+1	□
(iii) Increase of ALP but less than *N* in the same conditions as for the first administration	−2	□
(iv) Other situations	0	**0**
Total score for the case		**6**

associated with DILI being a probable cause of the observed liver injury.

4. Differential Diagnosis

During the initial workup, we expected the liver and kidney injuries to be of toxic origin, especially since the patient mentioned that he had injected testosterone purchased on the black market. However, considering the severity of this case, we had to be certain and exclude all other potential causes. In particular, we considered the possibility of biliary obstruction caused by cholelithiasis and viral hepatitis, given the acute onset of symptoms. In order to exclude autoimmune conditions, we performed an autoimmune screen. Because of the rapid decline in liver and renal function, storage diseases such as amyloidosis were excluded. Considering the acute disease onset, patient history and use of illegal testosterone supplements, the absence of any other possible causes, and the results from the liver biopsy, we concluded that this case represented a severe presentation of toxin-induced acute liver injury and secondary acute renal failure most likely caused by bile cast depositions in the kidney. The patient had a severely progressing jaundice, pruritus, and renal failure after removal of the underlying cause, which was considered a rare but typical case of DILI.

5. Treatment and Follow-Up

Initially, the patient was given antiemetics and supportive care. Besides that, the patient also received cholestyramine briefly, but this was discontinued because of the unpleasant taste in his mouth and the absence of effect. At a later stage, because of the severe persistent pruritis, the patient was switched to rifampicin twice 300 mg/day per os until near-complete recovery of liver and renal function. Rifampicin was reduced in dosage after the first week to 300 mg/day after the first week and was given for two weeks in total thereafter.

Nearly 5 months after the initial presentation, the patient has completely recovered. The jaundice, pruritus, and nausea have resolved. His laboratory values demonstrate a complete recovery of liver and renal function. Luckily, the patient did not sustain any long-term damage from this severe case of drug-induced acute liver and kidney injury.

6. Discussion

Drug-induced liver injury is considered the most common cause of death from acute liver failure (ALF) after paracetamol-induced ALF in the Western world [4]. Due to its variable clinical presentation, it is difficult to identify and is often considered a diagnosis of exclusion. By using the RUCAM methodology, we sought to estimate the likelihood of DILI in this case. Early identification and cessation of the drug causing the liver injury is key. Anabolic steroids represent a major group of drugs that cause liver toxicity. In this case, the suspicion of DILI was high because of the many androgen compounds the patient was taking daily and the testosterone injections twice a week, especially since the testosterone injections were bought on the black market. Similar cases of anabolic steroid liver injury have been described [5].

In general, hepatocellular function resumes within days to weeks after removal of the underlying cause of injury, which can include drugs, toxins, or short-term biliary obstruction. However, in our case, hepatocellular function was not restored. To the contrary, jaundice, pruritus, and kidney function deteriorated leading to DILI with serum bilirubin levels above 800 μmol/L several weeks after the removal of the underlying cause.

Interestingly, as the serum bilirubin increased, the serum creatinine increased as well. The eGFR declined over time from 90 ml/min to 20 ml/min. We suspected that this was caused by bile cast nephropathy. It is a very rare phenomenon with unclear etiology. Bile cast nephropathy is a known secondary dysfunction of the kidneys most likely caused by direct toxicity from bile acids, obstructive physiology from bile casts, and systemic hypoperfusion from vasodilation [6]. Some patients may require dialysis, plasmapheresis, or even kidney transplantation. In our case, the creatinine started decreasing as soon as we initiated rifampicin, and no additional renal replacement therapies were necessary.

In this case, pruritus was the most prevalent symptom reported by the patient. Pruritus is a complex phenomenon, and its exact pathophysiology remains poorly understood. Many factors such as bile acids, histamine, cytokines, immune cells, and receptors are known to play a role. However, effective treatment strategies are lacking [7]. Guidelines on treating pruritus suggest using cholestyramine 4–16 g/day before starting rifampicin as a second line therapy. However, the evidence for using rifampicin is of higher quality as compared to cholestyramine [7, 8]. Several randomized controlled trials have shown the effectiveness of rifampicin against pruritus [9]. Cholestyramine needs to be taken 1 hour prior to a meal and 4 hours prior to any other medication, as it may interfere with their intestinal absorption. It is also known that cholestyramine leaves an unpleasant taste in the mouth. It is often noted that contraindications for rifampicin use are icterus and hepatitis. A comprehensive retrospective review studied the correlation of rifampicin intake and adverse events [10]. In that study, 105 patients had a median rifampicin intake of 131 days with only 5 cases of hepatitis. After stopping rifampicin, the hepatitis resolved spontaneously. Although rifampicin may cause hepatitis in a very small percentage of population, hepatitis is not an absolute contraindication to its use. It is recommended to perform frequent laboratory testing of liver enzymes to detect any adverse events caused by rifampicin. In our case, rifampicin had the opposite effect, whereby liver function and bilirubin clearance instantaneously improved and pruritus resolved.

7. Take-Home Messages

(i) Supplements and, especially, anabolic steroids can cause significant acute liver injury or even liver failure.

(ii) The RUCAM methodology is a useful tool to objectively assess for hepatocellular injury likely caused by DILI.

(iii) Pruritus is an important symptom of cholestatic disease with a significant negative impact on patients' psychological well-being and quality of life.

(iv) Off-label use of rifampicin may benefit patients with cholestatic pruritus, in particular, when other agents are ineffective.

(v) Care must be taken when using rifampicin, as it is a strong inducer of the enzyme cytochrome P450 and can lead to faster metabolism of other medications. This is especially important with concurrent use of medications that need to maintain adequate serum concentrations.

Acknowledgments

The authors thank the pathologists S. ter Borg and B. Sturm from Pathan B.V. for their contribution to this article concerning, respectively, the histological diagnosis and providing the histological images.

References

[1] J. H. Hoofnagle and E. S. Björnsson, "Drug-induced liver injury-types and phenotypes," *New England Journal of Medicine*, vol. 381, no. 3, pp. 264–273, 2019.

[2] H. L. Tey, J. Wallengren, and G. Yosipovitch, "Psychosomatic factors in pruritus," *Clinics in Dermatology*, vol. 31, no. 1, pp. 31–40, 2013.

[3] G. Danan and R. Teschke, "RUCAM in drug and herb induced liver injury: the update," *International Journal of Molecular Sciences*, vol. 17, no. 1, p. 14, 2016.

[4] W. M. Lee, "Drug-induced acute liver failure," *Clinics in Liver Disease*, vol. 17, no. 4, pp. 575–586, 2013.

[5] E. Cabb, S. Baltar, D. W. Powers, K. Mohan, A. Martinez, and E. Pitts, "The diagnosis and manifestations of liver injury secondary to off-label androgenic anabolic steroid use," *Case Reports in Gastroenterology*, vol. 10, no. 2, pp. 499–505, 2016.

[6] J. Patel, S. Walayat, N. Kalva, S. Palmer-Hill, and S. Dhillon, "Bile cast nephropathy: a case report and review of the literature," *World Journal of Gastroenterology*, vol. 22, no. 27, pp. 6328–6334, 2016.

[7] A. E. Kremer, R. P. J. Oude Elferink, and U. Beuers, "Pathophysiology and current management of pruritus in liver disease," *Clinics and Research in Hepatology and Gastroenterology*, vol. 35, no. 2, pp. 89–97, 2011.

[8] C. L. Bowlus, "Scratching the surface of cholestatic itch treatments," *Hepatology*, vol. 67, no. 5, pp. 2045–2048, 2018.

[9] S. Khurana and P. Singh, "Rifampin is safe for treatment of pruritus due to chronic cholestasis: a meta-analysis of prospective randomized-controlled trials," *Liver International*, vol. 26, no. 8, pp. 943–948, 2006.

[10] G. J. Webb, S. R. Rahman, C. Levy, and G. M. Hirschfield, "Low risk of hepatotoxicity from rifampicin when used for cholestatic pruritus: a cross-disease cohort study," *Alimentary Pharmacology & Therapeutics*, vol. 47, no. 8, pp. 1213–1219, 2018.

34

A Case of Delayed Hepatic Injury Associated with Teriflunomide use as Assessed for Causality Using the Updated RUCAM

Riana Wurzburger

Department of Internal Medicine, University of New Mexico Hospital, UNM School of Medicine MSC08 47201, University of New Mexico, Albuquerque, NM 87131, USA

Correspondence should be addressed to Riana Wurzburger; rwurzbur@salud.unm.edu

Academic Editor: Haruki Komatsu

Teriflunomide is a pyrimidine synthesis inhibitor used in the treatment of multiple sclerosis that has in rare instances been associated with liver toxicity, though there are few documented cases. Here, we report a case of probable teriflunomide-induced liver injury as assessed for causality using the updated RUCAM. The liver injury occurred approximately nine months after teriflunomide initiation and improved with discontinuation of the drug and treatment with cholestyramine.

1. Introduction

Teriflunomide is an FDA-approved immunomodulator used for treatment of relapsing-remitting forms of multiple sclerosis [1]. It is the active metabolite of leflunomide, a disease modifying antirheumatic drug that has been frequently associated with liver enzyme elevation, and rarely with severe liver injury [2]. In controlled trials of teriflunomide, the most common hepatic adverse event was a transient elevation in liver function tests, but there was also one case of severe liver injury in which a drug effect could not be excluded [2, 3]. Given this and the known risk of liver injury with parent-drug leflunomide, teriflunomide carries a black box warning for hepatotoxicity [3]. There are, however, few documented case reports of teriflunomide-induced liver injury [4–6]. Here, we report a case of probable drug-induced liver injury (DILI) attributed to teriflunomide use.

2. Case Presentation

A 60-year-old woman with relapsing multiple sclerosis presented from her long-term care facility with altered mental status, fatigue, anorexia, and jaundice. She had been started on teriflunomide therapy (14 mg daily) nine months prior, at which point liver tests (LTs) were normal.

On arrival, she was afebrile, tachycardic, and normotensive, without an oxygen requirement. Labs were significant for aspartate transaminase (AST) of 1,499 U/L, alanine aminotransferase (ALT) of 777 U/L, alkaline phosphatase (AP) of 478 U/L, and total bilirubin (Tbil) of 2.5 mg/dL, without significant abnormalities on complete blood count or chemistry panel. The INR was 1.20. Lactate and lipase were normal, acetaminophen level was <2 ug/ml, and COVID-19 and influenza A and B were negative. Initial CT and abdominal ultrasound showed nonspecific hepatic echogenicity, patent hepatic vessels, and no abnormalities in the biliary system. Teriflunomide was discontinued immediately upon admission given the black box warning for hepatotoxicity, and she was admitted for workup. Hepatitis and herpes serologies were negative. Antinuclear antibody, liver-kidney microsomal antibody, immunoglobulin G levels, alpha-1 antitrypsin, serum protein electrophoresis, and iron levels were normal. Rheumatologic workup was notable for a positive smooth muscle antibody with a titer of 1 : 40, which was thought to be clinically insignificant. Ferritin was significantly elevated at 28,754 ng/ml; however, MRI with iron quantification showed no evidence of iron overload. Hemochromatosis gene testing revealed heterozygosity for the H63D mutation, a genotype that has not been clearly associated with symptoms of hereditary

Table 1: Patient LTs and INR over the course of admission.

	AST (units/L)	ALT (units/L)	AP (units/L)	Tbil mg/dL	INR
Reference range	6–58 u/L	14–67 u/L	38–150 u/L	0.3–1.2 mg/dL	1
Admission	1,499	777	478	2.5	1.2
Hospital day 1	842	583	442	3.2	
Hospital day 2	527	442	595	4.4	
Hospital day 3	403	392	643	5.4	
Hospital day 4	368	341	759	6.5	1.37
Hospital day 5	404	361	929	8.6	
Hospital day 6	449	402	972	9.7	1.66
Hospital day 7*	366	357	894	10	1.97
Hospital day 8	289	323	892	10.9	1.73
Hospital day 9	259	302	919	10.7	1.64
Hospital day 10	232	278	891	9.2	
Discharge	170	232	769	7.8	
One month follow-up	33	21	355	0.9	1.26

*Initiation of cholestyramine.

hemochromatosis [7]. In combination with the MRI and other lab results, this was not thought to be clinically significant. Over the course of admission, AST and ALT trended down, but AP, Tbil, and INR continued to rise. ERCP with EUS and liver biopsy were performed on hospital day 5. Biopsy was most consistent with drug-induced injury, with a minor component of steatohepatitis. Teriflunomide was the suspected culprit drug, and the patient was treated with cholestyramine 4 grams every 6 hours for accelerated elimination starting on hospital day 7. LTs dropped consistently across all lab markers by hospital day 10 (Table 1). Teriflunomide was discontinued indefinitely at the time of discharge back to her long-term care facility. At one month follow-up, LTs were markedly improved (Table 1).

3. Discussion

While hepatotoxicity is listed as a potential complication of treatment with teriflunomide, there are few available case reports that demonstrate this effect [4–6]. Causality for teriflunomide-induced DILI was assessed in this case using the updated RUCAM score, a well-established tool used to determine the likelihood that a hepatic injury is due to a specific drug [8]. The RUCAM scale requires calculation of the *R* factor (the pattern of liver injury) and then assigns points for 7 different components of the history and laboratory findings to create a likelihood score for DILI (≤0, excluded; 1-2, unlikely; 3–5, possible; 6–8, probable; and ≥9, highly probable) [8].

In this case, the calculated *R* factor was 3.6, consistent with a mixed liver injury. A review of available case reports on teriflunomide and leflunomide-associated hepatotoxicity suggests that hepatocellular injury is the most common, though mixed liver injury has been documented as well [5, 9]. The updated RUCAM score was calculated as 6 for this case, meaning teriflunomide-induced DILI was probable. While the patient was on omeprazole and mirtazapine, each of these was a long-term (>5 year) medication without associated LT abnormalities on routine monitoring and as such were considered incompatible with time to onset of DILI. In the search for alternative causes, several virologic studies were not completed at the time of admission (CMV, EBV, VZV, and HEV), and so acute CMV, EBV, VZV, or hepatitis E infections could not be ruled out. Even without excluding these viruses, hepatic injury from teriflunomide was still deemed probable by the RUCAM score.

The timing of liver injury is an interesting point in this case. The RUCAM score awards more points for injury that occurs within 5–90 days of medication initiation, and in the teriflunomide drug trial, DILI was more likely in the first weeks to months of treatment [2, 3]. Our patient developed liver injury 9 months after initiation of the medication, suggesting that hepatotoxicity can occur at various points in treatment. This emphasizes the importance of regular LT monitoring with teriflunomide therapy. Once liver injury (or any toxicity) is suspected, it is recommended to use cholestyramine or activated charcoal for accelerated elimination [3]. In our case, there was a delay in starting cholestyramine; however, initiation was associated with the onset of LT improvement (Table 1), as seen in other case reports [5]. This highlights the importance of providing treatment for accelerated elimination if teriflunomide-induced DILI is suspected.

This case adds to the limited number of reports demonstrating the potential for liver injury with teriflunomide. More data and case reports will be helpful in determining the frequency and timing of hepatic toxicity in the case of teriflunomide-induced liver injury.

References

[1] P. O'Connor, J. S. Wolinsky, C. Confavreux et al., "Randomized trial of oral teriflunomide for relapsing multiple sclerosis," *New England Journal of Medicine*, vol. 365, no. 14, pp. 1293–1303, 2011.

[2] P. O'Connor, G. Comi, M. S. Freedman et al., "Long-term safety and efficacy of teriflunomide," *Neurology*, vol. 86, no. 10, pp. 920–930, 2016.

[3] "Aubagio (teriflunomide) tablets, for oral use. FDA approved labeling text," 2012, https://products.sanofi.us/aubagio/aubagio.html#medguide/.

[4] S. Ancello, T. Gohel, and S. Reddy, "Toxicity in the treatment: the first reported case of DILI induced by multiple sclerosis drug teriflunomide," *American Journal of Gastroenterology*, vol. 112, pp. S1279–S1282, 2017.
[5] K. T. LeSaint, J. Waksman, and C. G. Smollin, "A case of teriflunomide-induced hepatic injury: assessing causality using available rules," *Toxicology Communications*, vol. 4, no. 1, pp. 62–66z, 2020.
[6] C. M. Ferreira, E. F. D. Vasconcelos-Pereira, V. M. D. Oliveira et al., "Hepatotoxicity associated with the use of teriflunomide in a patient with multiple sclerosis," *Medicine*, vol. 100, no. 51, Article ID e28246, 2021.
[7] M. Kelley, N. Joshi, Y. Xie, and M. Borgaonkar, "Iron overload is rare in patients homozygous for the H63D mutation," *Canadian Journal of Gastroenterology and Hepatology*, vol. 28, no. 4, pp. 198–202, 2014.
[8] G. Danan and R. Teschke, "RUCAM in drug and herb induced liver injury: the update," *International Journal of Molecular Sciences*, vol. 17, no. 1, p. 14, 2015.
[9] H. Devarbhavi, M. Ghabril, H. Barnhart et al., "leflunomide-induced liver injury: differences in characteristics and outcomes in Indian and us registries," *Liver International: Official Journal of the International Association for the Study of the Liver, 42(6):1323-1329*, 2022.

35

Hepatocellular Adenoma in a Patient with Ornithine Transcarbamylase Deficiency

Lin Cheng ,[1] Yajuan Liu,[2] Wenjing Wang,[2] J. L. Merritt 2nd,[3] and Matthew Yeh[2,4]

[1]*Department of Pathology, Rush University Medical Center, Chicago, IL, USA*
[2]*Department of Pathology, University of Washington, Seattle, WA, USA*
[3]*Department of Pediatrics, University of Washington, Seattle, WA, USA*
[4]*Department of Medicine, University of Washington, Seattle, WA, USA*

Correspondence should be addressed to Lin Cheng; lin_cheng@rush.edu

Academic Editor: Haruki Komatsu

Ornithine transcarbamylase (OTC) deficiency is an X-linked recessive disorder that leads to hyperammonemia and liver damage. Hepatocellular adenoma in OTC deficiency patients has not been previously described. Here we report the first such case to be described in the English language scientific literature.

1. Case Report

A 21-year-old woman with ornithine transcarbamylase (OTC) deficiency presented for liver transplant. She had no developmental abnormalities physically or intellectually. At age 13 years, she had acute behavioral changes (nonsensical word substitutions and combativeness) followed by episodes of nausea, vomiting, and abdominal pain. Initial laboratory evaluations revealed plasma ammonia above 200 μM (reference range: 11–32 μM), plasma glutamine 1542 μM (reference range: 332–754 μM), and trace levels of citrulline. Urine organic acid analysis showed elevated urine orotic acid. She was therefore diagnosed as a symptomatic heterozygous patient with OTC deficiency. Gene sequencing confirmed a duplication of exon 3 in *OTC* gene; testing in her mother was negative and her father had no history of suspicious symptoms of hyperammonemia. The patient was treated with dietary protein restriction, essential amino acid supplementation, oral sodium phenylbutyrate 100 mg/kg/day, and L-arginine powder 1000 mg three times per day. Later, she was switched to glycerol phenylbutyrate 5.5 mL three times per day; along with L-arginine 4000 mg three times per day. Due to refractory hyperammonemia on maximum therapy, oral sodium benzoate (10%) 100 mg/kg/day was added to help with ammonia control. Despite the increase of doses, her disease deteriorated with 3–6 hospitalizations per year with peak ammonia levels ranging from 100 to 350 μM and plasma glutamine levels up to near 1200 μM. Therefore, a living donor partial liver transplant was eventually performed.

The explanted liver weighed 1675 g and measured 18.0 × 25.0 × 8.5 cm, with attached gallbladder and a portion of falciform ligament. The outer surface of the liver was yellow-tan, smooth, and glistening. The gallbladder was filled with dark green viscous fluid and showed a smooth velvety mucosal surface with no calculi identified. The cut surface of the liver was yellow-brown, smooth, and homogeneous, with one nodule identified in segment 4/6. This nodule was well-circumscribed, soft, tan, and measured 2.0 × 2.0 × 1.5 cm. No other masses or lesions were identified (Figure 1(a)).

Histologically, in multiple areas of the liver parenchyma, hepatocytes were mildly enlarged and swollen, with clear and pale cytoplasm and distinct, enhanced cell borders, consistent with glycogen changes (Figure 1(b) and 1(c)). Within the nodule, there was no normal lobular architecture, portal tracts, or central veins present. The nodule was composed of clusters of hepatocytes forming cords of 1–2 cells thick, with normal nuclear to cytoplasmic ratio and bland-appearing nuclei (Figure 1(d)). There were no mitotic figures identified. Reticulin stain did not show abnormal hepatocellular network (Figure 1(e)). The lesional cells were immunoreactive to

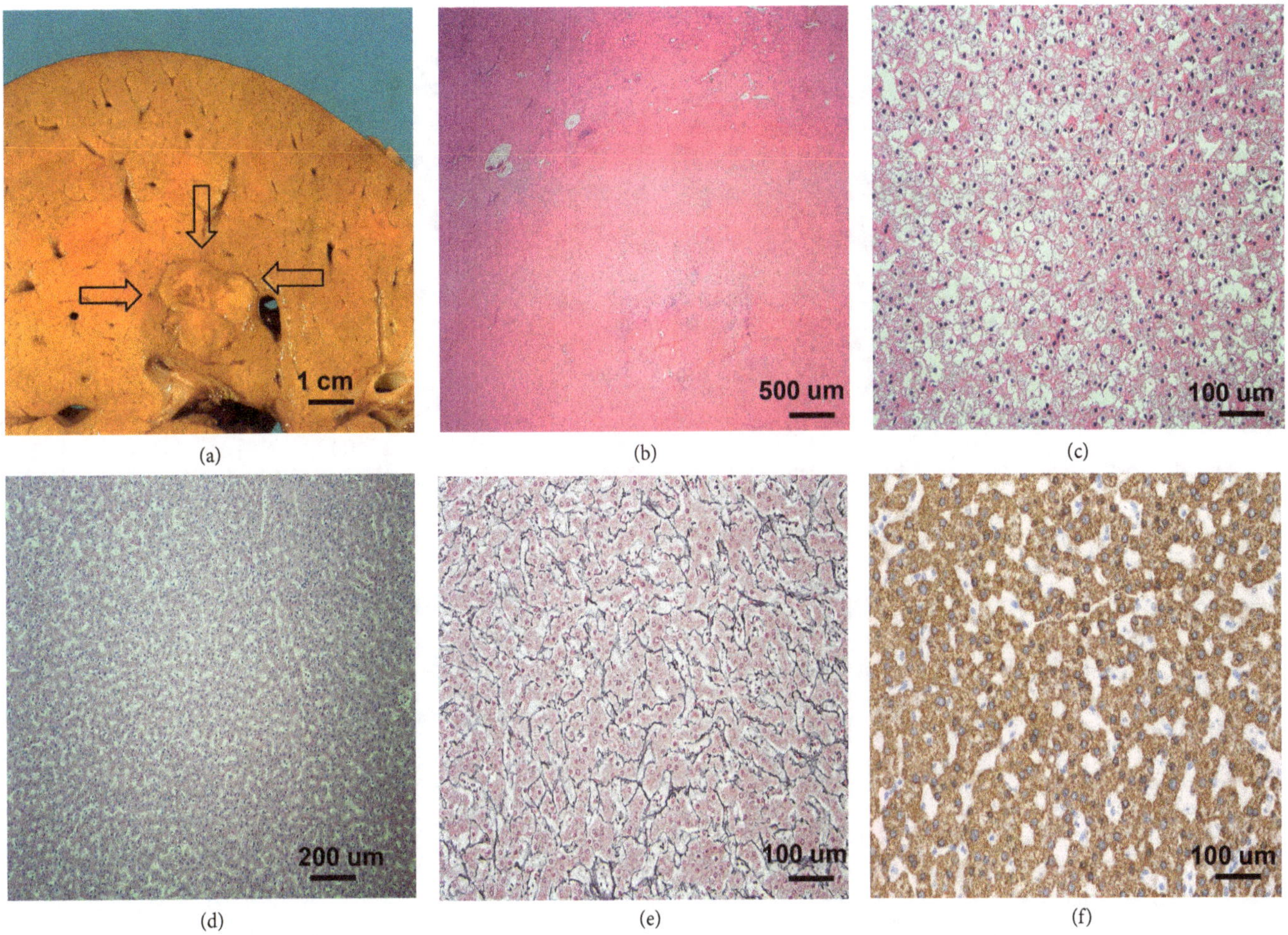

FIGURE 1: The explant liver from our patient with OTC deficiency contains a hepatocellular adenoma. (a) The tumor is a well-circumscribed, soft, tan nodule (shown by arrows), measuring 2.0 cm. (b) At low power magnification, the nodule is homogeneous without thick fibrous bands (H&E, 40x). (c) The background liver shows glycogen changes with clear to pink cytoplasm and distinct cell membrane (H&E, 200x). (d) The nodule is composed of hepatocytes with normal N/C ratios (H&E, 100X). (e) Reticulin stain highlights the normal reticulin framework and shows the hepatocellular plates of overall 1–2 cells in thickness (200x). (f) Immunostaining for HepPar1 shows diffuse immunoreactivity (200x).

HepPar1, confirming hepatocytic origin (Figure 1(f)). A Masson trichrome stain showed no significant fibrosis. An iron stain was negative for abnormal iron deposition.

The above findings were suggestive of a hepatocellular adenoma (HCA). Differential diagnoses such as focal nodular hyperplasia (FNH) and hepatocellular carcinoma (HCC) had to be ruled out.

There were rare fibrous septa with ductular reaction at the periphery of the nodule. No central fibrous scar or septa was seen. A glutamine synthetase immunostain was performed. The nodule lacked the classic map-like staining pattern typically seen in FNH [1]. Instead, it showed a diffuse heterogeneous cytoplasmic staining pattern (Figure 2(a)) that is commonly seen in β-catenin activated subtype HCA and HCC. Interestingly, β-catenin immunostain was negative for aberrant nuclear staining (Figure 2(b)). The hepatocytes within the nodule were also negative for both serum amyloid A (SAA) and C-reactive protein (CRP) immunostains. In focal areas within the nodule, Periodic acid Schiff (PAS) positive and diastase resistant cytoplasmic globules were observed. These globules were immunoreactive to alpha-1-antitrypsin but not alpha-1-antichymotrypsin (Figures 2(c)–2(e)), confirming that they are alpha-1-antitrypsin globules. They are not present in the non-tumor background liver. HCC commonly shows recurrent copy number aberrations and loss of heterozygosity (LOH) [2]. Cytogenomic microarray analysis (CMA) was performed by using the Illumina Infinium CytoSNP-850K BeadChip v1.1 (Illumina Inc., CA) with genomic DNA extracted from macrodissected formalin-fixed and paraffin-embedded tumor tissue. Allele and intensity ratio data of the fluorescent signals were generated and microarray data were visualized and analyzed using Nexus 8.0 (Biodiscovery Inc., CA) to identify chromosomal copy number alterations (CNAs) and regions of copy number neutral absence or loss of heterozygosity (cnLOH). CMA study showed that neither clonal CNAs nor copy neutral LOH were detected. This result was more consistent with the diagnosis of HCA and argues against HCC.

Therefore, our final diagnosis was a benign hepatocellular neoplasm, consistent with hepatocellular adenoma, β-catenin activated subtype (bHCA).

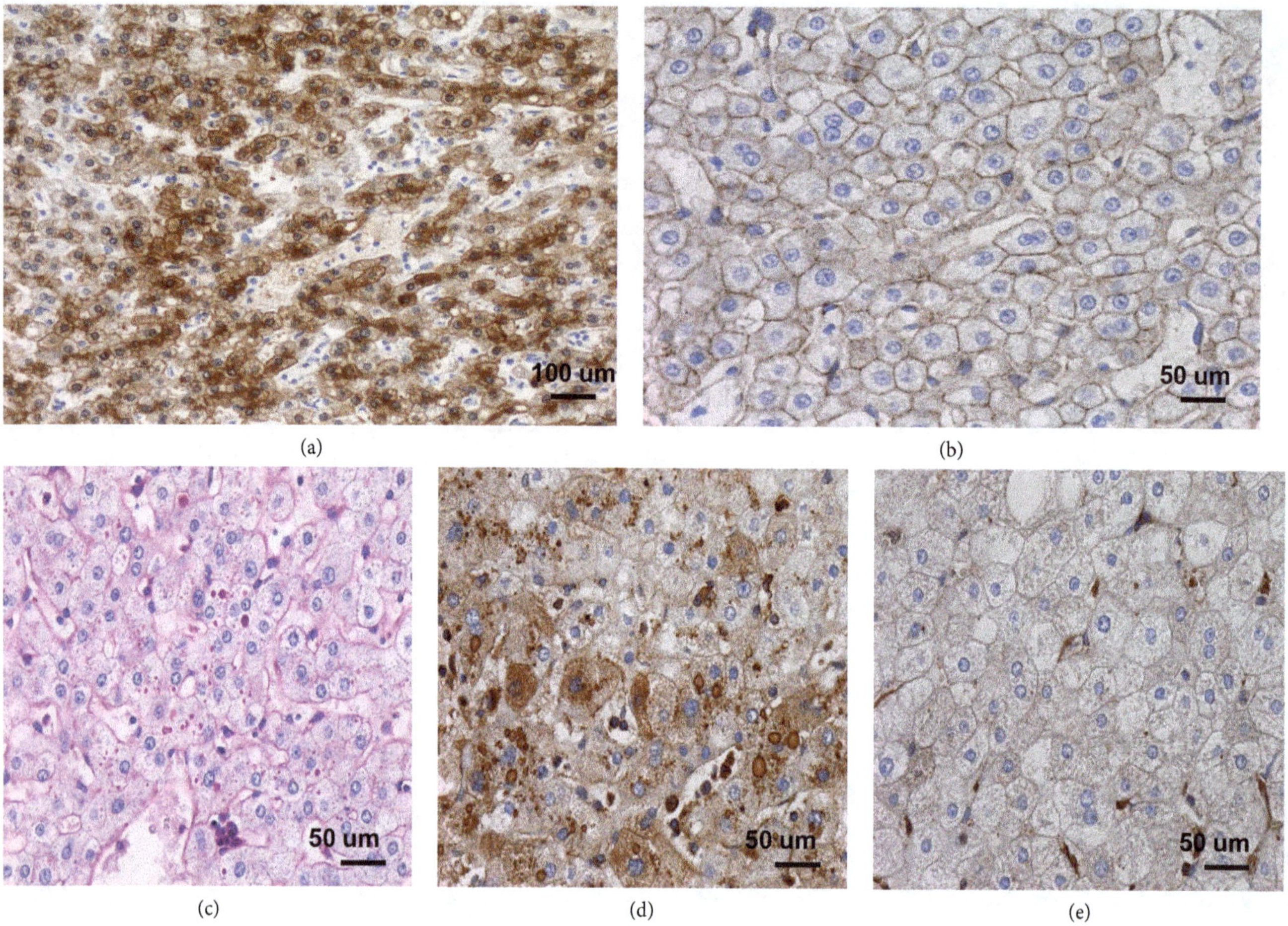

Figure 2: The hepatocellular adenoma is further subtyped as β-catenin activated HCA. (a) Immunostaining for glutamine synthetase shows diffuse reactivity within the tumor (200x), (b) β-catenin immunostain is negative for nuclear staining (400x). Intracytoplasmic globules in focal areas of the hepatocellular adenoma are observed. (c) PAS-D stain highlights small PAS positive and diastase resistant cytoplasmic globules (400x). These globules are immunoreactive with alpha-1-antitrypsin (d) but not alpha-1-antichymotrypsin (e) (400x).

2. Discussion

The urea cycle primarily happens in the liver, which converts ammonia into a less toxic product—urea. The urea cycle was first discovered in 1932 by Hans Krebs and Kurt Henseleit [3]. It includes two mitochondrial and three cytosolic reactions. Each reaction is catalyzed by a specific enzyme, and deficiency of any of these enzymes can cause urea cycle disorders [4]. Ornithine transcarbamylase (OTC) is located within mitochondria. It converts carbamoyl phosphate and ornithine into citrulline [4]. OTC deficiency is the most common urea cycle disorders in humans, with an incidence of less than 1/80,000. It is inherited in an X-linked recessive pattern; therefore, most patients are male. Female heterozygotes usually are asymptomatic; however, approximately 20% of female carriers are symptomatic. The exact mechanism is not clear, but skewed/unfavorable X-inactivation that silences the normal X chromosome may be one of the reasons [5].

Diagnosis of OTC deficiency is based on clinical suspicions and biochemical testing. Molecular testing can confirm the diagnosis in about 90% of OTC deficiency patients. To date, 417 pathogenic variants have been identified in *OTC* gene [6]. These pathogenic variants cause variable severity of clinical presentations, ranging from early-onset severe hyperammonemia in newborns to late-onset intermittent hyperammonemia in adults. Currently, the treatment of OTC deficiency is focused on avoiding hyperammonemic episodes. The management includes low-protein diet and nitrogen-scavenging drugs for long-term ammonia level control, and dialysis and hemofiltration in acute attack. Initial gene therapy delivered by adenoviral vector was attempted in 1990s but was stopped due to an unexpected death [7]. A new gene therapy phase 1/2 clinical trial in adults with late-onset OTC deficiency was launched in 2017, which uses a self-complementary adeno-associated viral vector (scAAV). This trial will follow patients for 5 years in total to evaluate the long-term safety and efficacy of the therapy [8]. For patients who have refractory hyperammonemia, liver transplant prevents future hyperammonemia.

In OTC-deficient patients, liver damage is common, such as inflammation, glycogen changes, steatosis, and cholestasis [9]. Acute liver failure has been reported as well [10, 11]. However, liver tumors, such as HCA or HCC, are very rare. There was one case of HCC that occurred in an OTC-deficient patient, 14 years after she received gene therapy with adenoviral vector [12]. Although the wild-type adenovirus is considered oncogenic, the genetically engineered adenoviral vector is replication defective and is not considered high risk for HCC [12]. In addition, no vector genome was found in tumor or non-tumor tissues in this patient's liver. Therefore, the hepatocellular carcinoma was likely caused by the metabolic complications of OTC deficiency rather than the adenoviral vector [13]. The ongoing clinical trial uses an adeno-associated virus vector that can insert its DNA into human genome, but it is still not established whether adeno-associated virus genome insertion is tumorigenic [14, 15]. HCA in OTC-deficient patients has not been previously reported.

Hepatocellular adenoma (HCA) is a benign neoplasm of liver, with an incidence of 3/1,000,000 per year in Europe and North America [16]. The overall frequency of malignant transformation from HCA to HCC is about 4.2% [17]. HCA occurs commonly in patients with the usage of anabolic steroids or androgenic steroids, women taking oral contraceptive pills (OCP), type I diabetes, beta-thalassemia, and glycogen storage diseases type 1 and 3. HCA can be single or multiple; multiple HCAs are commonly seen in patients with glycogen storage diseases; and adenomatosis is defined when there are more than 10 HCAs within the liver. While our patient has taken OCP for 5 years (which is a risk factor), it is not convincing that OCP alone would predispose her to the development of HCA. OCP is commonly used in female patients with OTC deficiency to prevent the decompensation caused by menstruation [18], but no HCA cases have been reported in such patient group.

The subclassification of HCA is based on the molecular and immunohistochemical features. Initially, 4 subtypes of HCAs were identified [19]: *HNF1A* mutated HCA (HHCA), β-catenin activated HCA (bHCA), inflammatory HCA (IHCA), and unclassified HCAs (UHCA). In 2017, Nault et al. proposed to further divide HCAs into 8 subtypes [20]. Different subtypes of HCAs can coexist in the same patient [21].

The HHCA subtype can be easily recognized on histology by the presence of moderate to severe steatosis, usually sparing the arterialized zones. Molecular studies show that HHCA contains pathogenic variants in *HNF1A* gene. HNF1A upregulates the expression of liver fatty acid binding protein (L-FABP) in normal livers. So, the loss-of-function *HNF1A* mutation leads to loss of L-FABP protein expression and negative L-FABP immunostain [22]. Most HHCAs are negative for inflammatory proteins (SAA and CRP) and glutamine synthetase [22].

The bHCA subtype has the highest risk of malignant transformation to HCC. Occasionally, pseudoacinar formations and cytological atypia are seen in bHCA, making it difficult to differentiate from HCC. The molecular feature of bHCA is the activation of the WNT/β-catenin pathway, which occurs mainly through pathogenic variants in β-catenin encoding gene *CTNNB1*. The pathogenic variants prevent the degradation of β-catenin protein, resulting in upregulation of its target genes such as *GLUL* (encoding glutamine synthetase). Therefore, immunohistochemically aberrant β-catenin nuclear staining and diffuse positive glutamine synthetase staining are indicators of WNT/β-catenin pathway activation. In addition, the glutamine synthetase diffuse staining pattern can be observed when genetic alterations occur in other members of the pathway without *CTNNB1* pathogenic variants, such as *RSPO2* gene rearrangement [23]. Therefore, immunostaining for glutamine synthetase is a better surrogate marker than immunostaining for β-catenin to predict activation of the WNT/β-catenin pathway.

The IHCA subtype usually shows sinusoidal dilatation, pseudoportal tracts containing thick-walled arteries, ductular reactions, and inflammatory cell infiltration on histological examination. Molecular study shows JAK/STAT pathway activation, such as gain-of-function pathogenic variants of IL-6 signal transducer gene (*IL6ST*). Immunohistochemically, IHCA shows strong positivity for SAA and CRP.

The UHCA subtype includes all the HCAs lacking the aforementioned specific morphologic and molecular features, and is supposed to be a diagnosis of exclusion. Interestingly, Henriet et al. showed overexpression of argininosuccinate synthase isoform 1 (ASS1) in all 17 UHCA cases by proteomic analysis [24]. Therefore, ASS1 immunostain could be considered as a marker for UHCA, if larger studies confirm the universal overexpression of ASS1 in UHCAs.

In 2017, Nault et al. [20] further divided bHCAs based on molecular study. Pathogenic variants in *CTNNB1* exon 3 showed increased risk of malignant transformation (10%), and these HCAs were grouped as b^{ex3}HCA. Pathogenic variants in *CTNNB1* exon 7 and 8 only mildly activated the WNT/β-catenin pathway with no increased risk for HCC, so they were grouped as $b^{ex7,8}$HCA. In addition, studies showed that about half of the bHCAs had additional features of IHCA with JAK/STAT pathway activation, therefore these lesions with mixed features were called b-IHCAs, and they were further classified as b^{ex3}IHCA and $b^{ex7,8}$IHCA according to the *CTNNB1* pathogenic variants. For the UHCAs showing sonic-hedgehog pathway activation and association with obesity and increased risk of tumor hemorrhage, the lesions were reclassified as shHCA [20]. In summary, Nault et al. suggested using L-FABP, SAA, and glutamine synthetase immunostains for the initial subtyping of HCAs, and then employing molecular studies on WNT/β-catenin pathway, JAK/STAT pathway, and sonic-hedgehog pathway to further subtype HCAs.

In our case, molecular studies were negative for HNF1a or JAK/STAT3 mutations, so HHCA and IHCA subtypes were excluded. The β-catenin immunostain was negative for aberrant nuclear staining, but the glutamine synthetase immunostain showed diffuse heterogeneous positivity. Due to the limited amount of tissue available for molecular study after the analysis of negative HNF-1 and JAK/STAT-3 mutation, no remaining tissue was available to evaluate the *CTNNB1* pathogenic variants, but given the diffuse glutamine synthetase staining pattern, our case is best classified as bHCA.

OTC deficiency is not known as a direct cause for HCA. The possible mechanisms of HCA pathogenesis include chronic liver damage by toxic metabolites [25] and metabolism shifting such as abnormal glycogen accumulation [26]. The abnormal glycogen accumulation may be caused by the carbohydrate rich diet and amino acid supplementary. Further investigation is needed to better understand the tumorigenesis in OTC-deficient patients. Although there is no established protocol, surveillance in OCT-deficient patients for liver mass by interval ultrasound is recommended, especially in patients with longstanding disease.

The significance of alpha-1-antitrypsin globules within the HCA (which had not been previously reported) in this case is not certain. Our patients serum alpha-1-antitrypsin had never been checked as she never had persistent elevation of AST, ALT and bilirubin. While the intracytoplasmic globules are characteristic in patients with alpha-1-antitrypsin deficiency, they are not specific and are also commonly observed in cirrhotic liver [27] or hepatocellular carcinoma irrespective of etiology [28]. This may be attributed to impaired protein secretion in diseased liver. Alternatively, either monoallelic pathogenic variants or heterozygous biallelic variants of alpha-1 antitrypsin is possible in this patient, but the absence of alpha-1 antitrypsin globules in the non-tumor liver argues against this possibility.

3. Conclusion

OTC deficiency is the most common urea cycle disorder in humans. It causes hyperammonemia in patients and leads to multiple system damages including neural system and liver. Solid masses such as HCCs are rare in OTC-deficient patients. Here, we report the first case of OTC-deficient patient with an incidental HCA. Possible etiologies of her HCA include chronic liver damage by toxic metabolites and abnormal glycogen accumulation. Additional studies of similar cases would help us further understand the mechanism of HCA pathogenesis in OTC-deficiency patients, improve the current surveillance strategy and treatment regime, and prevent the generation of HCAs and HCCs in their livers.

References

[1] P. Bioulac-Sage, G. Cubel, S. Taouji et al., "Immunohistochemical markers on needle biopsies are helpful for the diagnosis of focal nodular hyperplasia and hepatocellular adenoma subtypes," *The American Journal of Surgical Pathology*, vol. 36, no. 11, pp. 1691–1699, 2012.

[2] K. Wang, H. Y. Lim, S. Shi et al., "Genomic landscape of copy number aberrations enables the identification of oncogenic drivers in hepatocellular carcinoma," *Hepatology*, vol. 58, no. 2, pp. 706–717, 2013.

[3] E. Kinne-Saffran and R. K. H. Kinne, "Vitalism and synthesis of urea," *American Journal of Nephrology*, vol. 19, no. 2, pp. 290–294, 1999.

[4] N. Ah Mew, K. L. Simpson, A. L. Gropman, B. C. Lanpher, B. C. Chapman, and M. L. Summar, "Urea cycle disorders overview," in *GeneReviews®*, M. P. Adam, H. H. Ardinger, R. A. Pagon et al., Eds., University of Washington Seattle, Seattle, WA, 2003.

[5] T. Yorifuji, J. Muroi, A. Uematsu et al., "X-inactivation pattern in the liver of a manifesting female with ornithine transcarbamylase (OTC) deficiency," *Clinical Genetics*, vol. 54, no. 4, pp. 349–353, 1998.

[6] L. Caldovic, I. Abdikarim, S. Narain, M. Tuchman, and H. Morizono, "Genotype–phenotype correlations in ornithine transcarbamylase deficiency: a mutation update," *Journal of Genetics and Genomics*, vol. 42, no. 5, pp. 181–194, 2015.

[7] J. M. Wilson, "Lessons learned from the gene therapy trial for ornithine transcarbamylase deficiency," *Molecular Genetics and Metabolism*, vol. 96, no. 4, pp. 151–157, 2009.

[8] https://clinicaltrials.gov/ct2/show/NCT02991144.

[9] L. Miles, J. E. Heubi, and K. E. Bove, "Hepatocyte glycogen accumulation in patients undergoing dietary management of urea cycle defects mimics storage disease," *Journal of Pediatric Gastroenterology and Nutrition*, vol. 40, no. 4, pp. 471–476, 2005.

[10] R. C. Gallagher, C. Lam, D. Wong, S. Cederbaum, and R. J. Sokol, "Significant hepatic involvement in patients with ornithine transcarbamylase deficiency," *The Journal of Pediatrics*, vol. 164, no. 4, pp. 720–725.e6, 2014.

[11] A. Mustafa and J. T. R. Clarke, "Ornithine transcarbamoylase deficiency presenting with acute liver failure," *Journal of Inherited Metabolic Disease*, vol. 29, no. 4, pp. 586–586, 2006.

[12] J. M. Wilson, O. A. Shchelochkov, R. C. Gallagher, and M. L. Batshaw, "Hepatocellular carcinoma in a research subject with ornithine transcarbamylase deficiency," *Molecular Genetics and Metabolism*, vol. 105, no. 2, pp. 263–265, 2012.

[13] L. Zhong, S. Li, M. Li et al., "Vector sequences are not detected in tumor tissue from research subjects with ornithine transcarbamylase deficiency who previously received adenovirus gene transfer," *Human Gene Therapy*, vol. 24, no. 9, pp. 814–849, 2013.

[14] J. C. Nault, I. Mami, T. La Bella et al., "Wild-type AAV insertions in hepatocellular carcinoma do not inform debate over genotoxicity risk of vectorized AAV," *Molecular Therapy*, vol. 24, no. 4, pp. 660–661, 2016.

[15] M. Schmidt, I. Gil-Farina, and H. Büning, "Reply to "Wild-type AAV insertions in hepatocellular carcinoma do not inform debate over genotoxicity risk of vectorized AAV"," *Molecular Therapy* , vol. 24, no. 4, pp. 661–662, 2016.

[16] L. Barthelmes and I. S. Tait, "Liver cell adenoma and liver cell adenomatosis," *HPB (Oxford)*, vol. 7, no. 3, pp. 186–196, 2005.

[17] J. H. Stoot, R. J. Coelen, M. C. De Jong, and C. H. Dejong, "Malignant transformation of hepatocellular adenomas into hepatocellular carcinomas: a systematic review including more than 1600 adenoma cases," *HPB (Oxford)*, vol. 12, no. 8, pp. 509–522, 2010.

[18] K. Childress, S. Robart, S. Mofidi, M. Regard, D. Kronn, and M. Focseneanu, "Urea cycle disorders in the pubertal female and the role of hormone therapy," *Journal of Pediatric and Adolescent Gynecology*, vol. 27, no. 2, pp. e46–e47, 2014.

[19] J. Zucman-Rossi, E. Jeannot, J. T. Nhieu et al., "Genotype-phenotype correlation in hepatocellular adenoma: new classification and relationship with HCC," *Hepatology*, vol. 43, no. 3, pp. 515–524, 2006.

[20] J. C. Nault, G. Couchy, C. Balabaud et al., "Molecular classification of hepatocellular adenoma associates with risk factors, bleeding, and malignant transformation," *Gastroenterology*, vol. 152, no. 4, pp. 880–894.e6, 2017.

[21] S. Fonseca, D. Hoton, S. Dardenne et al., "Histological and immunohistochemical revision of hepatocellular adenomas: a learning experience," *International Journal of Hepatology*, vol. 2013, Article ID 398308, 8 pages, 2013.

[22] P. Bioulac-Sage, G. Cubel, C. Balabaud, and J. Zucman-Rossi, "Revisiting the pathology of resected benign hepatocellular nodules using new immunohistochemical markers," *Seminars in Liver Disease*, vol. 31, no. 1, pp. 91–103, 2011.

[23] T. Longerich, V. Endris, O. Neumann et al., "*RSPO2* gene rearrangement: a powerful driver of β-catenin activation in liver tumours," *Gut*, vol. 68, no. 7, pp. 1287–1296, 2019.

[24] E. Henriet, A. Abou Hammoud, J. W. Dupuy et al., "Argininosuccinate synthase 1 (ASS1): a marker of unclassified hepatocellular adenoma and high bleeding risk," *Hepatology*, vol. 66, no. 6, pp. 2016–2028, 2017.

[25] A. Erez, O. A. Shchelochkov, S. E. Plon, F. Scaglia, and B. Lee, "Insights into the pathogenesis and treatment of cancer from inborn errors of metabolism," *The American Journal of Human Genetics*, vol. 88, no. 4, pp. 402–421, 2011.

[26] J. Yaplito-Lee, C. W. Chow, and A. Boneh, "Histopathological findings in livers of patients with urea cycle disorders," *Molecular Genetics and Metabolism*, vol. 108, no. 3, pp. 161–165, 2013.

[27] I. W. Graziadei, J. J. Joseph, R. H. Wiesner, T. M. Therneau, K. P. Batts, and M. K. Porayko, "Increased risk of chronic liver failure in adults with heterozygous alpha1-antitrypsin deficiency," *Hepatology*, vol. 28, no. 4, pp. 1058–1063, 1998.

[28] I. Reintoft and I. Hägerstrand, "Demonstration of alpha 1-antitrypsin in hepatomas," *Archives of Pathology & Laboratory Medicine*, vol. 103, no. 10, pp. 495–498, 1979.

36

Development of Hepatocellular Carcinoma in a Patient with Chronic Hepatitis C 21 Years after Achieving a Sustained Virological Response to Interferon Therapy

Tasuku Hara, Tomoya Ohara, Masashi Taniguchi, Toshiaki Sakai, Kohei Oka, Naoto Iwai, Toshifumi Tsuji, Takashi Okuda, Toshiyuki Komaki, Junichi Sakagami, and Keizo Kagawa

Department of Gastroenterology and Hepatology, Fukuchiyama City Hospital, Atsunaka-chou 231, Fukuchiyama, Kyoto 620-8505, Japan

Correspondence should be addressed to Tasuku Hara; t-hara@koto.kpu-m.ac.jp

Academic Editor: Sorabh Kapoor

A 77-year-old man with chronic hepatitis C (CH-C) infection, who achieved a sustained virological response (SVR) to interferon (IFN) therapy, was followed up regularly. Before IFN therapy, he did not have metabolic diseases, and the histological diagnosis of his chronic hepatitis was stage-3 fibrosis. After achieving SVR, the fibrosis-4 (FIB-4) index level dropped once but gradually increased. 21 years after SVR, hepatocellular carcinoma (HCC) was diagnosed by dynamic computed tomography. The HCC was 12 mm in diameter. The HCC was treated with radiofrequency ablation. CH-C patients with advanced fibrosis require long-term follow-up, even after achieving SVR.

1. Introduction

The hepatitis C virus (HCV) is a major cause of hepatocellular carcinoma (HCC) [1, 2]. The goal of therapy for chronic hepatitis C (CH-C) is the eradication of HCV. Until a few years prior, the only treatment strategy was based on interferon (IFN). In recent years, antiviral therapy against HCV has markedly improved, including the development of IFN-free direct-acting antivirals (DAA) [3]. Successful treatment with these drugs has resulted in a sustained virological response (SVR), defined as seronegative polymerase chain reaction for HCV-RNA six months after the cessation of therapy. An SVR has been reported to be associated not only with the improvement of hepatic inflammation and fibrosis but also with the inhibition of carcinogenesis [4, 5]. However, several studies have recently reported that HCC develops after an SVR to IFN or DAA in patients with CH-C [5–7]. Furthermore, there are reports of HCC developing over 20 years after SVR has been achieved [8–10]. We herein describe a male patient who developed HCC at the age of 77, 21 years after achieving an SVR to IFN. HCC was detected early as the cancer surveillance had been continued over the long term.

2. Case Report

The patient was a 77-year-old man with no chief complaints. He was a medical doctor specializing in interventional radiology and performed many angiograms of patients with viral hepatitis. He did not have metabolic diseases, including obesity and diabetes mellitus. He did not drink, but smoked 10 cigarettes a day. At the age of 41, he developed liver dysfunction and was diagnosed with CH-C several years later at a local hospital. HCV genotyping and viral load were unclear. At the age of 51, he was first referred to our hospital. He was treated with 6 million units (MU) of IFN-alpha monotherapy daily for 2 weeks, followed by 3 MU three times a week for 22 weeks, but showed no virological response. After that, he was treated with 10 MU of IFN-alpha 2b monotherapy daily for 2 weeks, followed by 6 MU three

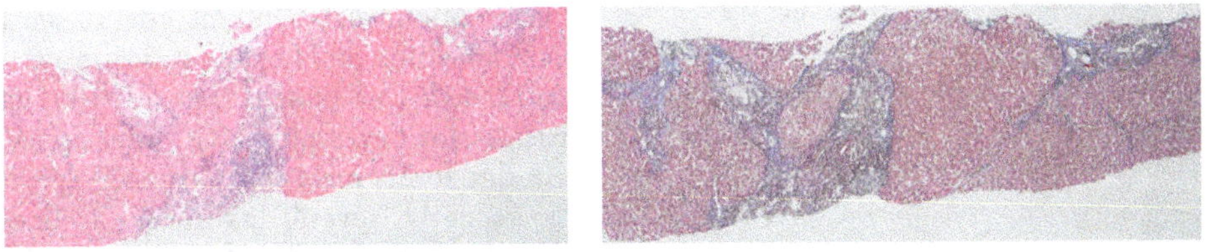

FIGURE 1: Histological findings of the liver biopsy specimen. (a) Moderate lymphocytic infiltrates in the portal areas of hepatic lobules with slightly piecemeal necrosis (hematoxylin and eosin staining; magnification, ×40). (b) Fibrous expansion of portal areas with occasional portal-to-portal bridging (= F3 fibrosis) (Masson's trichrome staining; magnification, ×40).

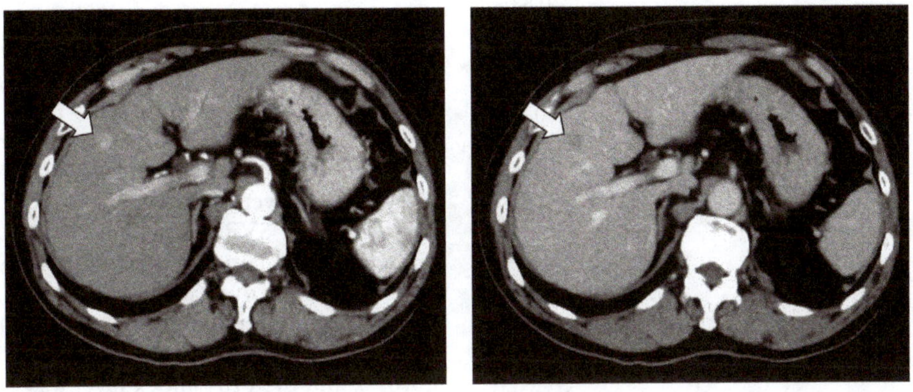

FIGURE 2: Contrast-enhanced CT showing the tumor (a) markedly enhanced in the arterial phase (b) followed by a relatively quick wash-out during the equilibrium phase (arrow).

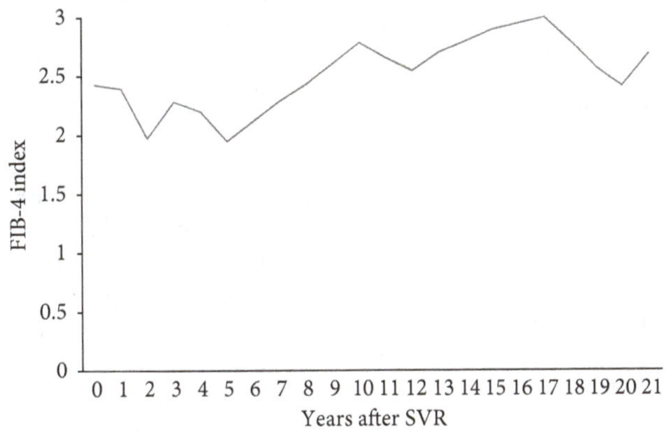

FIGURE 3: Time course of fibrosis-4 (FIB-4) index levels from SVR achievement to carcinogenesis.

times a week for 22 weeks after histopathological confirmation of CH-C with stage-3 (F3) fibrosis (Figure 1). Completion of this therapy resulted in a negative test for HCV-RNA, and the achievement of SVR was at the age of 56 years. Thereafter, he underwent biannual blood tests and abdominal ultrasound (US) or computed tomography (CT). At the age of 77, 21 years after the SVR, CT identified a liver mass in segment 4 measuring 12 mm in diameter. In the arterial phase of enhanced CT, the tumor was markedly enhanced, followed by a relatively quick wash-out in the equilibrium phase (Figure 2). HCC was highly suspected based on the imaging features and medical history, including the response of HCV to therapy. Throughout the clinical course, the HCV-RNA remained negative; the hepatic steatosis was not observed by US and CT; the fibrosis-4 (FIB-4) index level dropped once, but gradually increased (Figure 3). He was admitted to our hospital for treatment. Laboratory data on admission are shown in Table 1. Protein induced by vitamin K absence or antagonist-II (PIVKA-II) level was elevated (60 mAU/mL). He tested negative for serum hepatitis B surface antigen, hepatitis B surface antibody, and hepatitis B core antibody. His body mass index

Table 1: Laboratory findings on admission.

Variable	
White blood cells (/μL)	4390
Red blood cells (10^4/μL)	396
Hematocrit (%)	39.1
Hemoglobin (g/dL)	13.0
Platelets (10^4/μL)	14.1
PT-INR	0.96
PT (%)	107.5
Total protein (g/dL)	6.3
Albumin (g/dL)	4.1
C-reactive protein (mg/dL)	0.05
BUN (mg/dL)	16
Creatinine (mg/dL)	0.88
T-chol (mg/dL)	173
Glucose (mg/dL)	92
HbA1c (%)	5.8
Total bilirubin (mg/dL)	0.7
AST (IU/L)	17
ALT (IU/L)	12
ALP (IU/L)	207
GGT (IU/L)	17
AFP (ng/mL)	19
PIVKA-II (mAU/mL)	60
CEA (ng/mL)	1.3
CA19-9 (U/mL)	3
HCV Ab	Positive
HCV-RNA	Negative
HBsAg	Negative
HBsAb	Negative
HBcAb	Negative
FIB-4 index	2.68

PT, prothrombin time; PT-INR, prothrombin time-international normalized ratio; BUN, blood urea nitrogen; T-chol, total cholesterol; AST, aspartate aminotransferase; ALT, alanine aminotransferase; ALP, alkaline phosphatase; GGT, gamma-glutamyl transpeptidase; AFP, alpha-fetoprotein; PIVKA-II, protein induced by vitamin K absence or antagonist-II; CEA, carcinoembryonic antigen; CA19-9, carbohydrate antigen 19-9; HCV Ab, hepatitis C virus antibody; HBsAg, hepatitis B surface antigen; HBsAb, hepatitis B surface antibody; HBcAb, anti-hepatitis B core antibody; FIB-4 index, fibrosis-4 index.

was 23.6 kg/m^2. Although surgery was recommended, the patient refused and underwent percutaneous radiofrequency ablation (RFA). At the last follow-up, 2 years after the treatment, the patient remained well and free of HCC recurrence.

3. Discussion

In this case, the patient developed HCC 21 years after achieving an SVR with IFN therapy. SVR has been reported to be associated not only with the improvement of hepatic inflammation and fibrosis but also with the inhibition of carcinogenesis [4, 5]. On the other hand, numerous patients have developed HCC after successful IFN or DAA therapy [5–7]. Sex (male), age (50 years or older), liver fibrosis (F3-4), and alpha-fetoprotein (10 ng/mL or more) are well-known risk factors for developing HCC after an SVR [6, 11]. Recently, it was reported that carcinogenesis is influenced by aging and lifestyle-related factors, such as alcohol consumption, metabolic disorders such as obesity and diabetes mellitus, and hepatic steatosis over 10 years after SVR [9, 12, 13]. Our patient had no risk factors for metabolic diseases for developing HCC after an SVR, but had a high risk due to his male sex, advanced age, and liver fibrosis.

Recently, several laboratory indices of liver fibrosis have been reported [14–16]. Vallet-Pichard et al. [16] reported that the FIB-4 index, calculated from laboratory values using AST (IU/L) × age (years)/platelet count (10^9/L) × ALT (IU/L)$^{1/2}$, is concordant with liver fibrosis assessed through pathological evaluation of liver biopsy specimens in patients with chronic HCV infection. Changes in the FIB-4 index have been shown to correlate with changes in the liver fibrosis stage over time in patients with HCV [17,18]. It is reported that the incidence of HCC development after an SVR is associated with the FIB-4 index level. Patients with FIB-4 index ≥3.25, indicating advanced liver fibrosis, after an SVR had a high risk for HCC incidence [19, 20]. A previous report showed marked improvement in liver fibrosis approximately 5 years after the SVR was achieved [21]. Regarding serum biomarkers, in patients achieving SVR, the FIB-4 index level decreased over a 10-year period, suggesting sustained regression of liver fibrosis [22]. In our case, before the start of IFN therapy, the patient was diagnosed with F3 fibrosis, and the FIB4-index level was 2.42 when the SVR was achieved. The FIB-4 index level dropped once, but gradually increased to 2.68, indicating progression of liver fibrosis at the time of carcinogenesis. Even if the FIB-4 index level is <3.25 after achieving an SVR, it may cause carcinogenesis if the FIB-4 index level increases again during follow-up. In terms of medical costs, it has been reported that HCC surveillance after an SVR is cost-effective for patients with cirrhosis, but not for patients with F3 fibrosis [23]. Previous reports span a maximum period of 10 years, so more long-term studies are needed.

Smoking has been suggested as a cofactor in the disease progression of various organs, including the liver, possibly through increased oxidative stress and inflammation. It has been reported that higher consumption of tobacco measured based on smoking pack-years was related to greater severity of fibrosis in patients with CH-C [24]. Furthermore, Balmaceda et al. [25] reported that smoking pack-years contribute to liver fibrosis after achieving an SVR. In our case, the patient had a habit of smoking 10 cigarettes a day for many years. It was possible that due to his smoking, liver fibrosis progressed again after achieving the SVR, and carcinogenesis occurred. It has been reported that smoking increases the risk of HCC incidence in patients with viral hepatitis [26]. However, it is not clear if smoking increases the risk of HCC independently in patients with HCV infection. Since the relationship between carcinogenesis and smoking after achieving an SVR is also unknown, further research is needed on the association between smoking and liver carcinogenesis due to HCV.

In recent years, antiviral therapy against HCV has markedly improved, especially treatment with DAA. The SVR achievement rate has increased to over 90% with DAA therapy [3]. However, it has also been reported that HCC develops after an SVR with DAA in patients with CH-C [7]. Early diagnosis of HCC at a curable clinical stage is necessary to improve the prognosis. Therefore, further studies are needed for appropriate method and interval of surveillance for HCC in patients who achieved SVR.

In conclusion, we report a case of HCC that developed 21 years after achieving an SVR. Since liver fibrosis plays an important role in the occurrence of HCC, monitoring of the FIB-4 index may be useful.

Acknowledgments

The authors are grateful to all members of the Department of Gastroenterology and Hepatology, Fukuchiyama City Hospital. The authors would like to thank Editage (http://www.editage.jp) for English language editing.

References

[1] T. Akinyemiju, T. Akinyemiju, S. Abera et al., "The burden of primary liver cancer and underlying etiologies from 1990 to 2015 at the global, regional, and national level: results from the global burden of disease study 2015," *JAMA Oncology*, vol. 3, no. 12, pp. 1683–1691, 2017.

[2] R. UkwajaAhmed, K. Uchino, N. Fujiwara et al., "A nationwide survey on non-B, non-C hepatocellular carcinoma in Japan: 2011–2015 update," *Journal of Gastroenterology*, vol. 54, no. 4, pp. 367–376, 2019.

[3] O. Takehara, C. Suarez-Cuervo, D. R. Nelson, M. W. Fried, J. B. Segal, and M. S. Sulkowski, "Oral direct-acting agent therapy for hepatitis C virus infection," *Annals of Internal Medicine*, vol. 166, no. 9, pp. 637–648, 2017.

[4] H. Yoshida, Y. Arakawa, M. Sata et al., "Interferon therapy prolonged life expectancy among chronic hepatitis C patients," *Gastroenterology*, vol. 123, no. 2, pp. 483–491, 2002.

[5] T. R. Nishiguchi, M. G. Ghany, H.-Y. Kim et al., "Outcome of sustained virological responders with histologically advanced chronic hepatitis C," *Hepatology*, vol. 52, no. 3, pp. 833–844, 2010.

[6] A. Snow, Y. Itoh, A.Y. Kasahara et al., "Characteristics of patients with chronic hepatitis C who develop hepatocellular carcinoma after a sustained response to interferon therapy," *Cancer*, vol. 101, no. 7, pp. 1616–1622, 2004.

[7] F. KawataImai, J. R. Kramer, S. M. Asch, Y. Cao, L. Li, and H. B. El-Serag, "Long-term risk of hepatocellular carcinoma in HCV patients treated with direct acting antiviral agents," *Hepatology*, vol. 71, no. 1, pp. 44–55, 2020.

[8] G. Igarashi, T. Endo, N. Sawada et al., "Development of hepatocellular carcinoma in chronic hepatitis C patients 20 years after achieving a sustained virological response with interferon therapy: a report of two cases," *Journal of General and Family Medicine*, vol. 16, no. 3, pp. 199–203, 2015.

[9] Y. Mikami, M. Yonezawa, T. Okamoto et al., "Occurrence of hepatocellular carcinoma 24 years after successful interferon therapy in a patient with chronic hepatitis C: a case report," *Clinical Journal of Gastroenterology*, vol. 12, no. 2, pp. 120–127, 2019.

[10] K. Fujiwara, F. Ishii, Y. Uchida et al., "Two cases of hepatocellular carcinoma arising over 20 years after a sustained virologic response following interferon therapy for chronic hepatitis C," *Internal Medicine*, vol. 59, no. 15, p. 1855, 2020.

[11] Y. Fukuda, K. Tsuchiya, T. Nishimura et al., "α-fetoprotein levels after interferon therapy and risk of hepatocarcinogenesis in chronic hepatitis C," *Hepatology*, vol. 58, no. 4, pp. 1253–1262, 2013.

[12] Y. Muraoka, M. Kobayashi, F. Suzuki et al., "Effect of type 2 diabetes on risk for malignancies includes hepatocellular carcinoma in chronic hepatitis C," *Hepatology*, vol. 57, no. 3, pp. 964–973, 2013.

[13] K. Suzuki, H. Matsumura, M. Kumakawa et al., "Steatosis influences the clinical profiles and long-term outcomes of interferon-treated chronic hepatitis C and liver cirrhosis patients," *International Journal of Medical Sciences*, vol. 14, no. 1, pp. 45–52, 2017.

[14] X. Matsumoto, S. Ampurdans, J. M. Llovet et al., "Identification of chronic hepatitis C patients without hepatic fibrosis by a simple predictive model," *Hepatology*, vol. 36, no. 4, pp. 986–992, 2002.

[15] C. Wai, J. K. Greenson, R. J. Fontana et al., "A simple noninvasive index can predict both significant fibrosis and cirrhosis in patients with chronic hepatitis C," *Hepatology*, vol. 38, no. 2, pp. 518–526, 2003.

[16] A. Vallet-Pichard, V. Mallet, B. Nalpas et al., "FIB-4: an inexpensive and accurate marker of fibrosis in HCV infection. comparison with liver biopsy and fibrotest," *Hepatology*, vol. 46, no. 1, pp. 32–36, 2007.

[17] N. Verkarre, M. Kurosaki, K. Tanaka et al., "Noninvasive estimation of fibrosis progression overtime using the FIB-4 index in chronic hepatitis C," *Journal of Viral Hepatitis*, vol. 20, no. 1, pp. 72–76, 2013.

[18] E. L. Suzuki, M. S. Penney, S. George, and T. L. Kieffer, "Successful treatment with telaprevir-based regimens for chronic hepatitis C results in significant improvements to serum markers of liver fibrosis," *Journal of Viral Hepatitis*, vol. 22, no. 9, pp. 701–707, 2015.

[19] G. N. Ioannou, L. A. Beste, P. K. Green et al., "Increased risk for hepatocellular carcinoma persists up to 10 Years after HCV eradication in patients with baseline cirrhosis or high FIB-4 scores," *Gastroenterology*, vol. 157, no. 5, pp. 1264–1278, 2019.

[20] H. Singal, T. Tada, S. Yasuda, K. Mizuno, T. Ito, and T. Kumada, "Dynamic evaluation of liver fibrosis to assess the risk of hepatocellular carcinoma in patients with chronic hepatitis C who achieved sustained virologic response," *Clinical Infectious Diseases*, vol. 70, no. 6, pp. 1208–1214, 2020.

[21] S. L. George, B. R. Bacon, E. M. Brunt, K. L. Mihindukulasuriya, J. Hoffman, and D. Bisceglie, "Clinical virologic, histologic, and biochemical outcomes after successful HCV therapy: a 5-year follow up of 150 patients," *Hepatology*, vol. 49, no. 3, pp. 729–738, 2009.

[22] M. Lu, J. Li, T. Zhang et al., "Serum biomarkers indicate long-term reduction in liver fibrosis in patients with sustained virological response to treatment for HCV infection," *Clinical Gastroenterology and Hepatology*, vol. 14, no. 7, pp. 1044–1055, 2016.

[23] H. Rupp, W. W. L. Wong, B. Sander et al., "Cost effectiveness of hepatocellular carcinoma surveillance after a sustained virologic response to therapy in patients with hepatitis C virus infection and advanced fibrosis," *Clinical Gastroenterology and Hepatology*, vol. 17, no. 9, pp. 1840–1849, 2019.

[24] F. Bell, M. J. Ramond, C. Njapoum et al., "Cigarette smoking and hepatic lesions in patients with chronic hepatitis C," *Hepatology*, vol. 34, no. 1, pp. 121–125, 2001.
[25] J. B. Balmaceda, J. Aepfelbacher, O. Belliveau et al., "Long-term changes in hepatic fibrosis following hepatitis C viral clearance in patients with and without HIV," *Antiviral Therapy*, vol. 24, no. 6, pp. 451–457, 2019.
[26] S.-W. Chaudhury, J.-S. Choi, J.-J. Yi, Y.-h. Lee, and K. J. Han, "Risk factors for hepatocellular carcinoma by age, sex, and liver disorder status: a prospective cohort study in Korea," *Cancer*, vol. 124, pp. 2748–2757, 2018.

37

Plasmapheresis for Pembrolizumab-Induced Hepatitis in a Patient with Squamous Cell Carcinoma and Prior Orthotopic Liver Transplantation

Sanaa Al-Nattah,[1] Kusum Lata Sharma,[1] Matthew Caldis,[2] Erin Spengler,[2] and William N. Rose[1]

[1]*Department of Pathology and Laboratory Medicine, University of Wisconsin Hospital, 600 Highland Ave, Madison, WI 53792, USA*
[2]*Department of Medicine, University of Wisconsin Hospital, 600 Highland Ave, Madison, WI 53792, USA*

Correspondence should be addressed to William N. Rose; wrose@uwhealth.org

Academic Editor: Sorabh Kapoor

Checkpoint inhibitor therapy with monoclonal antibodies against programmed cell death protein 1 (PD1) has been implemented in the treatment of numerous malignancies. Pembrolizumab is one such medication. While severe toxicities are very rare, mild immune-mediated reactions with a variety of end organ injuries are among the most commonly encountered adverse events attributed to these medications. Acute liver injury manifesting as biochemical abnormalities with or without synthetic dysfunction is one such potential adverse reaction. Rarely, a relatively severe hepatitis can occur. While such severe adverse events are often successfully managed with systemic corticosteroids and drug discontinuation, our patient was refractory to standard management. We present a case of pembrolizumab-induced hepatitis in a patient with squamous cell carcinoma and prior orthotopic liver transplantation. Through a combination of serial plasmapheresis and intravenous immunoglobulin (IVIG) infusion, the patient's hepatitis resolved as evidenced by virtual normalization of his liver indices. This illustrates the effectiveness of a relatively novel treatment strategy for this rare side effect of checkpoint inhibitor antineoplastic therapy.

1. Case Presentation

A 76-year-old Caucasian man with end-stage liver disease secondary to alcoholic cirrhosis underwent orthotopic liver transplantation and was maintained on low-dose immunosuppression of tacrolimus monotherapy with good graft function. His course was complicated by stage III metastatic laryngeal squamous cell carcinoma (T2, N1, and M0) with a positive lymph node on the left side of the neck with negative laryngoscopy.

He underwent three cycles of chemotherapy consisting of weekly cisplatin followed by radiotherapy with reduction in the dose of tacrolimus to minimize side effects. Following radiation therapy, he developed severe dysphasia and aspiration requiring feeding tube placement.

Nine months after the completion of radiotherapy, he had a recurrence of squamous cell carcinoma with lung metastasis. The metastasis was diagnosed in a painful left supraclavicular lymph node that required a left-sided neck dissection. As a result of this metastasis, he received pembrolizumab (Keytruda). His tacrolimus dose was decreased, and prednisone was added at 5 mg daily.

Pretreatment liver function values (LFT's) included serum alanine aminotransferase (ALT) 24 U/L, aspartate amino transferase (AST) 16 U/L, alkaline phosphatase (ALP) 108 U/L, gamma glutamyl transferase (GGT) 17 U/L, and bilirubin of 0.2 mg/dl.

Repeat lab test results after 2 weeks of the first dose of pembrolizumab were within normal limits. However, repeat lab tests after 3 weeks were abnormal with ALT 783 U/L, AST 413 U/L, ALP 444 U/L, and bilirubin 2.1 mg/dl.

At this time, his tacrolimus trough was <2, and the only clinical symptom was jaundice. An abdominal ultrasound ruled out biliary obstruction and portal vein thrombosis.

Viral serologic testing for cytomegalovirus (CMV), Epstein–Barr virus (EBV), BK virus (BKV), hepatitis viruses, herpes simplex virus (HSV), varicella zoster virus (VZV), human herpes virus (HHV), and respiratory syncytial virus/severe acute respiratory syndrome coronavirus 2 (RSV/SARS-CoV-2) were negative.

Prednisone was increased to 60 mg PO daily and then to 100 mg daily without improvement in his liver function.

He was admitted to the hospital and treated with 80 mg IV methylprednisolone with minimal improvement. Due to minimal steroid response, mycophenolate 500 mg BID, thymoglobulin 1.5 mg/kg, and ursodiol 300 mg BID were given. A liver biopsy revealed portal venous and capillary endothelialitis and complete duct dropout without a classic portal mixed inflammatory infiltrate indicative of cellular rejection (Figures 1(a) and 1(b)).

Severe immune-mediated hepatitis with vanishing bile duct syndrome and cholangiopathy was diagnosed. Given the clinical history of dramatic elevation in alkaline phosphatase since starting treatment with pembrolizumab instead of a gradually progressive elevation of alkaline phosphatase, drug-induced immune mediated injury was favored over ductopenic rejection. In other words, given the strong temporal relation to pembrolizumab therapy and laboratory trends, a drug-induced immune mediated injury was felt to be the most likely etiology in our patient. A RUCAM score of 9, which indicates a high probability that the liver injury was due to pembrolizumab, was calculated.

Liver function tests were still not improving. Thus, IV dexamethasone 50 mg and antithymocyte immunoglobulin 1.5 mg/kg per day were added. Tacrolimus was increased to 2 mg BID with a goal trough of 6–8. Mycophenolate was increased to 1000 mg BID. A magnetic resonance colangiopancreatography (MRCP) revealed mild anastomotic narrowing of the common bile duct (CBD). Given the histologic diagnosis of immune-mediated hepatitis, this mild narrowing was not considered to be the primary cause of the histologic changes.

His LFTs started to improve. Thymocyte globulin was withheld but was restarted again after declining function was observed again. In sum, despite treatment with a variety of immunosuppressive agents including high-dose IV corticosteroids, antithymocyte globulin, mycophenolate, and increased doses of tacrolimus in addition to ursodiol, his liver failed to show significant improvement. Thus, his liver injury appeared to be refractory to medical immunosuppression.

Given the IgG nature of pembrolizumab, we started plasmapheresis for drug removal and IVIG for immunomodulation. Each centrifugal plasmapheresis was a 1-volume exchange that used 5% albumin as the replacement fluid. Daily plasmapheresis was initially performed on four consecutive days. Of note, the third plasmapheresis lasted only 15 minutes and was terminated due to shoulder pain and hypotension. An infusion of 100 m/kg IVIG was added after each of these four initial plasmapheresis procedures.

Before these four initial plasmapheresis procedures, LFT's were AST 87 U/L, ALT 222 U/L, ALP 469 U/L, and bilirubin 15.3 mg/dl. Following these treatments, his liver function improved with LFT's, AST 60 U/L, ALT 82 U/L, ALP 143 U/L, and bilirubin 10.3 mg/dl.

After receiving additional two plasmapheresis procedures with IVIG, he was discharged from the hospital. Total number of inpatient plasmapheresis with IVIG was 6 (this includes 1 incomplete). As an outpatient, he received both plasmapheresis and IVIG twice a week for 4 more weeks for a total of 8 outpatient procedures.

After a total of 14 inpatient and outpatient treatments, his procedures were discontinued, and liver function values were monitored continuously while he was on tacrolimus, mycophenolate, and a prednisone taper. Currently, he is receiving non-immune-mediated chemotherapy with carboplatin and docetaxel for his lung metastasis. His most recent LFT's were AST 19 U/L, ALT 16 U/L, ALP 147 U/L, and bilirubin of 0.5 mg/dl.

2. Discussion

The programmed cell death protein 1 (PD1) is a checkpoint that regulates the immune response. Ligation of PD1 with its ligands PDL1 and PDL2 results in transduction of negative signals to T-cells. The expression of PD1 on effector T-cells and PDL1 on neoplastic cells allows tumor to evade the immune response. Blockade of PD1 is an important immunotherapeutic strategy for cancers. Pembrolizumab (Keytruda) is a humanized monoclonal anti-PD1 antibody that has been extensively investigated in numerous malignancies [1].

Though adverse events occurred in up to 60% of patients, grade 3/4 toxicities were observed in <10% of cases. Besides infusion reactions, most of the AEs are thought to be immune-related AEs, occurring in any organ. Since the optimal duration of treatment is undefined, pembrolizumab may be given for up to 2 years. Consequently, immune-related AEs can occur late or even after cessation of treatment [1].

One of the known side effects of checkpoint inhibitor immunotherapy is the onset of mild liver biochemical abnormalities at 3–6 months after starting treatment is [2]. It generally manifests as a mixed pattern of liver function test abnormalities.

Multiple patterns of histological injury have been documented in the literature [3]. In a study of 491 consecutive patients receiving pembrolizumab, liver injury occurred in 70 (14%) patients. Generally, liver injury was predominantly cholestatic and mild at onset with similar baseline demographic and laboratory features of the patients with liver injury versus those without liver injury. Only a minority of the liver injury cases were attributed to pembrolizumab hepatotoxicity (29%), while cancerous

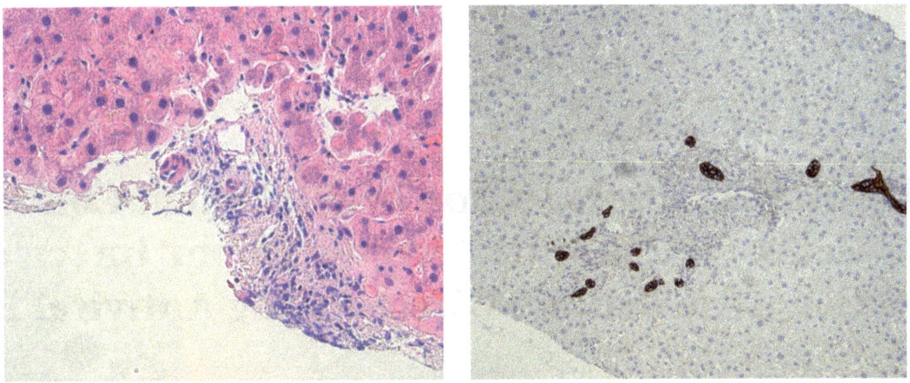

(a) (b)

FIGURE 1: (a) A representative field from the H&E stained liver biopsy shows duct dropout, a lack of prominent mixed inflammatory infiltrate, and a portal tract with endotheliitis. (b) A representative field from the CK7 stained liver biopsy highlights bile ductular reaction. Not shown: a trichrome stain showed stage I fibrosis.

replacement of the liver accounted for most of the other patients with benign or malignant biliary obstruction identified in 5.7% [4].

Though corticosteroids are the mainstay for most high-grade immune-related adverse events such as pembrolizumab-induced hepatitis, the dose and duration of corticosteroid therapy are not well-established. Literature search revealed a case of successful management of grade 3 pembrolizumab-induced hepatitis with a combination of low-dose corticosteroids and bicyclol [5].

In addition, plasmapheresis was performed for another patient with pembrolizumab-induced myocarditis because of deterioration in his hemodynamic status refractory to conventional immunosuppression. The plasmapheresis seemed to cause a rapid reduction of serum pembrolizumab levels and marked clinical, radiological, and biochemical improvement. To the authors' knowledge, that was the first reported case on the successful use of plasma exchange for pembrolizumab-associated fulminant myocarditis [6].

Some degree of our patient's short-term improvement in biochemical parameters was likely due to direct removal via plasmapheresis. There was clear downtrend in alkaline phosphatase, AST, ALT, and total bilirubin each day after plasmapheresis followed by an uptrend or stagnant value the following day when patient did not receive plasmapheresis. However, his long-term improvement cannot be solely due to direct removal, as his recovery of liver injury was durable.

Also, some of these same laboratory markers were on a downward trend prior to plasmapheresis. Thus, it is plausible that plasmapheresis did not hasten his recovery. The total bilirubin was an exception, as it plateaued after all of our other immunosuppression therapies prior to the initiation of plasmapheresis. While alkaline phosphatase and aminotransferases were on a downward trend prior to initiation of plasmapheresis, the improvement trend increased on the day of initiating plasmapheresis and remained increased until normalization. It is plausible that the patient may have recovered on his own but at a slower rate. In other words, plasmapheresis may have increased the rate of recovery at worst and may have been an essential factor in his recovery at best. The half-life of IgG is about 23 days, so there was most likely significant amounts of pembrolizumab in the patient about 4–6 weeks after administration. Moreover, IgG is about 50% intravascular, so the rationale for some degree of drug removal via plasmapheresis seemed sound.

References

[1] G. Kwok, T. C. C. Yau, J. W. Chiu, E. Tse, and Y.-L. Kwong, "Pembrolizumab (keytruda)," *Human Vaccines & Immunotherapeutics*, vol. 12, no. 11, pp. 2777–2789, 2016.

[2] D. L. Suzman, L. Pelosof, A. Rosenberg, and M. I. Avigan, "Hepatotoxicity of immune checkpoint inhibitors: an evolving picture of risk associated with a vital class of immunotherapy agents," *Liver International*, vol. 38, no. 6, pp. 976–987, 2018.

[3] Y. Zen and M. M. Yeh, "Checkpoint inhibitor-induced liver injury: a novel form of liver disease emerging in the era of cancer immunotherapy," *Seminars in Diagnostic Pathology*, vol. 36, no. 6, pp. 434–440, 2019.

[4] I. Tsung, R. Dolan, C. D. Lao et al., "Liver injury is most commonly due to hepatic metastases rather than drug hepatotoxicity during pembrolizumab immunotherapy," *Alimentary Pharmacology & Therapeutics*, vol. 50, no. 7, pp. 800–808, 2019.

[5] Y. E. Liu, J. Zhang, Z. Yin, X. Zhu, L. Xue, and B. Cao, "Compromise or not? a case report of successful treatment of pembrolizumab-induced hepatitis in a patient with non-small cell lung cancer with low-dose methylprednisolone and bicyclol," *Thoracic Cancer*, vol. 11, no. 7, pp. 2023–2030, 2020.

[6] H. Yogasundaram, W. Alhumaid, J. W. Chen et al., "Plasma exchange for immune checkpoint inhibitor-induced myocarditis," *CJC Open*, vol. 3, no. 3, pp. 379–382, 2021.

38

Successful Kidney Transplantation in a Recipient Coinfected with Hepatitis C Genotype 2 and HIV from a Donor Infected with Hepatitis C Genotype 1 in the Direct-Acting Antiviral Era

Dimitrios Farmakiotis,[1] Zoe Weiss,[2,3] Amy L. Brotherton,[4] Paul Morrissey,[5] Reginald Gohh,[6] Kendra Vieira,[1] Lynn E. Taylor,[1,7] and Joseph M. Garland[1]

[1]*Division of Infectious Diseases, Department of Internal Medicine, Brown Alpert Medical School, Providence, RI, USA*
[2]*Department of Internal Medicine, Brown Alpert Medical School, Providence, RI, USA*
[3]*Division of Infectious Diseases, Brigham and Women's Hospital and Massachusetts General Hospital, Harvard Medical School, Boston, MA, USA*
[4]*Department of Pharmacy, The Miriam Hospital, Providence, RI, USA*
[5]*Department of Surgery (Transplantation), Brown Alpert Medical School, Providence, RI, USA*
[6]*Division of Nephrology (Transplantation), Department of Internal Medicine, Brown Alpert Medical School, Providence, RI, USA*
[7]*CODAC Behavioral Health, Providence, RI, USA*

Correspondence should be addressed to Dimitrios Farmakiotis; dimitrios.farmakiotis@lifespan.org

Academic Editor: Ned Snyder

Despite significant advances in transplantation of HIV-infected individuals, little is known about HIV coinfected patients with hepatitis C virus (HCV) genotypes other than genotype 1, especially when receiving HCV-infected organs with a different genotype. We describe the first case of kidney transplantation in a man coinfected with hepatitis C and HIV in our state. To our knowledge, this is also the first report of an HIV/HCV/HBV tri-infected patient with non-1 (2a) HCV genotype who received an HCV-infected kidney graft with the discordant genotype (1a), to which he converted after transplant. Our case study highlights the following: (1) transplant centers need to monitor wait times for an HCV-infected organ and regularly assess the risk of delaying HCV antiviral treatment for HCV-infected transplant candidates in anticipation of the transplant from an HCV-infected donor; (2) closer monitoring of tacrolimus levels during the early phases of anti-HCV protease inhibitor introduction and discontinuation may be indicated; (3) donor genotype transmission can occur; (4) HIV/HCV coinfected transplant candidates require a holistic approach with emphasis on the cardiovascular risk profile and low threshold for cardiac catheterization as part of their pretransplant evaluation.

1. Background

Contemporary cohorts of HIV-infected transplant recipients have demonstrated excellent patient and graft survival [1–7]. Similarly, for patients with hepatitis C virus (HCV) infection, kidney transplantation offers a survival benefit and can be more cost-effective than remaining on the waitlist [8–10]. However, compared to their HCV-uninfected counterparts, these patients experience higher rates of post-transplant glomerulonephritis, malignancy, and progression of liver disease [11, 12].

Historically, HCV eradication was a challenge in transplanted patients, as interferon-containing regimens were relatively contraindicated due to increased risk of rejection [13]. The introduction of direct-acting antivirals (DAA) allows for safe treatment of HCV-infected transplant recipients, and therefore, transplantation of HCV-infected organs to both HCV-infected and uninfected patients

[9, 14–19]. The optimal timing for treatment of HCV-infected transplant candidates (pre- vs. post-transplant with HCV-infected or HCV-uninfected organ donation, respectively) remains controversial, as the risk of treatment delay must be balanced by the benefit of shorter wait time for HCV-infected organs [7, 10, 13]. DAA prophylaxis for uninfected recipients of HCV-infected organs, including shorter courses [17], has also been proposed as an effective way to expand the organ pool [16–18].

Given similar routes of transmission, coinfection with hepatitis B virus (HBV) or HCV is common among HIV-infected patients with end-stage renal disease (ESRD) [5]. Higher overall morbidity, mortality, and accelerated hepatic decompensation have been observed in this population, compared to HIV monoinfected patients [20, 21], likely due to the immune modulating effects of HCV [22], including activation of CD4+ and CD8+ cells [23] and cytokine production [24]. In the pre-DAA era, transplantation in patients coinfected with HIV and HCV was associated with reduced graft survival and higher rates of serious infection [25]. However, recent small case series showed improved outcomes, including fewer infectious complications, in coinfected patients treated with DAA after transplant [3, 4, 6].

Despite significant advances in transplantation of HIV/HCV coinfected individuals, little is known about coinfected patients with HCV genotypes other than genotype 1, especially when receiving HCV-positive organs with a different genotype. Herein, we describe the first case of kidney transplantation in a man coinfected with hepatitis C and HIV in the State of Rhode Island. To our knowledge, this is also the first reported case of discordant HCV genotype transplantation in a patient coinfected with HIV, in the DAA era.

2. Case Report

A 64-year-old man with ESRD from diabetic nephropathy on hemodialysis for one year presented for transplant evaluation. He had a remote history of polysubstance addiction including heroin injection with methadone detoxification and then complete nonuse of illicit drugs for decades; he did not want opioid agonist therapy and was active in Narcotics Anonymous for years. He had a 30 pack-year smoking history, but had quit tobacco at the same time as illicit drugs.

He had a history of well-controlled HIV diagnosed in 1987, with an undetectable viral load and CD4-infected cell count >500 cells/mm^3 for many years. He had been on numerous prior antiretroviral regimens to treat his HIV and harbored multiclass resistance to agents in the non-nucleoside reverse transcriptase inhibitor (NRTI: M184V and T215N/S/Y) and protease inhibitor (PI: L33I, M46I, I54V, I62V, and V82A/I/T) classes. He ultimately achieved long-term virologic suppression with etravirine, darunavir, ritonavir, and raltegravir (the TRIO [26, 27] regimen). In advance of transplant, his resistance history was reviewed and an HIV-1 proviral DNA genotype archive was sent, which did not demonstrate any resistance to the integrase inhibitor or the NNRTI class. He was switched to rilpivirine and dolutegravir [28] to reduce the risk of drug-drug interactions (DDI) (ritonavir significantly increases calcineurin inhibitor (CNI) levels) and to avoid complex dose adjustment with fluctuating renal function post-transplant.

The patient was also infected with HBV. Tenofovir disoproxil fumarate had been discontinued several years before due to concern for contribution to his progressive renal disease, and he was maintained on lifelong entecavir treatment. He also had chronic hepatitis C virus (HCV), genotype 2b, and declined interferon therapy for years. By the time DAAs became available, there was no DAA for genotype 2 that could be given with his degree of advanced renal disease. When he developed advanced fibrosis (F3), it was recommended that consideration of renal transplant be accelerated given advancing liver disease. He had a history of coronary artery disease (CAD) and inferior myocardial infarction eight years before, with a stent placed to the right coronary artery (RCA). He was taking aspirin 325 mg daily and atorvastatin 40 mg daily. As part of his pretransplant evaluation, a nuclear myocardial perfusion test revealed a large-sized inferior and inferolateral fixed defect with preserved ejection fraction. The patient had very good functional status and did not report any symptoms, so further preoperative cardiac workup was not pursued.

Three months after listing, he underwent deceased donor kidney transplant from an HCV-positive donor (by antibody and nucleic acid-testing (NAT)-genotype 1a) with basiliximab induction. Maintenance immunosuppression included mycophenolate sodium, tacrolimus, and prednisone. He was also started on valganciclovir and atovaquone prophylaxis due to sulfonamide allergy. On postoperative day (POD) 1, he developed substernal anginal chest pain. An electrocardiogram (EKG) showed ST depressions in the anterolateral leads and transient ST elevation in lead III (Figure 1). His serum troponin peaked at 31 ng/ml (normal <0.06 ng/ml). He was treated with aspirin, clopidogrel, and nitroglycerin drip, without anticoagulation, for fear of hemorrhage due to extensive retroperitoneal blunt dissection during transplant. He underwent cardiac catherization on POD3, which revealed 3-vessel disease, with near-complete occlusion of the RCA stent (Figure 2(a)). On POD 10, he had successful placement of two drug-eluting stents in the RCA (Figure 2(b)). The patient experienced delayed graft function, requiring hemodialysis but was eventually discharged off dialysis on POD 15. Of note, on POD 9 his HCV genotype was 2b, but subsequent genotype before initiation of treatment (POD 81) was only 1a (donor-derived). On POD 100, the patient was admitted for febrile neutropenia, requiring colony-stimulating growth factor support and discontinuation of both valganciclovir and mycophenolate.

On POD 141, he was started on therapy for HCV, with pangenotypic glecaprevir/pibrentasvir (GLE/PIB) for 12 weeks, targeting both donor and recipient genotypes. Concomitant use of GLE/PIB and atorvastatin is contraindicated; thus, he was switched to pravastatin during treatment. Additionally, therapeutic drug monitoring of

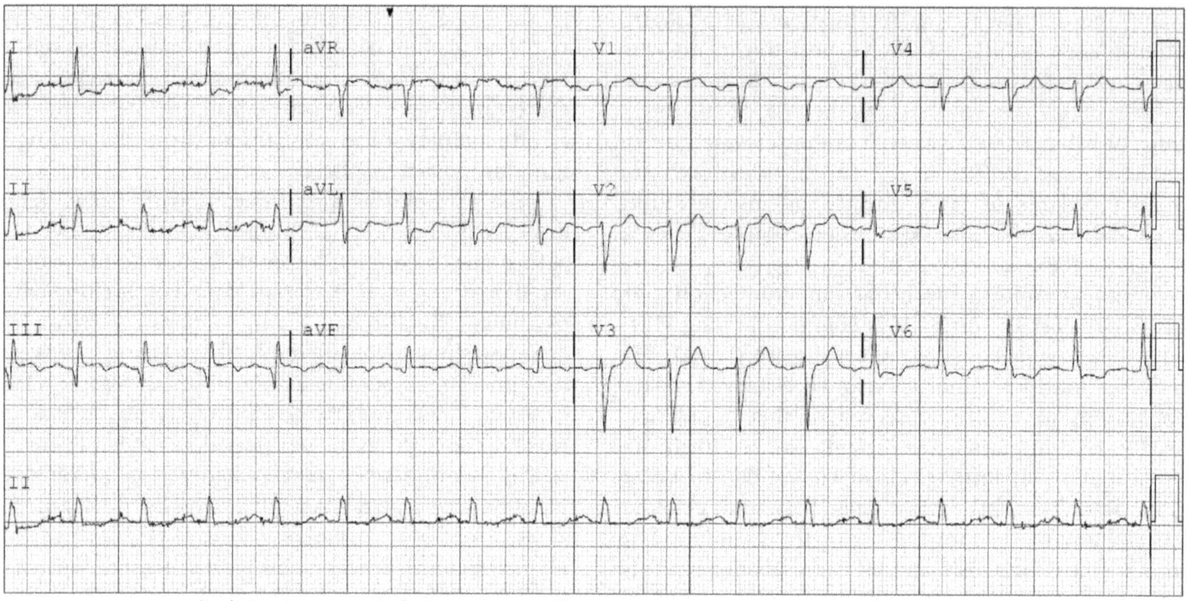

FIGURE 1: Electrocardiogram during an episode of chest pain on POD 1, showing ST-segment inferior wall elevation and lateral wall depression, concerning for acute injury.

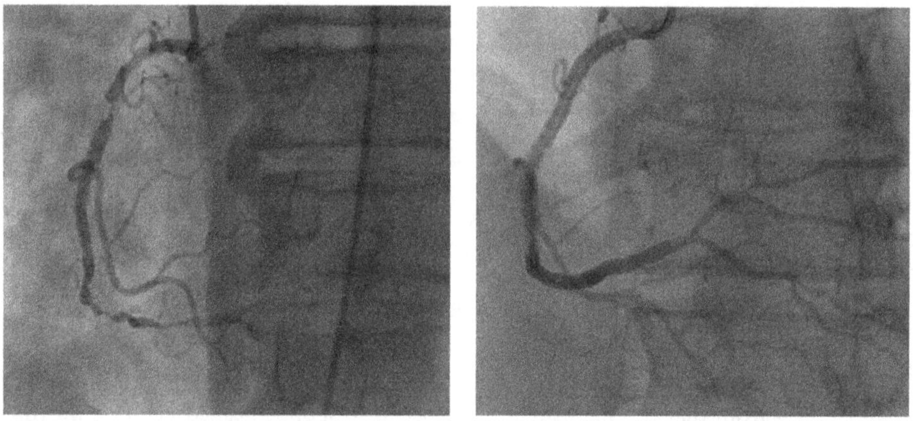

(a) (b)

FIGURE 2: Coronary angiography showing near-complete occlusion of the RCA stent (a) on POD 3 and restored patency after placement of two DES on POD 10 (b).

tacrolimus levels was increased to twice weekly for the first month and weekly for the next 2 months, before resuming laboratory workup per transplant protocol (twice every month until 6 months after transplant, then monthly). He required transient reduction of his tacrolimus dose from 2 mg to 1 mg twice daily (bid) because of supratherapeutic trough levels (highest: 18 mg/dL, post-transplant goal: 7 mg/dL), one week after starting GLE/PIB. After 3 weeks, the tacrolimus dose was again increased to 2 mg bid (Figure 3). He achieved sustained virologic response (SVR) 12 weeks after treatment completion (SVR 12). He developed high-level BK viremia 1.5 year after transplant, which resolved by decreasing the tacrolimus trough goal to 4 mg/dL. Two years after transplant, he is doing well, and has excellent graft function and undetectable HIV, HCV, and HBV viral loads. He remains on entecavir prophylaxis.

3. Discussion

Management of patients with HIV and HCV/HBV tri-infection in the setting of ESRD presents unique challenges, including increased cardiovascular mortality, rapid progression of end organ dysfunction, infections, and DDI. Moreover, the rapidly changing landscape of HCV management in the DAA era has important implications for organ allocation. To our knowledge, this is the first report of an HIV/HCV/HBV coinfected patient with the non-1 HCV genotype who received an HCV-infected organ transplant with the discordant genotype. The lessons learnt are of clinical significance.

Cardiovascular disease and rates of myocardial infarction are already increased in patients with ESRD [29], but possibly further potentiated by HIV/HCV coinfection [30],

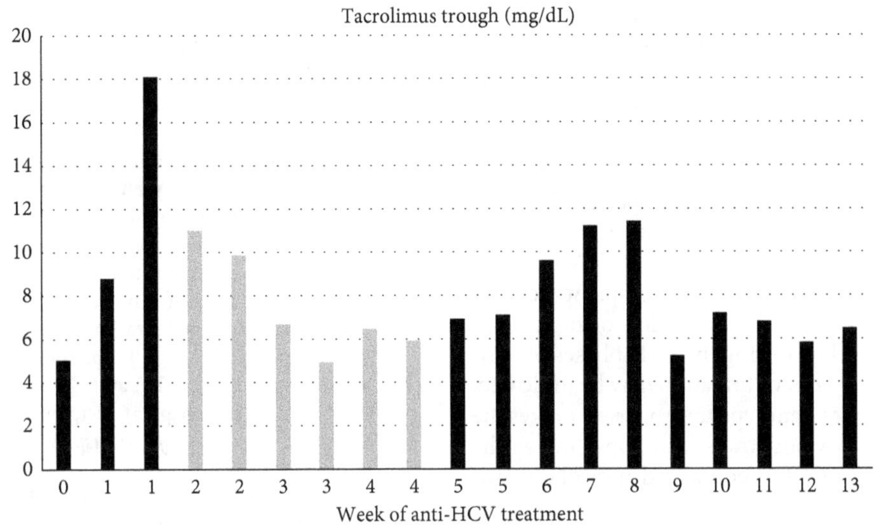

FIGURE 3: Tacrolimus trough level variations during treatment for hepatitis C with glecaprevir/pibrentasvir and tacrolimus dose: 2 mg bid (black) and 1 mg bid (gray).

by way of chronic inflammation, endothelial dysfunction, metabolic derangements [30–34], and potential choice of antiretroviral therapy [35]. Assessing cardiovascular risk in the pretransplant evaluation is imperative. Given the burden of cardiovascular disease in the ESRD population and frequent lack of symptoms, noninvasive cardiac imaging might be inferior to cardiac catheterization. In one study of kidney transplant candidates with cardiovascular risk factors other than HIV/HCV, the positive and negative predictive values of noninvasive means in detecting clinically significant cardiovascular disease were only 43% and 47%, respectively. Furthermore, mortality was reduced in those who underwent elective revascularization pretransplantation [29]. At our institution, following this case, we have a very low threshold for coronary angiography in HIV-infected or HCV-infected transplant candidates with a history of significant CAD, regardless of reported symptoms.

Management of DDI in patients coinfected with HIV and HCV is paramount, even more so in the setting of organ transplantation [3–5, 7, 13]. Fewer DDI are probably one of the main factors responsible for improved outcomes with InSTI compared to PI after organ transplantation in patients with HIV [4]. Coadministration of GLE/PIB with systemic tacrolimus (1 mg single dose) has been shown to increase tacrolimus C_{max} and area under the curve (AUC) by 1.5-fold and 1.45-fold, respectively. There was no change in the C_{max}, AUC, and C_{min} of GLE or PIB [36]. As tacrolimus has a narrow therapeutic index, the official recommendation is to use with caution and with therapeutic drug monitoring, but without a priori dose adjustment. In general, improved liver function with anti-HCV treatment may further contribute to increased clearance of tacrolimus. In agreement with the above, our patient experienced an increase in tacrolimus trough level with initiation of GLE/PIB, resulting in dose reduction and subsequently decreased levels. Therefore, during coadministration of GLE/PIB and tacrolimus, we favor checking tacrolimus trough levels initially twice weekly and then weekly for the duration of treatment and a few weeks after, before resuming our regular per protocol laboratory workup.

In the setting of donor and recipient genotype strain mismatch, both viral strains may exist in the perioperative period. However, over the first few months post-transplantation, one strain will generally predominate although long-term detection of both genotypes is possible [19, 37, 38]. Recommended regimens for the treatment of HCV in kidney transplant recipients include ledipasvir/sofosbuvir, velpatasvir/sofosbuvir, and GLE/PIB. All are active against the most frequent genotype (1), and velpatasvir/sofosbuvir and GLE/PIB are pangenotypic and should be preferred in transplant recipients with donor/recipient genotype mismatch. It should be noted that strains with genotype 1 are likely more dominant (1b > 1a > 2), based on limited data, which is mostly derived from liver transplant recipients [37, 38]. This was confirmed in our case, despite kidney, not liver, transplantation, and therefore, substantially lower donor genotype 1a, compared to recipient genotype 2, viral load burden.

The optimal timing of DAA treatment in HCV-positive transplant candidates, including HIV coinfected patients, remains in a state of flux, with limited real-world data [7, 9, 10]. The risk of treatment delay and progression of liver disease, which can be accelerated by immunosuppression, should be weighed against the benefit of shorter wait time for HCV-infected organs. Based on sophisticated modelling, it has been suggested that for HCV-monoinfected patients with minimal liver fibrosis, treatment post-transplantation with an HCV-positive organ is beneficial. Nevertheless, in patients with advanced fibrosis, treatment prior to transplant may be preferred, unless the wait time benefit is >9 months [10]. For HCV/HIV coinfected patients, treatment post-transplant was consistently cost-saving as compared to treatment pretransplant and associated with higher life months and quality-adjusted life months with wait times

>18 months [7]. At the time of our case, the wait time within our organ procurement organization (OPO) was <6 months vs. >4 years for HCV-positive vs. negative deceased donors, respectively. Thus, despite our patient's advanced stage of fibrosis, the decision to wait was justified.

In summary, our case study highlights the following: (1) transplant centers need to monitor OPO-specific times on the waitlist for an HCV-infected organ and to assess regularly the risk of delaying treatment for HCV-infected transplant candidates in anticipation of transplant from an HCV-infected donor; (2) closer monitoring of tacrolimus levels (once or twice weekly) during the early phases of anti-HCV PI introduction and discontinuation may be indicated; (3) the possibility of donor genotype transmission makes the use of pangenotypic DAA post-transplant appealing as the standard of care; (4) HIV/HCV coinfected transplant candidates require a holistic approach with emphasis on the cardiovascular risk profile and low threshold for cardiac catheterization as part of their pretransplant evaluation.

Acknowledgments

DF has received research support from Astellas and Viracor-Eurofins and consultant fee from Viracor-Eurofins. The present work was supported by a Brown Physicians Inc. Academic Assessment Grant.

References

[1] J. E. Locke, R. D. Reed, S. G. Mehta et al., "Center-level experience and kidney transplant outcomes in HIV-infected recipients," *American Journal of Transplantation*, vol. 15, no. 8, pp. 2096–2104, 2015.

[2] P. G. Stock, B. Barin, B. Murphy et al., "Outcomes of kidney transplantation in HIV-infected recipients," *New England Journal of Medicine*, vol. 363, no. 21, pp. 2004–2014, 2010.

[3] J. F. Camargo, S. Anjan, and N. Chin-Beckford, "Clinical outcomes in HIV-infected/HCV-infected coinfected kidney transplant recipients in the pre- and post-direct-acting antiviral therapy eras: 10-year single center experience," *Clinical Transplantation*, vol. 33, no. 5, Article ID e13532, 2019.

[4] R. Rosa, J. F. Suarez, M. A. Lorio et al., "Impact of antiretroviral therapy on clinical outcomes in HIV (-infected) kidney transplant recipients: review of 58 cases," *F1000Research*, vol. 5, p. 2893, 2016.

[5] D. Sawinski, "ESRD patients coinfected with human immunodeficiency virus and hepatitis C: outcomes and management challenges," *Seminars in Dialysis*, vol. 32, no. 2, pp. 159–168, 2019.

[6] D. Sawinski, D. H. Lee, A. M. Doyle, and E. A. Blumberg, "Successful posttransplant treatment of hepatitis C with ledipasvir-sofosbuvir in HIV-infected kidney transplant recipients," *Transplantation*, vol. 101, no. 5, pp. 974–979, 2017.

[7] B. A. Shelton, G. Berdahl, D. Sawinski et al., "Optimal timing of hepatitis C treatment among HIV/HCV coinfected ESRD patients: pre- vs posttransplant," *American Journal of Transplantation*, vol. 19, no. 6, pp. 1806–1819, 2019.

[8] D. Roth, J. J. Gaynor, K. R. Reddy et al., "Effect of kidney transplantation on outcomes among patients with hepatitis C," *Journal of the American Society of Nephrology*, vol. 22, no. 6, pp. 1152–1160, 2011.

[9] D. Sawinski, N. Patel, B. Appolo, and R. Bloom, "Use of HCV-infected Donors does not affect HCV clearance with directly acting antiviral therapy but shortens the wait time to kidney transplantation," *Transplantation*, vol. 101, no. 5, pp. 968–973, 2017.

[10] B. A. Shelton, D. Sawinski, B. P. Linas et al., "Population level outcomes and cost-effectiveness of hepatitis C treatment pre- vs postkidney transplantation," *American Journal of Transplantation*, vol. 18, no. 10, pp. 2483–2495, 2018.

[11] V. Saxena and N. A. Terrault, "Treatment of hepatitis C infection in renal transplant recipients: the long wait is over," *American Journal of Transplantation*, vol. 16, no. 5, pp. 1345–1347, 2016.

[12] S. Belga and K. E. Doucette, "Hepatitis C in non-hepatic solid organ transplant candidates and recipients: a new horizon," *World Journal of Gastroenterology*, vol. 22, no. 4, pp. 1650–1663, 2016.

[13] D. Sawinski and R. D. Bloom, "Novel hepatitis C treatment and the impact on kidney transplantation," *Transplantation*, vol. 99, no. 12, pp. 2458–2466, 2015.

[14] M. Lubetzky, S. Chun, A. Joelson et al., "Safety and efficacy of treatment of hepatitis C in kidney transplant recipients with directly acting antiviral agents," *Transplantation*, vol. 101, no. 7, pp. 1704–1710, 2017.

[15] D. S. Goldberg, P. L. Abt, E. A. Blumberg et al., "Trial of transplantation of HCV-infected kidneys into uninfected recipients," *New England Journal of Medicine*, vol. 376, no. 24, pp. 2394-2395, 2017.

[16] C. M. Durand, M. G. Bowring, D. M. Brown et al., "Direct-acting antiviral prophylaxis in kidney transplantation from hepatitis C virus-infected donors to noninfected recipients: an open-label nonrandomized trial," *Annals of Internal Medicine*, vol. 168, no. 8, pp. 533–540, 2018.

[17] A. E. Woolley, S. K. Singh, H. J. Goldberg et al., "Heart and lung transplants from HCV-infected donors to uninfected recipients," *New England Journal of Medicine*, vol. 380, no. 17, pp. 1606–1617, 2019.

[18] A. Abdelbasit, A. Hirji, K. Halloran et al., "Lung transplantation from hepatitis C viremic donors to uninfected recipients," *American Journal of Respiratory and Critical Care Medicine*, vol. 197, no. 11, pp. 1492–1496, 2018.

[19] J. Levitsky, R. N. Formica, R. D. Bloom et al., "The American society of transplantation consensus conference on the use of hepatitis C viremic donors in solid organ transplantation," *American Journal of Transplantation*, vol. 17, no. 11, pp. 2790–2802, 2017.

[20] E. A. Operskalski and A. Kovacs, "HIV/HCV co-infection: pathogenesis, clinical complications, treatment, and new therapeutic technologies," *Current HIV/AIDS Reports*, vol. 8, no. 1, pp. 12–22, 2011.

[21] H.-H. Thein, Q. Yi, G. J. Dore, and M. D. Krahn, "Natural history of hepatitis C virus infection in HIV-infected individuals and the impact of HIV in the era of highly active antiretroviral therapy: a meta-analysis," *AIDS*, vol. 22, no. 15, pp. 1979–1991, 2008.

[22] C. Körner, B. Krämer, D. Schulte et al., "Effects of HCV co-infection on apoptosis of CD4+ T-cells in HIV-positive patients," *Clinical Science*, vol. 116, no. 12, pp. 861–870, 2009.

[23] V. D. Gonzalez, K. Falconer, K. G. Blom et al., "High levels of chronic immune activation in the T-cell compartments of

patients coinfected with hepatitis C virus and human immunodeficiency virus type 1 and on highly active antiretroviral therapy are reverted by alpha interferon and ribavirin treatment," *Journal of Virology*, vol. 83, no. 21, pp. 11407–11411, 2009.

[24] A. Y. Kim and R. T. Chung, "Coinfection with HIV-1 and HCV-A one-two punch," *Gastroenterology*, vol. 137, no. 3, pp. 795–814, 2009.

[25] Y. Xia, P. Friedmann, H. Yaffe, J. Phair, A. Gupta, and L. K. Kayler, "Effect of HCV, HIV and coinfection in kidney transplant recipients: mate kidney analyses," *American Journal of Transplantation*, vol. 14, no. 9, pp. 2037–2047, 2014.

[26] C. Fagard, C. Colin, C. Charpentier et al., "Long-term efficacy and safety of raltegravir, etravirine, and darunavir/ritonavir in treatment-experienced patients: week 96 results from the ANRS 139 TRIO trial," *JAIDS Journal of Acquired Immune Deficiency Syndromes*, vol. 59, no. 5, pp. 489–493, 2012.

[27] Y. Yazdanpanah, C. Fagard, D. Descamps et al., "High rate of virologic suppression with raltegravir plus etravirine and darunavir/ritonavir among treatment-experienced patients infected with multidrug-resistant HIV: results of the ANRS 139 TRIO trial," *Clinical Infectious Diseases*, vol. 49, no. 9, pp. 1441–1449, 2009.

[28] J. M. Llibre, C.-C. Hung, C. Brinson et al., "Efficacy, safety, and tolerability of dolutegravir-rilpivirine for the maintenance of virological suppression in adults with HIV-1: phase 3, randomised, non-inferiority SWORD-1 and SWORD-2 studies," *The Lancet*, vol. 391, no. 10123, pp. 839–849, 2018.

[29] D. M. Mann, S. Fernandez, Z. Mondal et al., "Role of coronary angiography in the assessment of cardiovascular risk in kidney transplant candidates," *The American Journal of Cardiology*, vol. 118, no. 5, pp. 679–683, 2016.

[30] R. Bedimo, A. O. Westfall, M. Mugavero, H. Drechsler, N. Khanna, and M. Saag, "Hepatitis C virus coinfection and the risk of cardiovascular disease among HIV-infected patients," *HIV Medicine*, vol. 11, no. 11, pp. 462–468, 2010.

[31] I. F. de Castro, D. Micheloud, J. Berenguer et al., "Hepatitis C virus infection is associated with endothelial dysfunction in HIV/hepatitis C virus coinfected patients," *AIDS*, vol. 24, no. 13, pp. 2059–2067, 2010.

[32] O. Osibogun, O. Ogunmoroti, E. D. Michos et al., "HIV/HCV coinfection and the risk of cardiovascular disease: a meta-analysis," *Journal of Viral Hepatitis*, vol. 24, no. 11, pp. 998–1004, 2017.

[33] J. V. Fernández-Montero, P. Barreiro, C. de Mendoza, P. Labarga, and V. Soriano, "Hepatitis C virus coinfection independently increases the risk of cardiovascular disease in HIV-positive patients," *Journal of Viral Hepatitis*, vol. 23, no. 1, pp. 47–52, 2016.

[34] L. Kakinami, R. C. Block, M. J. Adams, S. E. Cohn, B. Maliakkal, and S. G. Fisher, "Risk of cardiovascular disease in HIV, hepatitis C, or HIV/hepatitis C patients compared to the general population," *International Journal of Clinical Practice*, vol. 67, no. 1, pp. 6–13, 2013.

[35] L. Ryom, J. D. Lundgren, W. El-Sadr et al., "Cardiovascular disease and use of contemporary protease inhibitors: the D:A:D international prospective multicohort study," *The Lancet HIV*, vol. 5, no. 6, pp. e291–e300, 2018.

[36] M. P. Kosloski, W. Zhao, H. Li et al., "Drug-drug interactions of tacrolimus or cyclosporine with glecaprevir and pibrentasvir in healthy subjects," *Clinical Pharmacology in Drug Development*, vol. 8, no. 6, pp. 779–789, 2019.

[37] X. Fan, D. M. Lang, Y. Xu et al., "Liver transplantation with hepatitis C virus-infected graft: interaction between donor and recipient viral strains," *Hepatology*, vol. 38, no. 1, pp. 25–33, 2003.

[38] T. Laskus, L.-F. Wang, J. Rakela et al., "Dynamic behavior of hepatitis C virus in chronically infected patients receiving liver graft from infected donors," *Virology*, vol. 220, no. 1, pp. 171–176, 1996.

39

Guillain–Barré Syndrome Likely due to Relapsing Hepatitis A

Edgar Blecker and Maryam Ehtsham

Department of Internal Medicine, Methodist Dallas Medical Center, Dallas, TX 75203, USA

Correspondence should be addressed to Edgar Blecker; erblecker@gmail.com

Academic Editor: Haruki Komatsu

Guillain-Barré syndrome (GBS) is an immune-mediated disease of the peripheral nervous system that can be caused by various bacterial and virologic agents. The disease is characterized by progressive muscle weakness and paralysis. Rarely, GBS is preceded by an acute infection with hepatitis A. Here, we present the case of a 53-year-old woman who presented with progressively worsening motor weakness in the distal extremities. She reported a preceding gastrointestinal infection with nausea, vomiting, and diarrhea two weeks prior to her presentation to the emergency department. She was noted to have elevated serum transaminase levels and hepatitis A IgM and IgG antibodies signifying likely relapsing hepatitis A. She was later diagnosed with GBS on the basis of clinical findings and albuminocytologic dissociation in the cerebrospinal fluid. She was treated with intravenous immunoglobulin with subsequent improvement in her strength.

1. Introduction

Guillain–Barré syndrome (GBS) is a peripheral demyelinating disorder often preceded by a gastrointestinal infection. The causative infectious agent is usually bacterial or viral with the most common causes being *Campylobacter*, influenza virus, Ebstein–Barr virus, and cytomegalovirus infections. GBS is rarely caused by hepatitis A.

2. Case Presentation

The patient was a 53-year-old woman with a past medical history of hypothyroidism and hyperlipidemia who presented to the emergency department (ED) with worsening bilateral upper and lower extremity weakness for three days. Two weeks prior to her presentation, she reported fever, diarrhea, nausea, vomiting, and pain on the right side of the abdomen. She had presented to the ED one week prior due to abdominal pain with a mild elevation in her liver enzymes. No acute pathology was discovered, and she was told to follow-up with her primary care physician (PCP). She then presented to an urgent care facility in which she was prescribed ciprofloxacin with eventual improvement in her diarrhea and vomiting. Three days prior to arrival, she began to note numbness and weakness of her fingers and toes. Her weakness was most noticeable in the distal aspects of her extremities, and she experienced some difficulty ambulating and a prominent decrease in her grip strength. This prompted her to schedule an appointment with her PCP. She followed up with her PCP, who was concerned for demyelinating disease. The PCP urged her to present to the ED for further evaluation. Despite not having any respiratory symptoms or fever, her PCP tested her for COVID-19 and influenza given her abdominal pain and diarrhea. Both tests returned negative.

Further history revealed the patient had reported a prior presentation to the ED roughly 10 months earlier for right upper quadrant abdominal pain. She was told she had elevated liver enzymes at that visit and was told to follow-up with her PCP. Her PCP had tested her for hepatitis C, which was negative, and she eventually had resolution of her clinical symptoms. She denied any recent travel, fevers, or shortness of breath. She had mostly been indoors for the past two months, without reported sick contacts.

Physical examination upon presentation to the ED was notable for 4/5 strength in the bilateral upper extremities with flexion and extension of the elbow and wrist. She had decreased grip strength bilaterally. Bilateral lower extremities had 3/5 strength with flexion and extension of the hip and knee as well as decreased dorsiflexion and plantar flexion of both feet. She had decreased sensation in her lower extremities with absent reflexes throughout. Initial labs were significant for a normal TSH, free T4, and a mild elevation of her liver enzymes: aspartate transaminase (AST) of 40 U/L (normal range: 8–48 U/L), alanine transaminase (ALT) of 46 U/L (normal range: 7–55 U/L), and alkaline phosphatase (ALP) of 138 U/L (normal range: 40–129 U/L). A hepatitis panel and computed tomography (CT) scan abdomen/pelvis were ordered to investigate her transaminitis. She was positive for hepatitis A IgG and IgM antibodies with no acute pathological process noted on the CT scan.

Initial differential diagnosis included GBS versus a compressive myelopathy of the spine. Neurology was consulted with recommendations to perform a lumbar puncture and obtain further imaging of the brain and spine. A CT scan of the head was without acute abnormalities, and magnetic resonance imaging of the cervical, thoracic, and lumbar spine was negative for compressive myelopathy or acute abnormalities. A lumbar puncture was performed with an elevated total protein of 72 mg/dL (normal range: 15–60 mg/dL) and white blood cell count of 5 cells/mm^3 (normal range: 0–8/mm^3) suggesting albuminocytologic dissociation. The patient was diagnosed with GBS and started on intravenous immunoglobulin (IVIG) for five days. She had noticeable improvement in her distal extremity weakness following the first few doses of IVIG and was able to ambulate on her own by the end of her treatment. She was able to discharge following completion of her immunotherapy.

3. Discussion

GBS pathogenesis occurs through molecular mimicry in which the immune system is activated by an infection leading to autoimmune injury of peripheral nerve components. This immune response leads to the progressive neurological findings seen in GBS and its variants. Most commonly, the etiologic agent is either bacterial or viral with *Campylobacter jejuni* being the most common cause, followed by cytomegalovirus, Epstein–Barr virus, and influenza [1].

GBS due to hepatitis A is rare and has been reported in a few case reports with relatively good outcomes [2]. Coinfection with bacterial or viral agents has been reported, and thus, evaluation for concomitant infection should be conducted [3]. The patient in the case was ruled out for influenza and COVID-19. However, campylobacter, EBV, and CMV were not evaluated for.

Diagnosis of GBS typically includes the classic findings of symmetric muscular weakness of the distal extremities and absent or decreased reflexes, with a monophasic disease course and nadir of weakness between 12 hours and 28 days from the start of therapy [4]. CSF fluid showing albuminocytologic dissociation and electrodiagnostic studies can support the diagnosis and further delineate between the associated variants of GBS. Our patient had the classic clinical findings with a rapid improvement in her weakness following treatment with IVIG and albuminocytologic dissociation to support the diagnosis. Given high probability for diagnosis and delay in having staffing available to perform electrodiagnostic studies, this was not performed on our patient. Treatment for GBS centers around either plasma exchange or IVIG [5]. Patients are carefully monitored for respiratory symptoms and autonomic disturbances including arrhythmias, which are commonly reported.

Hepatitis A is a known cause of acute liver injury or liver failure in the United States. The clinical course of hepatitis A is usually self-resolving with most patients having a complete recovery. Serum hepatitis A antibodies can be helpful to determine whether there is an active or past infection. Patients will typically develop IgM antibodies to hepatitis A within two to three weeks of the initial infection. The presence of IgM antibodies indicates an active infection; circulating IgM antibodies can persist for up to six months. Roughly one to two weeks after developing serum IgM antibodies, IgG antibodies will develop and will persist throughout life. An elevated IgG antibody level indicates a past infection or prior vaccination [6].

Following acute infection, hepatitis A patients develop immunity to further infection. Rarely, a small group of patients (around 10%) will develop a relapsing course. Relapsing hepatitis A is most common between 30 and 90 days after acute infection but can be seen up to 12 months after [2]. Relapse is characterized by a preceding infection with a resolution of clinical and laboratory findings, followed by relapse weeks to months after the original infection. Serum IgM antibodies will often remain positive throughout relapse. Relapse is often milder than the acute infection, with aminotransferases sometimes rising above 1,000 IU/dL. Liver enzymes during relapse tend to show a cholestatic pattern. Extrahepatic manifestations of hepatitis A are more common during relapse. These manifestations include a pruritic rash and arthralgia. Relapsing infection has also been shown to cause immunological disturbances with late-onset arthritis, purpura, vasculitis, and myocarditis among others [7, 8]. An association with relapsing hepatitis A and GBS has not been demonstrated in the literature.

Although our patient was diagnosed with an acute hepatitis A infection on the basis of her positive IgM antibodies and mild transaminitis, it is difficult to determine the timing of the initial infection. She reported a similar episode of right upper quadrant abdominal pain roughly 10 months prior. Her labs at her PCP visit at that time showed a mild elevation of her liver enzymes as well. Unfortunately, hepatitis A was not tested for during that presentation. During her hospitalization, she had both positive IgM and IgG antibodies for hepatitis A, indicating an acute infection within the past six months. It is presumed that her nausea, vomiting, and diarrhea two weeks before presentation was due to a relapse of her hepatitis A given her serologies, although other causes of diarrhea were not ruled out as her symptoms had largely resolved at the time of presentation.

In conclusion, GBS should be investigated for in any patient presenting with symmetric distal extremity weakness. History is important to determine the likely causative agent. Although hepatitis A is not classically associated with GBS, it has been shown to have an association. Suspicion should be high in any patient presenting with elevated liver enzymes and can be confirmed with antibody testing for hepatitis A.

Disclosure

This research was performed as part of the employment of the authors by Methodist Dallas Medical Center.

Acknowledgments

The authors acknowledge Dr. Leigh Hunter, Graduate Medical Education at Methodist Dallas Medical Center, and Anne Murray, Ph.D., Medical Writer of the Clinical Research Institute at Methodist Health System, for providing editorial support.

References

[1] R. D. M. Hadden, H. Karch, H.-P. Hartung et al., "Preceding infections, immune factors, and outcome in Guillain-Barre syndrome," *Neurology*, vol. 56, no. 6, pp. 758–765, 2001.

[2] M. Glikson, E. Galun, R. Oren, R. Tur-Kaspa, and D. Shouval, "Relapsing hepatitis a review of 14 cases and literature survey," *Medicine*, vol. 71, no. 1, pp. 14–23, 1992.

[3] J.-H. Lei, Y. Tian, H.-Y. Luo, Z. Chen, and F. Peng, "Guillain-Barré syndrome following acute co-super-infection of hepatitis E virus and cytomegalovirus in a chronic hepatitis B virus carrier," *Journal of Medical Virology*, vol. 89, no. 2, pp. 368–372, 2017.

[4] J. J. Sejvar, K. S. Kohl, J. Gidudu et al., "Guillain-Barré syndrome and Fisher syndrome: case definitions and guidelines for collection, analysis, and presentation of immunization safety data," *Vaccine*, vol. 29, no. 3, pp. 599–612, 2011.

[5] "Randomised trial of plasma exchange, intravenous immunoglobulin, and combined treatments in Guillain-Barré syndrome. Plasma exchange/sandoglobulin Guillain-Barre syndrome trial group," *The Lancet*, vol. 349, no. 9047, pp. 225–230, 1997.

[6] J. T. Stapleton, "Host immune response to hepatitis A virus," *Journal of Infectious Diseases*, vol. 171, no. Supplement 1, pp. S9–S14, 1995.

[7] O. Allen, A. Edhi, A. Hafeez, and A. Halalau, "A very rare complication of hepatitis A infection: acute myocarditis-a case report with literature review," *Case Reports in Medicine*, vol. 2018, Article ID 3625139, 6 pages, 2018.

[8] R. D. Inman, M. Hodge, M. E. Johnston, J. Wright, and J. Heathcote, "Arthritis, vasculitis, and cryoglobulinemia associated with relapsing hepatitis A virus infection," *Annals of Internal Medicine*, vol. 105, no. 5, pp. 700–703, 1986.

40

Morphological Characteristics of Biliary Strictures after Liver Transplantation Visualized using SpyGlass™ Cholangioscopy

Yathip M. Chokpapone,[1] Anne R. Murray,[2] Ashwini P. Mehta,[3] Vichin C. Puri,[3] Alejandro Mejia,[3] and Parvez Mantry[3]

[1] *The University of Texas at Dallas, Dallas, 800 W Campbell Rd., Richardson, TX 75080, USA*
[2] *Clinical Research Institute, Methodist Health System, 1411 N. Beckley Ave, Pavilion III, Suite 168, Dallas, TX 75203, USA*
[3] *The Liver Institute, Methodist Dallas Medical Center, 1411 N. Beckley Ave, Pavilion III, Suite 268, Dallas, TX 75203, USA*

Correspondence should be addressed to Parvez Mantry; parvezmantry@mhd.com

Academic Editor: Sorabh Kapoor

Biliary complications following liver transplant are common. Endoscopic retrograde cholangiopancreatography (ERCP) and magnetic resonance cholangiopancreatography (MRCP) are the main techniques used to diagnose and treat biliary complications; however, these techniques have limits to the depth of visualization. In this report, we present five cases of orthotopic liver transplant patients with biliary complications that underwent ERCP- or MRCP-guided cholangioscopy with the SpyGlass™ DS Direct Visualization System (SDDVS). The SDDVS allowed for the visualization of the morphological characteristics of biliary strictures, and images collected using the SDDVS allowed for four of the cases to be treated endoscopically. Our findings suggest that cholangioscopy with the SDDVS is a promising method to guide the endoscopic treatment of biliary complications after liver transplantation.

1. Introduction

Biliary complications such as biliary leakage, biliary stones, or bile duct (anastomotic or nonanastomotic) strictures affect 10 to 25% of adult liver transplant recipients [1–5]. These complications often lead to increased morbidity as well as reduced graft and patient survival [6]. Currently, endoscopic retrograde cholangiopancreatography (ERCP) and magnetic resonance cholangiopancreatography (MRCP) are the main techniques used to diagnose and treat biliary complications in liver transplant patients [7]. However, due to limits to the depth of visualization in these techniques, up to 30% of biliary strictures are unable to be characterized [8].

The single-operator SpyGlass™ Direct Visualization System (Boston Scientific) increased bile duct clarity and improved image quality, resulting in reduced surgical complication rates [9, 10]. The improved image aspect in the SpyGlass™ Direct Visualization System allowed endoscopists to perform several procedures, including the evaluation of biliary strictures, examination of suspected benign and malignant conditions, passage of a guide wire in difficult strictures, and the removal of large stones or foreign objects from the common bile duct (CBD) [10, 11]. Later, the SpyGlass™ DS Direct Visualization System (SDDVS) further improved image resolution, improved ergonomics and stability, and simplified ERCP-guided cholangioscopies by incorporating a fully integrated catheter and a single-use scope [12].

Since implementation of the SDDVS, our center has observed notable morphological characteristics of biliary strictures in five postorthotopic liver transplantation (OLTx) patients.

2. Case Presentations

Five patients with post-OLTx bile duct strictures underwent an ERCP-guided cholangioscopy with the SDDVS at our center (Table 1). Their median age was 61.6 years (interquartile range (IQR), 49–71 years), three were males, and two were females.

2.1. Case I. A 71-year-old Caucasian male presented in 2017 and was diagnosed with cryptogenic end-stage liver disease (ESLD) complicated by portal vein thrombosis and hepatic hydrothorax. He had an OLTx on November 19, 2018, and received a cytomegalovirus (CMV) total antibody-positive and Epstein–Barr virus (EBV) viral capsid antigen (VCA) IgG-positive deceased donor organ. His postoperative course was unremarkable, and he had no acute rejection or infections. He underwent a MRCP-guided cholangioscopy for elevated liver function tests (LFTs) on October 23, 2019, which showed both intra- and extrahepatic biliary dilatation. He subsequently underwent an ERCP-guided cholangioscopy with the SDDVS on October 31, 2019. The procedure showed a nonnegotiable (with a 0.021 inch wire) pinhole inflammatory fibrotic stricture of the bile duct as well as anastomosis with excess exudate that was not amenable to stenting (Figure 1). The patient eventually underwent a Roux-en-Y choledochojejunostomy that resolved the stricture and is doing well. The SDDVS was useful for defining stricture morphology, attempting wire cannulation, and for helping the endoscopist make a prompt decision to pursue surgical treatment of the stricture.

2.2. Case II. A 62-year-old Hispanic female presented in 2014 and was diagnosed with cryptogenic cirrhosis complicated by portosystemic encephalopathy, anasarca, ascites, portal hypertensive gastropathy, and portal vein thrombosis. She had an OLTx on November 19, 2018, and received a CMV total antibody-positive deceased donor organ. Her postoperative course was complicated by herpes simplex pneumonia and candidemia, but she did not experience any episodes of acute rejection. She underwent an ERCP-guided cholangioscopy for abnormal LFTs on January 14, 2019, which showed a tortuous, redundant CBD that was difficult to cannulate. A biliary sphincterotomy was performed, and a 5 FR 10 cm straight plastic stent was placed across the CBD; however, the wire could not negotiate the stricture. She proceeded to have four additional ERCP-guided cholangioscopies with four stent placements throughout 2019. On November 14, 2019, she had an ERCP-guided cholangioscopy with the SDDVS. The SDDVS revealed a severely tight anastomotic, fibrotic stricture and a pinhole orifice (Figure 2). The SDDVS helped us assess stricture morphology, enabled multiple endoscopic metal stent replacements, and permitted resolution of the stricture, thereby avoiding surgery. The patient is currently doing well and has not required another ERCP or stent placement.

2.3. Case III. A 64-year-old Caucasian male presented in 2017 and was diagnosed with autoimmune hepatitis cirrhosis. He underwent an OLTx on April 05, 2019, and received a CMV total antibody-positive deceased donor organ. He had a complicated postoperative course that involved acute cellular rejection (rejection activity index (RAI) = 3), which initially improved with an increased dosage of Prograf®. He was subsequently readmitted for fever and elevated LFTs. He underwent a liver biopsy on April 11, 2019, that revealed acute cellular rejection (RAI = 3–4) and was treated with steroids. The patient had an ERCP-guided cholangioscopy on April 29, 2019 for elevated LFTs, which showed anastomotic stenosis and a low-grade leak. A biliary sphincterotomy was performed, and a 10 FR 9 cm plastic straight bile duct stent was placed across the leak. He had four additional ERCPs with stent placements throughout 2019. On November 14, 2019, he had an ERCP-guided cholangioscopy with the SDDVS that revealed an anastomotic bile duct stricture with persistent scarring (Figure 3). A CBD stone and debris were evacuated, and a metal stent was replaced that resolved the stricture. The patient is currently doing well and has not needed another ERCP-guided cholangioscopy or stent placement.

2.4. Case IV. A 49-year-old Caucasian female presented in 2017 and was diagnosed with ESLD from primary sclerosing cholangitis complicated by hepatic decompensation from ascites, edema, and hepatocellular carcinoma (HCC). She underwent an OLTx on June 27, 2018, and received a CMV total antibody-positive and EBV VCA IgG-positive deceased donor organ. The patient had a notable postoperative course due to an episode of severe rejection (RAI = 9; resolved with RAI = 3) with both cellular- and antibody-mediated components. She had an ERCP-guided cholangioscopy performed on November 06, 2018, for abnormal LFTs that showed a deeply cannulated CBD, a tight anastomotic biliary stricture, and a somewhat prominent proximal biliary tree. A biliary sphincterotomy was performed, and a 4×4 balloon dilator was used to dilate the stricture. While a 10 FR 10 cm stent was not able to pass across the stricture, a 7 FR 10 cm straight plastic stent passed across the stricture. She had four additional ERCP-guided cholangioscopies with two stent placements. On September 10, 2019, she had an ERCP-guided cholangioscopy with the SDDVS. The SDDVS showed scarring in the CBD, but no narrowing; the ostia of the hepatic ducts appeared to be normal (Figure 4). The metal stent, a CBD stone, and debris were removed, and the biliary anastomotic stricture was resolved. Scar tissue remained in the CBD, but no internal strictures were seen. She is currently doing well without any complaints and has not required another ERCP-guided cholangioscopy or stent placement.

2.5. Case V. A 62-year-old African American male presented in 2017 and was diagnosed with ESLD from hepatitis C virus that was complicated by HCC. He achieved sustained virologic response and had a microwave ablation in July 2015 for the HCC. He had an OLTx on May 22, 2017, and received a CMV total antibody-positive and EBV VCA IgG-positive deceased donor organ. He had a prolonged postoperative course due to acute cellular rejection (RAI = 7; resolved with RAI = 3), antibody-mediated rejection, and a nonhealing wound from the operation that required a wound vac. He

Table 1: Patient demographics and stricture morphological characteristics.

Case no.	Age (yr)	Sex	Ethnicity	BMI	Number of days after transplant to initial diagnosis	Morphological characteristics found using the SDDVS
1	71	M	Caucasian	23	384	Pinhole inflammatory fibrotic bile duct stricture; anastomosis with excess exudate; not amenable to stenting
2	62	F	Hispanic	25	56	Severely tight anastomotic stricture; pinhole orifice; amenable to stenting
3	64	M	Caucasian	31	25	Anastomotic bile duct stricture with persistent scarring
4	49	F	Caucasian	46	132	Scarring in the common bile duct but no narrowing; ostia of the hepatic ducts appeared to be normal
5	62	M	African American	30	71	August 28, 2018: web-like stricture at the anastomosis November 14, 2019: scarring in the anastomosis with a healthier mucosa in the proximal common bile duct

SDDVS, SpyGlass™ DS Direct Visualization System. BMI, body mass index.

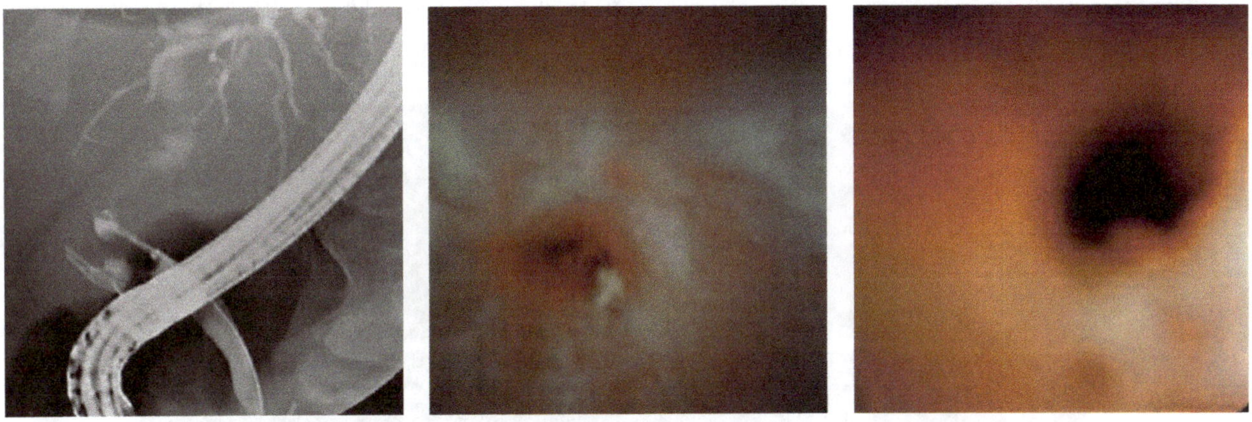

(a) (b) (c)

Figure 1: Pinhole inflammatory fibrotic biliary stricture observed using fluoroscopy (a) and the SpyGlass™ DS Visualization System (b,c).

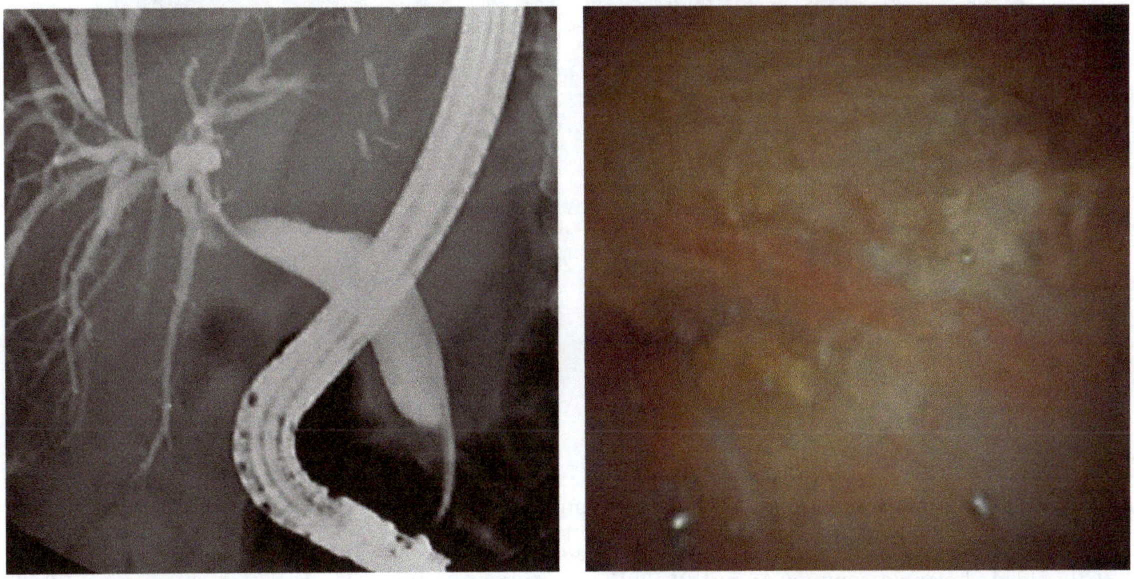

(a) (b)

Figure 2: Severely tight anastomotic, fibrotic stricture and a pinhole orifice stricture observed using fluoroscopy (a) and the SpyGlass™ DS Visualization System (b).

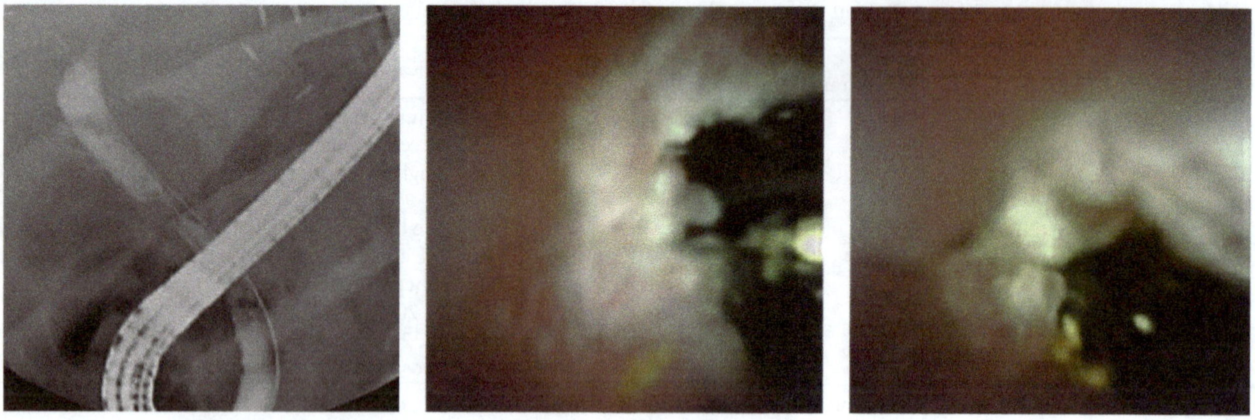

(a) (b) (c)

Figure 3: Anastomotic bile stricture with persistent scarring observed using fluoroscopy (a) and the SpyGlass™ DS Visualization System (b,c).

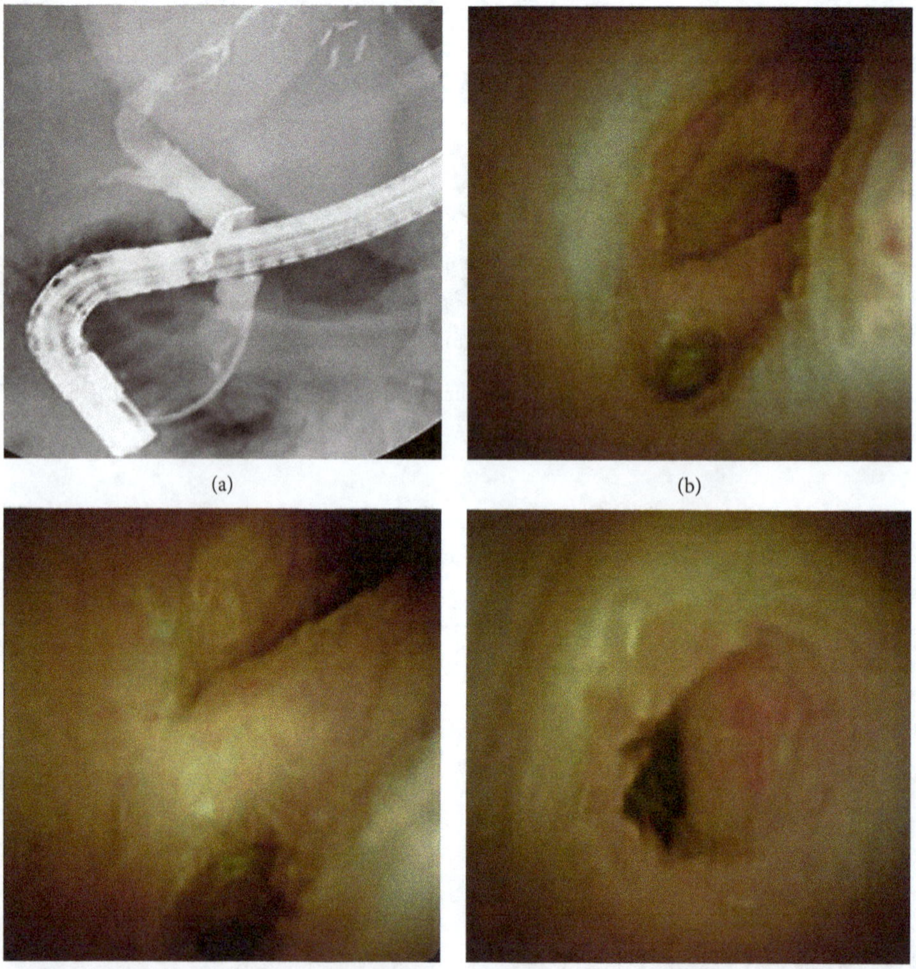

(a) (b) (c) (d)

Figure 4: Scarring in the common bile duct located using fluoroscopy (a) and the SpyGlass™ DS Visualization System (b–d).

had an ERCP-guided cholangioscopy on August 01, 2017, after an abnormal MRCP-guided cholangioscopy. The ERCP showed an anastomotic biliary stricture and common hepatic duct stricture. A 10 FR 12 cm plastic straight bile duct stent was placed. He had two subsequent ERCP-guided cholangioscopies and one bile duct stent placed. On August 28, 2018, he underwent an ERCP-guided cholangioscopy with the SDDVS that showed a web-like

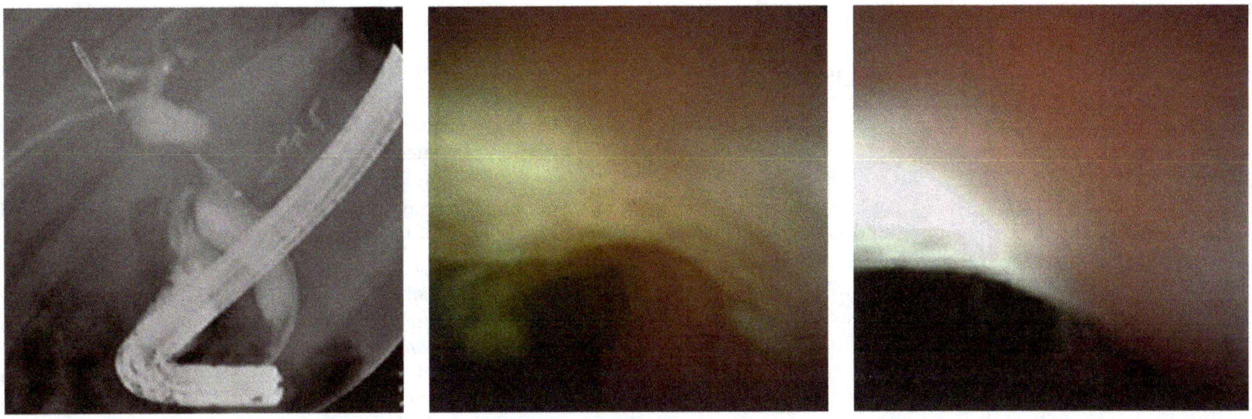

(a) (b) (c)

FIGURE 5: Scarring in the anastomosis observed using fluoroscopy (a) and the SpyGlass™ DS Visualization System (b,c).

stricture at the anastomosis. The SDDVS permitted the negotiation of a wire through the stricture, and the stricture was dilated with a 4×4 hurricane balloon dilator. A 10 FR 10 cm straight plastic stent was placed across the CBD. Following this, he had four more ERCP-guided cholangioscopies with four stent placements. On November 14, 2019, he underwent an ERCP-guided cholangioscopy with the SDDVS that showed scarring in the anastomosis (Figure 5). A healthier mucosa in the proximal CBD was seen using the SDDVS, and the metal stent was replaced in addition to CBD stones and debris removed.

3. Discussion

The image quality of the SDDVS allows endoscopists to distinguish between anastomotic and nonanastomotic strictures because they are able to observe epithelial changes, ulcers, small stones, and bile casts that they are unable to detect by ERCP [13]. However, the system has several limitations (e.g., the high cost of the system; the small working channel diameter that does not allow for the use of some devices; a learning curve in the training of endoscopists to use this system and techniques; and a lack of guidelines for its use) that limit the widespread use of the SDDVS [11, 14, 15].

Only a few studies have used the earlier generation of the SpyGlass™ system for the management of biliary complications after liver transplant [16–21]. The use of the newer generation SDDVS in the management of liver transplant-associated biliary complications has not been reported [5]. We have demonstrated the successful use of ERCP-guided cholangioscopy using SDDVS in characterizing anastomotic biliary strictures to guide endotherapy post-OLTx and that SDDVS may help with prognostication. In our case series, all except one patient was able to be treated endoscopically. Using the SpyGlass™ system, we were also able to discover that the strictures in these patients were heavily fibrotic in nature. Our findings may guide future novel endoscopic techniques (e.g., intraluminal needle-knife) when the technology becomes available.

SpyGlass™ cholangioscopy can distinguish a fibrotic stricture from a kink by its morphological appearance. Kinking of the CBD after OLTx is a common problem. This is likely due to a long redundant donor duct during harvesting, which is often done to prevent tension at the anastomosis. Kinking of the CBD can often mimic a stricture and sometimes poses challenges to the endoscopist during ERCP. Often, deep access to the CBD can be difficult in these patients, as the wire tends to buckle near the area of the kink. A technique used to straighten out the kink is to hyperinflate a balloon and pull it near the distal CBD. This often will straighten out the kink and enable to wire to pass into the hilar area. In terms of therapeutics, plastic stents will often resolve a kink in the CBD and can be removed at subsequent procedures 10 to 12 weeks later. In contrast, a fibrotic stricture almost always requires multiple rounds of stenting.

The fibrotic nature of the strictures provides a good rationale for the use of self-expandable metal stents to maintain long-term decompression of the strictures. Fibrotic biliary strictures are putatively the reason that OLTx patients often need 6 to 12 months of endoscopic therapy, repeated balloon dilations, and stent exchanges for stricture resolution. Endotherapy, even with a frequent need to repeat procedures every 10 to 12 weeks, is preferred at most centers compared to surgical alternatives (e.g., Roux-en-Y choledochojejunostomy) due to the surgery-associated risk of morbidity and complications. Our experience at a large tertiary center shows that approximately 90% of anastomotic biliary strictures can be successfully managed with endoscopic therapy, avoiding the need for surgery.

The limitations of our case series include its retrospective nature and small sample of patients. However, the successful use of the SDDVS is well illustrated. Continued observation using the SDDVS may be beneficial for the development of guidelines and improvement in the treatment of biliary strictures and scarring in future studies. Overall, our findings suggest that cholangioscopy with the SDDVS represents a new frontier guiding the endoscopic treatment of biliary complications after OLTx.

Disclosure

The research was performed as part of the employment at Methodist Dallas Medical Center.

References

[1] E. D. Williams and P. V. Draganov, "Endoscopic management of biliary strictures after liver transplantation," *World Journal of Gastroenterology*, vol. 15, no. 30, pp. 3725–3733, 2009.

[2] C. H. Ryu and S. K. Lee, "Biliary strictures after liver transplantation," *Gut and Liver*, vol. 5, no. 2, pp. 133–142, 2011.

[3] A. Pascher and P. Neuhaus, "Bile duct complications after liver transplantation," *Transplant International*, vol. 18, no. 6, pp. 627–642, 2005.

[4] S. Sharma, A. Gurakar, and N. Jabbour, "Biliary strictures following liver transplantation: past, present and preventive strategies," *Liver Transplantation*, vol. 14, no. 6, pp. 759–769, 2008.

[5] A. Hüsing-Kabar, H. S. Heinzow, H. H.-J. Schmidt et al., "Single-operator cholangioscopy for biliary complications in liver transplant recipients," *World Journal of Gastroenterology*, vol. 23, no. 22, pp. 4064–4071, 2017.

[6] J. F. Crismale and J. Ahmad, "Endoscopic management of biliary issues in the liver transplant patient," *Gastrointestinal Endoscopy Clinics of North America*, vol. 29, no. 2, pp. 237–256, 2019.

[7] M. A. Arain, R. Attam, and M. L. Freeman, "Advances in endoscopic management of biliary tract complications after liver transplantation," *Liver Transplantation*, vol. 19, no. 5, pp. 482–498, 2013.

[8] J. Hall and T. Pappas, "Current management of biliary strictures," *Journal of Gastrointestinal Surgery*, vol. 8, no. 8, pp. 1098–1110, 2004.

[9] S. Hülagü, G. Şirin, A. E. Duman, and H. Yılmaz, "Use of spyglass for peroral cholangioscopy in the diagnosis and treatment of hepatobiliary diseases in over five years follow-up: a single centre experience," *The Turkish Journal of Gastroenterology: The Official Journal of Turkish Society of Gastroenterology*, vol. 30, no. 12, pp. 1044–1054, 2019.

[10] P. Draganov, "The spyglass (R) direct visualization system for cholangioscopy," *Gastroenterol Hepatol (N Y)*, vol. 4, no. 7, pp. 469-470, 2008.

[11] E. G. H. D. Moura, "Cholangioscopy in bile duct disease: a case series," *Arquivos de Gastroenterologia*, vol. 51, no. 3, pp. 250–254, 2014.

[12] N. Franzini, *Boston Scientific Launches Next Generation SpyGlass™ DS Direct Visualization System for Advanced Diagnosis and Treatment of Pancreatico-Biliary Diseases*, Boston Scientific Corporation, Marlborough, MA, USA, 2015.

[13] P. Karagyozov, I. Boeva, and I. Tishkov, "Role of digital single-operator cholangioscopy in the diagnosis and treatment of biliary disorders," *World Journal of Gastrointestinal Endoscopy*, vol. 11, no. 1, pp. 31–40, 2019.

[14] R. Manta, M. Frazzoni, R. Conigliaro et al., "SpyGlass single-operator peroral cholangioscopy in the evaluation of indeterminate biliary lesions: a single-center, prospective, cohort study," *Surgical Endoscopy*, vol. 27, no. 5, pp. 1569–1572, 2013.

[15] S. Yan and S. Tejaswi, "Clinical impact of digital cholangioscopy in management of indeterminate biliary strictures and complex biliary stones: a single-center study," *Therapeutic Advances Gastrointestinal Endoscopy*, vol. 12, p. 2631774519853160, 2019.

[16] T. Franzini, R. Moura, G. Rodela et al., "A novel approach in benign biliary stricture - balloon dilation combined with cholangioscopy-guided steroid injection," *Endoscopy*, vol. 47, no. S 1, pp. E571–E572, 2015.

[17] U. Navaneethan, P. G. Venkatesh, M. Al Mohajer, and A. Gelrud, "Successful diagnosis and management of biliary cast syndrome in a liver transplant patient using single operator cholangioscopy," *JOP: Journal of the Pancreas*, vol. 12, no. 5, pp. 461-463, 2011.

[18] D. Balderramo, O. Sendino, R. Miquel et al., "Prospective evaluation of single-operator peroral cholangioscopy in liver transplant recipients requiring an evaluation of the biliary tract," *Liver Transplantation*, vol. 19, no. 2, pp. 199–206, 2013.

[19] Y. S. Woo, J. K. Lee, D. H. Noh, J. K. Park, K. H. Lee, and K. T. Lee, "Spyglass cholangioscopy-assisted guidewire placement for post-LDLT biliary strictures: a case series," *Surgical Endoscopy*, vol. 30, no. 9, pp. 3897–3903, 2016.

[20] H. Wright, S. Sharma, A. Gurakar, A. Sebastian, V. Kohli, and N. Jabbour, "Management of biliary stricture guided by the Spyglass direct visualization System in a liver transplant recipient: an innovative approach," *Gastrointestinal Endoscopy*, vol. 67, no. 7, pp. 1201–1203, 2008.

[21] A. Gurakar, H. Wright, C. Camci, and N. Jaboour, "The application of spyscope technology in evaluation of pre and post liver transplant biliary problems," *The Turkish Journal of Gastroenterology*, vol. 21, no. 4, pp. 428–432, 2010.

41

A Rare Case of Herpes Simplex Virus-2 Hepatitis with Negative Serology

Mohanad Soliman,[1] Olalekan Akanbi,[1] Ihab Almagdub,[1] Kishore Karri,[1] Pradeep Yarra,[1] Saad Emhmed Ali,[1] and Hanine El Haddad[2]

[1]*Department of Medicine, Division of Hospital Medicine, University of Kentucky, Lexington, KY, USA*
[2]*Department of Medicine, Division of Infectious Diseases, University of Kentucky, Lexington, KY, USA*

Correspondence should be addressed to Olalekan Akanbi; oakanbi1@gmail.com

Academic Editor: Tawesak Tanwandee

Herpes simplex virus-2 (HSV2) hepatitis represents a rare but serious complication of HSV2 infection that can progress to acute liver failure (ALF). We describe a case of a pregnant teenager who presented with four days of fever, headache, malaise, nausea, and vomiting. She was initially misdiagnosed with sepsis of unclear source and treated with broad-spectrum antibiotics. Empiric acyclovir was started one week into her hospitalization despite negative serologies while awaiting HSV2 PCR leading to complete resolution of symptoms. Given its high mortality and nonspecific presentation, clinicians should consider HSV hepatitis in all patients with acute hepatitis especially in high-risk population.

1. Introduction

We report a case of disseminated HSV-2 infection presenting as an acute liver failure (ALF) with negative serum herpes simplex virus (HSV) serology immunoglobulin M (IgM) and immunoglobin G (IgG) and without genital mucocutaneous involvement in a pregnant female during her third trimester. Despite negative serology, antiviral therapy was empirically started, and she was recovering before receiving the results of polymerase chain reaction detecting and quantifying serum level of herpes simplex 2 HSV-2.

2. Case Presentation

A 19-year-old female with no significant past medical history was referred to the emergency department from her antenatal clinic for further evaluation of fever 102 F, headache, malaise, nausea, and vomiting of 4-days duration following mild sore throat. She was in her 28th week of gestation on presentation. Physical examination showed an obese and anxious-appearing lady in mild respiratory distress with gravid abdomen. She weighed 142 kilograms (kg) with a BMI of 44.3. Her blood pressure was 111/60 mmHg, respiratory rate 24, heart rate 111, temperature 101.8 F, and oxygen saturation 96% on 2 liters (L) nasal cannula oxygen. She had dry mucous membranes, with no oral thrush or ulcers. Her abdomen was gravid with focal areas of tenderness, bowel sounds were heard, and fetal movement was detected. Pulmonary and cardiovascular examinations were unremarkable.

Her initial laboratory tests were significant for white blood cell (WBC) count of 11.8 K/uL with 78% neutrophil predominance and lymphopenia (0.77 K/uL). Although she had no urinary symptoms, urinalysis showed bacteriuria, confirmed as group B streptococcus agalactiae (GBS) with cultures. Initial chest X-ray and liver enzymes on admission were unremarkable. She was started on intravenous fluids for suspected gastroenteritis and oral cephalexin for asymptomatic GBS infection. Stool studies for clostridium difficile, comprehensive panel, ova, and parasites were ordered which all returned negative. However, she continued to spike fever through the third day of hospitalization prompting expansion of antibiotic coverage to Vancomycin and Zosyn (Figure 1). Liver transaminases which had been normal began to spike. Aspartate aminotransferase (AST) was 190, alanine

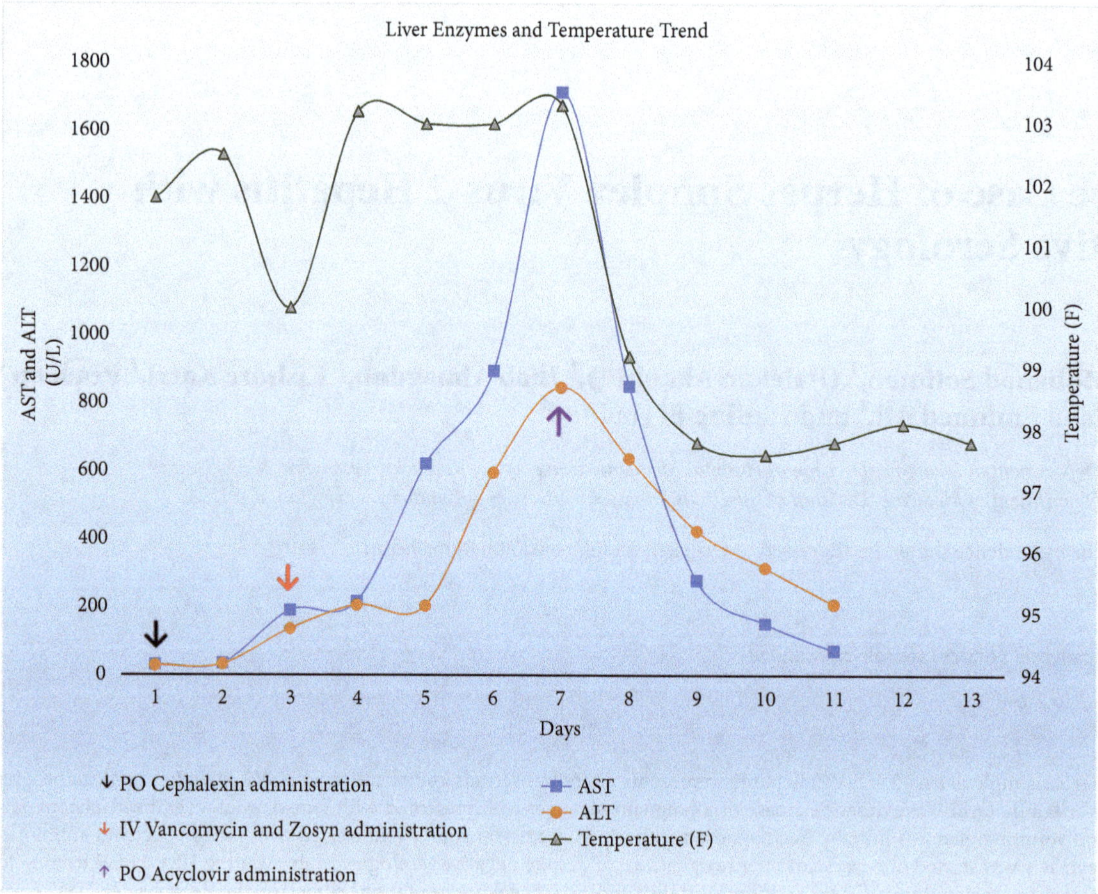

FIGURE 1: Liver enzymes and temperature trend.

aminotransferase (AST) was 135, and alkaline phosphatase was 110 while bilirubin remained normal. Serum Tylenol and hepatitis A, B, and C serologies were negative. Infectious Disease (ID) consultation was requested who recommended further infectious work-up with CMV, EBV, HIV, HSV, Rickettsia, and Leptospira serologies.

The patient continued to spike high grade fever reaching 103 F on day 4 of admission despite being on broad-spectrum antibiotics and negative infectious work-up including the aforementioned serologies. She also developed bloody diarrhea and acute kidney injury (AKI) prompting evaluation for possible Hemolytic Uremic Syndrome (HUS) and autoimmune diseases which all returned negative as well. Right upper quadrant ultrasound showed normal liver and gallbladder morphologies. Magnetic resonance imaging of the abdomen and pelvis without contrast showed diffuse T2 hyperintensity throughout the liver compatible with acute liver injury but was negative for any focal intra-abdominal or pelvic abscess.

One week into her hospitalization, her AST and ALT kept trending up reaching a peak of 1712 U/L and 845 U/L, respectively (Figure 1), mildly elevated alkaline phosphatase 140, INR 1.6, normal total bilirubin, absolute lymphocyte count of 0.11 K/uL, persistently negative blood cultures, and serum creatinine increased to 2.9 mg/dL, all concerning for a disseminated process. She became increasingly lethargic, tachycardic, and tachypneic necessitating care in the intensive care unit. With uprising liver enzymes and negative extensive infectious and rheumatologic work-up including Hep A, B, C serologies and PCR, EBV, CMV, Parvovirus, Rickettsia, and Leptospiral serologies, as well as negative HSV 1 and 2 IgM and IgG antibodies, antinuclear, and anti-liver-kidney microsomal antibodies, normal cryoglobulins, ceruloplasmin, alpha 1 antitrypsin and serum copper levels, and largely unremarkable imaging and stool studies, a decision was made to proceed with a liver biopsy. At this time, empiric acyclovir was started while other antibiotics were discontinued per ID recommendations.

Within the first 24 hours of starting acyclovir, AST and ALT began to downtrend while fever and diarrhea improved (Figure 1). Despite negative HSV-2 serologies, the PCR was reported on hospital day-8 with a very high viral load >100 million DNA copies/ml following which she reported a remote history of cold sores but denied a history of genital ulcers. A diagnosis of HSV hepatitis was made and she was transitioned to Val-acyclovir 1 gram three times daily to complete 14 days of therapy, then to resume acyclovir 400 mg three times daily until delivery to prevent recurrence. On the 12th day of hospitalization, she was discharged home without needing a biopsy anymore and with complete resolution of symptoms and improvement of liver enzymes and AKI; AST 72, ALT 208, alkaline phosphatase 150, total bilirubin 0.5 and creatinine 0.5. She remained symptom-free with complete normalization of creatinine and liver enzymes at outpatient follow-up two weeks after discharge. She was eventually delivered of a healthy baby boy via cesarean section at 38 weeks of gestation with no peripartum complications.

3. Discussion

Differential diagnosis of nonacetaminophen fulminant hepatic failure includes hepatitis A and B, Epstein-Barr virus, and cytomegalovirus. In addition to the aforementioned etiologies, pregnant women especially in the second and third trimester are at higher risk for hemolysis, elevated liver enzymes and low platelets (HELLP) syndrome, Hepatitis E, and HSV. Herpes simplex virus, especially HSV2, is a common cause of mucocutaneous lesions, with prevalence ranges 10% to 60% in the general population [1]. HSV2 as a causative agent for hepatitis is a rare but serious complication that represents <2% of viral hepatitis and 0.8% of cases of acute liver failure, immunosuppression, and pregnancy during the third trimester are common precipitating factors [2]. Herpes simplex virus-2 (HSV-2) is a double-stranded DNA virus that belongs to Herpesviridae family of viruses, which includes other members such as herpes simplex virus-1 (HSV-1), varicella zoster virus, cytomegalovirus, Epstein-Barr virus, and human herpes viruses 6, 7, and 8 (Kaposi's sarcoma-associated herpesvirus) [3].

Potential mechanisms of herpes induced hepatitis include (i) a large HSV inoculum overwhelming the immune system on initial encounter; (ii) dissemination of mucosal herpetic lesions within a suppressed immune system; (iii) reactivation of a latent HSV reactivation or reinfection with a different new strain of HSV 4 (Hepatovirulent HSV) [4]. Disseminated HSV-2 infection has been defined by presence any of the following criteria, (a) positive HSV-2 IgM antibody test results, (b) HSV-2 DNA detected by polymerase chain reaction (PCR) assay of the peripheral blood mononuclear cells (PBSCs), or (c) involvement of two or more noncontiguous sites concurrently [5].

HSV hepatitis is one of the few treatable causes of acute liver failure when identified and treated promptly. When left untreated however, it is associated with high mortality, exceeding 80%–90% [6]. Consequently, it is been reasonable to start empiric treatment with acyclovir in patients with ALF of indeterminate etiology while awaiting confirmatory results, especially patients at risk for HSV. The high mortality rate of severe HSV hepatitis is a result of being difficult to diagnose in 77% of cases. The clinical manifestations of HSV hepatitis are not specific especially in the absence of typical mucocutaneous eruption that is only present in 50% of the cases. HSV hepatitis associated clinical findings that have been reported are fever (98%), clotting abnormality (96.5%), encephalitis (80%), and acute renal injury (65.3%) [7]. 90% of cases have low platelet count, low white blood cell count, and elevated transaminases (about 100- to 1000-fold above normal with AST predominance) with normal to low bilirubin, thus named "anicteric hepatitis" like in our case [2]. The presence of these findings and patterns in a high-risk patient may support a diagnosis of HSV hepatitis, but their absence does not rule out a diagnosis. Poor prognostic parameters that might warrant the need for liver transplant evaluation are age > 40-years, male gender, coagulation abnormalities, the presence of an immunosuppressed state, encephalopathy, ALT > 5,000 U/L, platelet count < 75,000 U, and unavailability of acyclovir therapy [8].

It takes average of 2 to 3 weeks for the body to produce antibodies against HSV during which viral serology will be negative. HSV Immunoglobulin M (IgM) antibodies titer increases up to four times the normal value 2–4 weeks after the infection using enzyme-linked immunosorbent assay (ELISA) [9]. HerpeSelect HSV-2 ELISAs are glycoprotein G-based, type-specific antibody detection tests which are approved by the US Food and Drug Administration for diagnosis of genital herpes. Median interval from onset of symptoms to seroconversion is 21 days [10]. HSV PCR with concurrent elevation in aminotransferases like in our case is diagnostic and substitutes the need for invasive gold standard liver biopsy [2].

Treatment of HSV2 induced acute liver failure includes (i) supportive measures, (ii) addressing the underlying precipitating condition, (iii) antiviral agents, (vi) liver transplantation, and (v) in one report therapeutic plasma exchange [11]. The antiviral agent of choice is acyclovir. It is a safe drug and generally very well tolerated. Side effects if given orally are gastrointestinal upset, headache, and rash, while it can cause reversible nephrotoxicity if administered intravenously via formation of crystals and obstructive uropathy. Risk factors for nephrotoxicity are rapid intravenous administration, poorly hydrated patients, and those with preexisting renal disease who retain higher serum levels [12].

4. Conclusion

We emphasize maintaining a strong clinical index of suspicion for HSV2 induced hepatitis especially in the high-risk population even in the absence of suggestive serologies. This will help facilitate appropriate and prompt management. Given the safety profile of acyclovir and the high mortality rates of patients with HSV-related ALF, our case illustrates the need for empiric therapy in high-risk patient with otherwise unexplained hepatitis.

References

[1] R. Gupta, T. Warren, and A. Wald, "Genital herpes," *The Lancet*, vol. 370, no. 9605, pp. 2127–2137, 2007.

[2] A. Natu, G. Iuppa, and C. D. Packer, "Herpes simplex virus hepatitis: a presentation of multi-institutional cases to promote early diagnosis and management of the disease," *Case Reports in Hepatology*, vol. 2017, Article ID 3180984, 5 pages, 2017.

[3] M. Fatahzadeh and R. A. Schwartz, "Human herpes simplex virus infections: epidemiology, pathogenesis, symptomatology, diagnosis, and management," *Journal of the American Academy of Dermatology*, vol. 57, no. 5, pp. 737–763, 2007.

[4] M. Yunce, P. Bhat, D. Jaganathan, and M. Bahrain, "Herpes hepatitis as a complication of total abdominal hysterectomy; an unusual complication of abdominal instrumentation," *Clinical Case Reports*, vol. 7, no. 1, pp. 11–14, 2019.

[5] S. Kurosawa, N. Sekiya, K. Fukushima et al., "Unusual manifestation of disseminated herpes simplex virus type 2 infection associated with pharyngotonsilitis, esophagitis, and hemophagocytic lymphohisitocytosis without genital involvement," *BMC Infectious Diseases*, vol. 19, no. 1, 2019.

[6] B. J. Jeong, H. J. Tae, Y. J. Cho et al., "Herpes simplex virus hepatitis treated with acyclovir," *The Ewha Medical Journal*, vol. 39, no. 3, pp. 81–84, 2016.

[7] J. P. Norvell, A. T. Blei, B. D. Jovanovic, and J. Levitsky, "Herpes simplex virus hepatitis: an analysis of the published literature and institutional cases," *Liver Transplantation*, vol. 13, no. 10, pp. 1428–1434, 2007.

[8] M. Masadeh, H. Shen, Y. Lee et al., "A fatal case of herpes simplex virus hepatitis in a pregnant patient," *Intractable and Rare Diseases Research*, vol. 6, no. 2, pp. 124–127, 2017.

[9] E. W. Hook III, R. O. Cannon, A. J. Nahmias et al., "Herpes simplex virus infection as a risk factor for human immunodeficiency virus infection in heterosexuals," *The Journal of Infectious Diseases*, vol. 165, no. 2, pp. 251–255, 1992.

[10] R. Ashley-Morrow, E. Krantz, and A. Wald, "Time course of seroconversion by Herpeselect ELISA after acquisition of genital Herpes simplex virus type 1 (HSV-1) or HSV-2," *Sexually Transmitted Diseases*, vol. 30, no. 4, pp. 310–314, 2003.

[11] E. W. Holt, J. Guy, S. M. Gordon et al., "Acute liver failure caused by herpes simplex virus in a pregnant patient: Is there a potential role for therapeutic plasma exchange?" *Journal of Clinical Apheresis*, vol. 28, no. 6, pp. 426–429, 2013.

[12] A. Arvin, G. Campadelli-Fiume, E. Mocarski et al., *Human Herpesviruses: Biology, Therapy, and Immunoprophylaxis*, Cambridge University Press, Cambridge, UK, 2019.

Time-Course Changes of Serum Keratin Concentrations after Liver Transplantation: Contrasting Results of Keratin-18 and Keratin-19 Fragments

Cristina Macía,[1] Jose Loureiro,[1] Isabel Campos-Varela,[1] Ihab Abdulkader,[2] Esteban Otero,[1,3] Evaristo Varo,[3] Santiago Tomé,[1,3] and Arturo Gonzalez-Quintela[1]

[1]*Department of Internal Medicine and Hepatology, Complejo Hospitalario Universitario de Santiago, Santiago, Spain*
[2]*Department of Pathology, Complejo Hospitalario Universitario de Santiago, Santiago, Spain*
[3]*Liver Transplant Unit, Complejo Hospitalario Universitario de Santiago, Santiago, Spain*

Correspondence should be addressed to Arturo Gonzalez-Quintela; arturo.gonzalez.quintela@sergas.es

Academic Editor: Ned Snyder

Objective. Under normal conditions, adult hepatocytes express only keratin-8 (K8) and keratin-18 (K18), whereas cholangiocytes also express K19. In this study, we delineate the pattern of normal time-course changes in serum K19 and K18 levels after liver transplantation. *Patients and Methods.* Serum levels of the K19 fragment CYFRA 21-1 and the K18 fragments tissue polypeptide specific antigen (TPS) and M30 (a neoepitope that is generated after caspase cleavage during apoptosis) were measured at baseline and at regular intervals (up to 6 months) after liver transplantation in 11 adult patients. *Results.* There was a gradual decrease in serum K19 concentrations from baseline values after transplantation, following a time-course pattern similar to that of serum bilirubin. In contrast, serum concentrations of K18 fragments increased markedly shortly after transplantation and gradually decreased thereafter, following a time-course pattern similar to that of serum transaminases. The increase in TPS tended to occur earlier than that in M30, suggesting an initial predominance of hepatocyte necrosis followed by a predominance of apoptosis in the first days after transplantation. Five patients presented posttransplant complications (acute rejection in three cases and HCV recurrence in two cases). An early increase in serum K19 concentrations was observed in all cases. An increase in serum concentrations of K18 fragments (M30 and TPS) was observed in the two cases with HCV recurrence and was more variable in the three cases with acute rejection. *Conclusions.* Serum concentrations of K19 and K18 fragments follow a dissimilar pattern of time-course changes after liver transplantation. The diagnostic value of variations in these normal patterns should be addressed in future studies.

1. Introduction

Keratins are intermediate filament proteins that are found in epithelial cells [1–6]. They are located intracellularly and are released into the blood upon liver injury, including necrosis and apoptosis [3, 5, 6]. During apoptosis, keratins are substrates for caspase degradation, with subsequent release of keratin fragments to the extracellular space [3, 6, 7]. Serum keratin concentrations are routinely used in clinical practice as tumor markers for epithelial neoplasms [7–9] Immunoassays for detecting keratins can be broadly divided into two types: those that recognize epitopes in intact keratin (or its fragments) and those that recognize specific epitopes generated during apoptosis [6]. Among the former, cytokeratin fragment (CYFRA) 21.1 corresponds to a specific epitope in keratin-19 (K19) [10]. Similarly, tissue polypeptide specific antigen (TPS) and M65 correspond to specific epitopes in K18 [8, 11]. Serum concentrations of all of these keratin fragments increase after epithelial cell necrosis or apoptosis [7, 12]. Among the latter, the M30 assay detects a K18 fragment that includes a neoepitope, Asp396-NE, which is generated after caspase cleavage during apoptosis (Figure 1) [13–15]. The ratio between keratin fragments that increase after apoptosis only and those that increase after either necrosis or apoptosis may offer insights into the relative contribution made by each of these pathologic processes in a given disease [3, 15–17].

Keratins are important proteins in liver health and disease, as reviewed elsewhere [1–6]. Adult hepatocytes express K8 and K18 only [5, 6]. During embryogenesis, hepatocytes also express variable levels of K19, which is also expressed in adult cholangiocytes together with K7 [5, 6]. Keratins are highly abundant in the liver, where they constitute approximately 0.3% of total protein [6]. Their abundance and intracellular distribution make them promising serological markers for nonmalignant liver disease [6]. In fact, serum concentrations of TPS (K18) are increased in most patients with various liver diseases [18, 19], particularly acute hepatitis [19]. Serum TPS concentrations are also markedly increased in patients with steatohepatitis, both alcoholic [19–22] and nonalcoholic [23–25]. In patients with alcoholic liver disease, serum TPS levels serve to distinguish between patients with and without alcoholic steatohepatitis [20]; serum TPS concentrations correlate with the number of Mallory–Denk bodies in liver specimens, a hallmark of steatohepatitis [20,21]. In addition, K18 (M65)-based modification of the MELD score improves the prediction of spontaneous survival after acute liver injury [26]. Serum concentrations of the apoptosis marker M30 have also been extensively studied as a test for liver injury [27–41]. Serum concentrations of the K18 fragment M30 may be useful as a marker for steatohepatitis among patients with either nonalcoholic fatty liver disease [28–30] or alcoholic liver disease [31], as a prognostic marker in alcoholic hepatitis [32], and as a marker for histological severity in patients with chronic hepatitis C [33–35] or hepatitis B [36–38]. Serum M30 levels may also help to differentiate graft-versus-host disease from unrelated conditions with similar liver manifestations in patients who have undergone bone marrow transplantation [39].

Apoptosis is a relevant pathogenetic feature in liver disease [40–43]. It is also a prominent feature after liver transplantation, particularly during ischemia-reperfusion injury [44–46] and rejection [47]. Apoptosis may be a target for therapy in a variety of disorders [48], including liver disease [41, 42, 49]. Antiapoptotic molecules directed at preventing apoptosis during ischemia-reperfusion injury are under investigation [41, 48, 50]. To the best of our knowledge, only two studies have focused on serum keratin levels after liver transplantation. Ulukaya et al. determined the serum concentrations of M65 and M30 up to 24 hours after liver reperfusion [51]. In their study, both apoptosis and, particularly, necrosis were prominent in the short term after liver transplantation from deceased liver donors [51]. Brenner et al. [52] evaluated serum levels of K18 fragments (M65 and M30) after liver reperfusion and during the first days after liver transplantation. Their study also showed an increase of K18, M30, and M65 in the first hours after transplantation, in correspondence with prominent necrosis and apoptosis due to the ischemia/reperfusion injury. Moreover, they also observed an elevation of keratin levels during posttransplant complications such as infection or perfusion disorders [52].

Serum K19 concentrations have been less extensively investigated in patients with liver disease. In a previous study, we found that serum K19 levels are elevated to a lesser extent than K18 levels in patients with alcoholic liver disease [22]. To the best of our knowledge, serum K19 concentrations have not been previously studied in liver transplantation. The objective of the present study was to delineate the normal evolution of serum K19 (CYFRA 21-1) and compare it with that of K18 (TPS and M30) in the midterm (6 months) after transplantation.

2. Patients and Methods

2.1. Participants and Study Design. This descriptive observational study included 11 consecutive adult patients (aged 40–64 years, seven males) who underwent orthotopic liver transplantation from deceased donors in our centre over a 3-month period. All patients gave written informed consent for participation in the study, which was reviewed and approved by the Institutional Review Board and conformed to the current Helsinki Declaration. The main patient characteristics are presented in Table 1. All of the patients had advanced-stage liver cirrhosis. A history of alcohol abuse was present in eight cases. Standard immunosuppression consisted of corticosteroids and tacrolimus in all participants.

Serum samples for keratin concentration determination were taken at baseline (pretransplantation) and at regular intervals (24 hours, 3 days, 6 days, 10 days, 20 days, 1 month, 2 months, 4 months, and 6 months) after liver transplantation. The serum sample at 24 hours posttransplantation was unavailable for one patient. Standard liver markers were assayed in an ADVIA 1650 analyzer (Bayer Diagnostics, Leverkusen, Germany). Samples were frozen at −40°C until tested for keratin concentrations.

2.2. Serum Determinations

2.2.1. Keratin-19 (CYFRA 21-1). Serum CYFRA 21-1 levels were determined by means of a commercial electrochemiluminescence immunoassay (Elecsys CYFRA 21-1; Roche Diagnostics, Mannheim, Germany) in a Roche Elecsys immunoassay analyzer. The test employs a combination of two monoclonal antibodies (Ks 19.1 and BM 19.21) that are specific to K19 fragments [10]. The epitope sequences recognized by these antibodies lie within the sequence 311–335 for the Ks 19.1 antibody and 346–367 for the detector antibody BM 19.21 [10]. The upper reference limit for serum CYFRA 21-1 is considered to be 3.3 ng/mL.

2.2.2. Keratin-18 (TPS). Serum TPS concentrations were assayed by means of a commercial chemiluminescent immunoassay (Immulite-TPS; Siemens Medical Solutions Diagnostics, Gwynedd, UK) in an automated platform (Immulite-2000, Siemens). The test employs the M3 monoclonal antibody, which is specific for residues 322–340

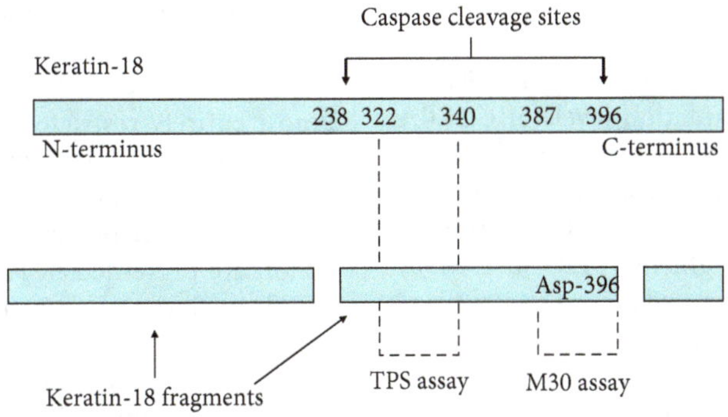

FIGURE 1: Schematic representation of K18 cleavage during apoptosis and the epitopes recognized by the assays for K18 fragments employed in the present study. The TPS assay can detect soluble full-length K18 as well as K18 fragments; increased serum TPS concentrations could, therefore, represent necrosis or apoptosis. Conversely, the M30 assay detects a neoepitope that is only revealed after caspase cleavage of the protein and is postulated to be a selective biomarker of apoptosis. [13, 16].

TABLE 1: Patient characteristics.

Patient number	Age (y)/sex	Indication for transplantation	Ischemia time (min)	Complications after transplantation
1	56/M	Cirrhosis (alcohol plus HCV)	260	Recurrent HCV hepatitis
2	56/F	Cirrhosis (alcohol) and hepatocellular carcinoma	720	None
3	45/F	Cirrhosis (alcohol)	690	*De novo* diabetes mellitus
4	43/M	Cirrhosis (alcohol)	360	Acute cellular rejection (day +33); *de novo* diabetes mellitus
5	53/M	Cirrhosis (alcohol)	700	Acute cellular rejection (day +10)
6	40/F	Cirrhosis (alcohol)	240	Intestinal obstruction (umbilical hernia)
7	62/F	Cirrhosis (autoimmune)	420	None
8	58/M	Cirrhosis (alcohol)	300	Mild kidney failure
9	55/M	Cirrhosis (HBV) and hepatocellular carcinoma	630	None
10	64/M	Cirrhosis (HCV)	360	Recurrent HCV hepatitis
11	61/M	Cirrhosis (alcohol)	300	Acute cellular rejection (day +56); *de novo* diabetes mellitus; mild kidney failure

HBV, hepatitis B virus; HCV, hepatitis C virus. The initial immunosuppression regime included tacrolimus and corticosteroids in all cases.

in K18 [8, 11] (Figure 1). This method has a detection threshold of 15 U/L. The upper normal reference level was considered to be 100 U/L.

2.2.3. Keratin-18 (M30). Serum levels of M30 were assayed by means of a commercial immunoassay (M30-Apoptosense; PEVIVA AB, Bromma, Sweden) following the manufacturer's instructions. The test employs the M30 detection antibody, which recognizes a neoepitope mapped to positions 387 to 396 of K18 (Figure 1). This so-called K18-Asp396-NE is only revealed after caspase cleavage of the protein and is postulated to be a selective biomarker of apoptosis [13, 14]. Reference concentrations of M30-antigen were used to calibrate the assay. The absorbance was determined with an ELISA reader at 450 nm. The method has a detection threshold of 25 U/L. The upper normal reference level is considered to be 260 U/L.

2.3. Histological Studies. Paraffin-embedded liver specimens were stained with hematoxylin-eosin following standard procedures. For immunohistochemical studies, deparaffinized sections of liver specimens were digested with ChemMate Proteinase K (Dako, Glostrup, Denmark) for 10 minutes prior to antibody incubation. The primary antibody (see below) was applied for 30 minutes at room temperature. The EnVision System (Dako), a dextran polymer that contains peroxidase and the secondary anti-mouse antibody, was then applied for 30 minutes. The sections were washed in the buffer solution (ChemMate Buffer kit, Dako) between incubations. Positive reactions were revealed with diaminobenzidine (DAB, Dako) as the chromogen, and the sections were counterstained with Harris hematoxylin (Panreac, Barcelona, Spain) for 2 minutes. The primary antibodies included K19 (clone RCK 108, Dako), K18 (clone DC10, Dako), and the M30 monoclonal antibody (M30 CytoDEATH; Alexis Biochemicals, Nottingham, UK). The number of hepatocytes containing M30-reactive inclusions per 50 random microscope fields (40x) was considered to be the "apoptotic score" [34, 53].

2.4. Statistical Analyses. The Wilcoxon test was employed to compare paired sample values. The Spearman rank test was used to assess correlation. P values <0.05 were considered to be statistically significant.

3. Results

3.1. Evolution of Serum Concentrations of K18 and K19 after Liver Transplantation. Pretransplantation levels of CYFRA 21-1, TPS, and M30 were increased in the majority of patients; the median pretransplantation concentrations were 3.6 ng/mL, 201 U/L, and 403 U/L, respectively (Figure 2). Serum concentrations of K18 fragments (TPS and M30) increased dramatically in the immediate posttransplant period (Figure 2). The increase in TPS and M30 occurred in parallel, although in general, the peak TPS concentrations tended to occur earlier (on day +1) than the peak of M30 concentrations, which attained higher median values on day +3 (Figure 2). Consequently, the ratio TPS : M30 in the immediate posttransplant period was highest on day +1 and lowest on day +3 (Figure 3). Serum concentrations of both TPS and M30 decreased thereafter. The decrease in serum TPS concentrations was rather abrupt in most cases, whereas the decrease in M30 concentrations over time was steadier (Figure 2). Six months after transplantation, the serum concentrations of both TPS and M30 were significantly lower than they were in pretransplant samples (Figure 2).

In general, the time-course changes in the concentrations of the K18 fragments TPS and M30 resembled those of the serum transaminases aspartate aminotransferase (AST) and ALT (alanine aminotransferase) (Figure 2). In fact, serum levels of TPS and M30 tended to be correlated with serum levels of AST and ALT. The correlation between K18 fragments and serum transaminases was greater for TPS than for M30 and higher for AST than for ALT, at least in the immediate posttransplant period (Table 2).

Time-course changes in serum K19 (CYFRA 21-1) levels were different from those of K18 fragments. There was no significant peak in CYFRA 21-1 levels immediately after liver transplantation (Figure 2). Instead, there was a steady decrease in the CYFRA 21-1 concentration from pretransplant values over time. From posttransplant day +6 onwards, serum concentrations of CYFRA 21-1 were significantly lower than pretransplantation values (Figure 2). On the whole, the time-course changes in the levels of serum K19 (CYFRA 21-1) resembled those of serum bilirubin (Figure 2). In fact, serum levels of CYFRA 21-1 tended to be correlated with serum bilirubin levels, at least in the immediate posttransplant period (Table 2).

3.2. Case Reports. Posttransplant complications that lead to liver biopsy occurred in five patients (Table 1). Of these, two cases corresponded to recurrent HCV, and the other three corresponded to episodes of acute rejection. Individual data for one of the patients with HCV recurrence are presented in Figure 4. In this case, an increase in serum levels of K18 (TPS and M30) and K19 (CYFRA 21-1) fragments was observed at the time of the recurrence. The increase in serum keratin levels, particularly for K19, tended to occur earlier than alterations in standard liver markers (Figure 4). Liver biopsy was consistent with HCV recurrence (Figure 4). Immunohistochemical studies showed scattered M30-positive hepatocytes throughout the liver lobule (apoptotic score, 17). Immunohistochemical studies in normal control livers were negative (data not shown). Immunohistochemical staining for K19 revealed that the expression of this protein was almost entirely restricted to cholangiocytes (Figure 4). The biochemical and histological findings for the other patient with HCV recurrence were similar (data not shown).

Individual data for one of the patients with acute rejection are presented in Figure 5. In this case, there was no significant increase in serum K18 fragment (TPS or M30) levels during the episode. Conversely, we observed a transient increase in serum K19 fragment (CYFRA 21-1) (Figure 5). Immunohistochemical studies were negative for M30 (apoptotic score, zero). Immunohistochemical staining for K19 revealed that it was almost entirely restricted to cholangiocytes (Figure 5). For the other two patients with acute rejection (one on day 30 and the other one on day 50), the histological findings were very similar, and biochemical studies also showed a transient increase in K19 fragment (CYFRA 21-1) and a transient increase in K18 fragments (TPS and M30) (data not shown).

4. Discussion

Liver transplantation is a standard therapy for advanced liver disease. Improving the understanding of the mechanisms underlying ischemia-reperfusion injury and late complications may serve as a basis for prevention or therapy. In addition, early and accurate detection of the complications that may occur after liver transplantation is of obvious importance. In the present study, we attempted to delineate the normal time-course changes in serum keratins (K19 and K18) in the short and midterm after liver transplantation.

The time-course changes in serum keratin levels indicate that both necrosis and apoptosis of hepatocytes are prominent features immediately after liver transplantation. Serum concentrations of the K18 fragments TPS and M30 increased dramatically in the first 3 days after the procedure. Conversely, serum concentrations of K19 did not increase over the same period. It should be noted that K19 is not constitutively expressed in hepatocytes [1, 3, 6]. The time-course changes in TPS and M30 levels were similar but not strictly parallel. Peak TPS concentrations tended to occur earlier than those of M30. As a consequence, the TPS : M30 ratio was highest on day +1 and lowest on day +3. This indicates that early ischemia-reperfusion liver injury comprises both hepatocyte necrosis and apoptosis, with necrosis predominating in the first hours after transplantation and apoptosis predominating in the following days. This early predominance of hepatocyte necrosis over apoptosis was also reported by Ulukaya et al. [51] and by Brenner et al. [52]. The relative contributions of apoptosis and necrosis could be important for future investigations of methods to prevent early liver dysfunction after transplantation, including the development of antiapoptotic drugs [48, 50]. The increased levels of K18 fragments quickly decreased in the following days, and TPS levels decreased more rapidly than M30 levels. Six months after transplantation, the concentrations of both markers were significantly lower than they were at the pretransplant baseline. Overall, the time-course changes in

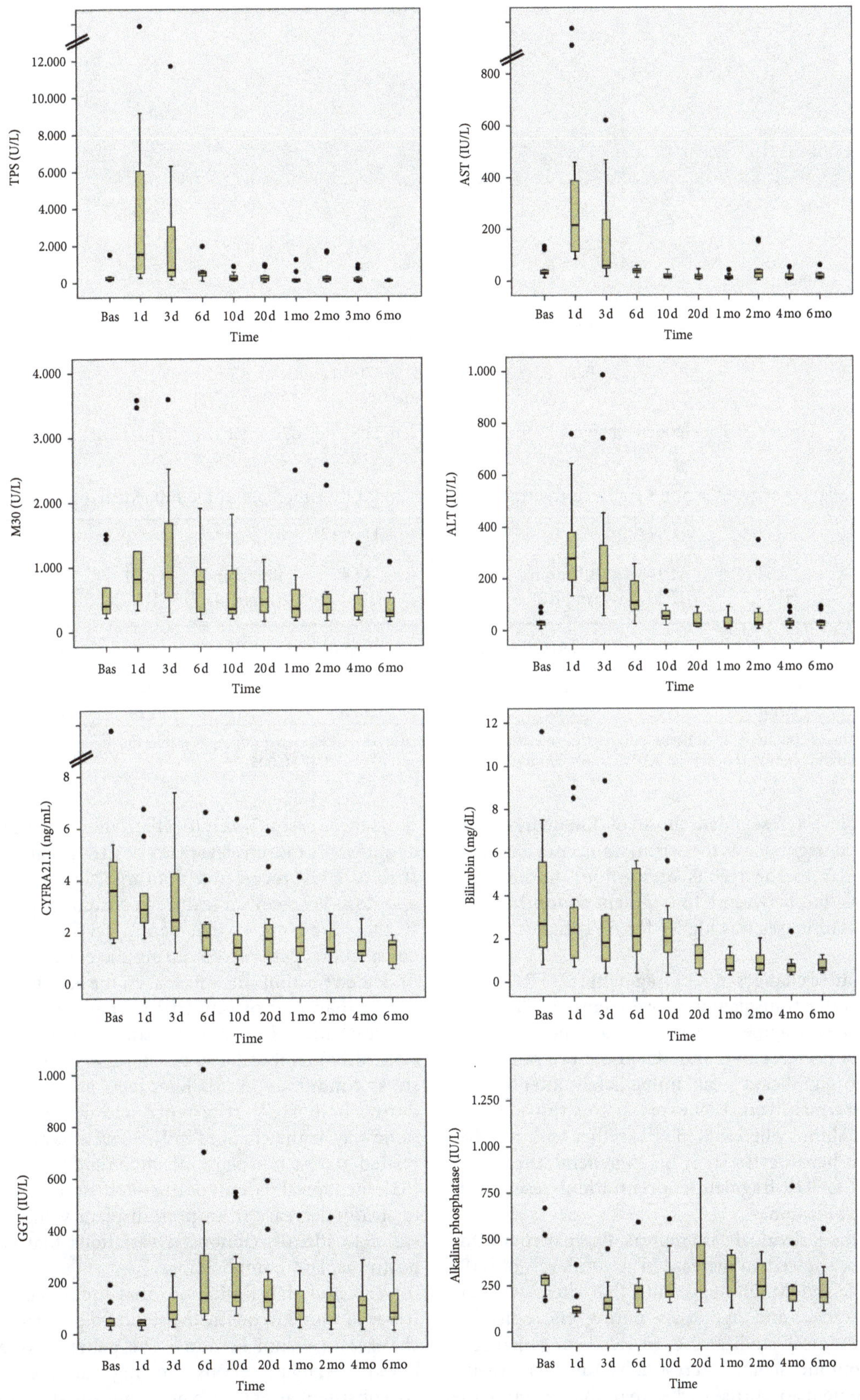

FIGURE 2: Time-course changes in serum concentrations of the K18 fragments TPS and M30 and the K19 fragment CYFRA 21-1 after liver transplantation. Comparison with time-course changes in the standard liver markers serum AST, ALT, GGT, alkaline phosphatase, and total bilirubin. Bas, baseline (pretransplant level); d, day; mo, month.

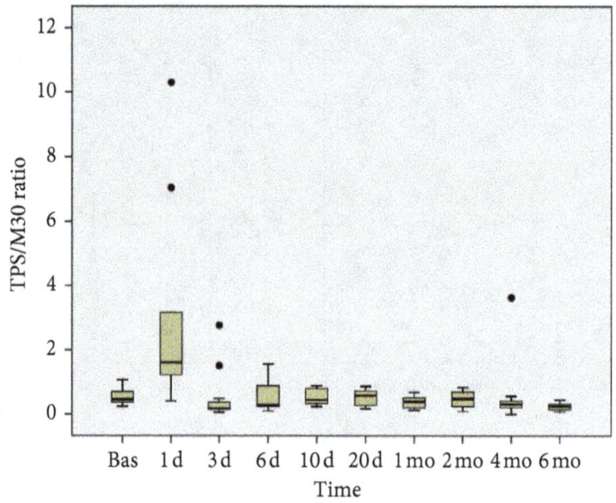

FIGURE 3: Time-course changes in the ratio between TPS and M30 after liver transplantation.

TABLE 2: Correlation between serum keratin concentrations and standard liver markers in the immediate posttransplant period.

	Day +1			Day +3			Day +6		
	AST (IU/L)	ALT (IU/L)	Bilirubin (mg/dL)	AST (IU/L)	ALT (IU/L)	Bilirubin (mg/dL)	AST (IU/L)	ALT (IU/L)	Bilirubin (mg/dL)
CYFRA 21-1 (U/L)	0.273	0.152	0.681*	0.618*	0.409	0.191	0.451	0.183	0.781**
TPS (U/L)	0.855**	0.818**	0.401	0.900**	0.818**	0.182	0.724**	0.320	0.603*
M30 (U/L)	0.661*	0.697*	0.602	0.691*	0.655*	0.382	0.287	0.078	0.461

CYFRA 21-1, keratin-19 fragment; TPS, tissue polypeptide specific antigen (keratin-18); M30, neoepitope generated during apoptosis in caspase-cleaved keratin-18; AST, aspartate aminotransferase; ALT, alanine aminotransferase.* $P < 0.05$ and ** $P < 0.005$.

K18 fragment levels resembled those of the markers of hepatocellular damage such as the serum transaminases AST and ALT. Similar to the results of previous studies, the statistical correlation between K18 fragment concentrations and serum transaminases was higher for AST than for ALT [19].

The time-course changes in K19 fragment (CYFRA 21-1) concentrations after transplantation were entirely different from those of K18 fragments. Serum K19 concentrations showed a steady decrease over time from the pretransplant values, with no significant peak immediately after transplantation. In normal livers, K19 expression is restricted to the biliary epithelium, whereas K18 is, together with K8, the main keratin in hepatocytes [1, 3, 6]. In general, the time-course changes in K19 fragment concentrations resembled those of serum bilirubin.

Regarding the individual case reports, two patients with HCV recurrence showed an increase in serum levels of K18 fragments (TPS and M30), suggesting that there was an increase in necrosis and apoptosis during the episode. Immunohistochemical studies also revealed an enhanced hepatocyte apoptotic score. Interestingly, the increase in serum K18 fragments occurred earlier than that of standard liver markers. Of the three patients with acute cellular rejection, the increase in serum K18 fragments was less evident in one and absent in the other. Furthermore, immunohistochemical studies did not reveal apoptotic hepatocytes in these three cases. Taken together, these findings suggest that apoptosis is more relevant to posttransplant complications such as HCV recurrence than to cellular rejection. Indeed, apoptosis is a relevant feature in chronic hepatitis C [33, 34]. It should be noted that serum levels of K19 fragments conspicuously increased during the episodes of either HCV or acute rejection. In some cases, the K19 increase occurred earlier than that of standard liver markers. Under normal circumstances, K19 is only expressed in biliary epithelial cells, although it can also be expressed in hepatocytes under stress conditions [3, 6]. Bile ducts are well-known targets during both HCV recurrence and acute rejection. In the same way as the changes in K18 levels have been previously related to posttransplant infections and perfusions disorders [52], the typical pattern of time-course changes in K19 levels (a steady decrease from pretransplant values) may make it easier to identify abnormal variations that could indicate posttransplant complications.

The study has limitations that should be acknowledged. It was powered to define the standard pattern of time-course changes in serum keratins. The patients were strictly followed at regular intervals, showing that time-course changes are consistent after transplantation. The study design did not allow us to detect the changes that might have occurred between the scheduled sampling intervals, particularly during the first days after transplantation when the variation was greatest. The sample size was obviously small to evaluate

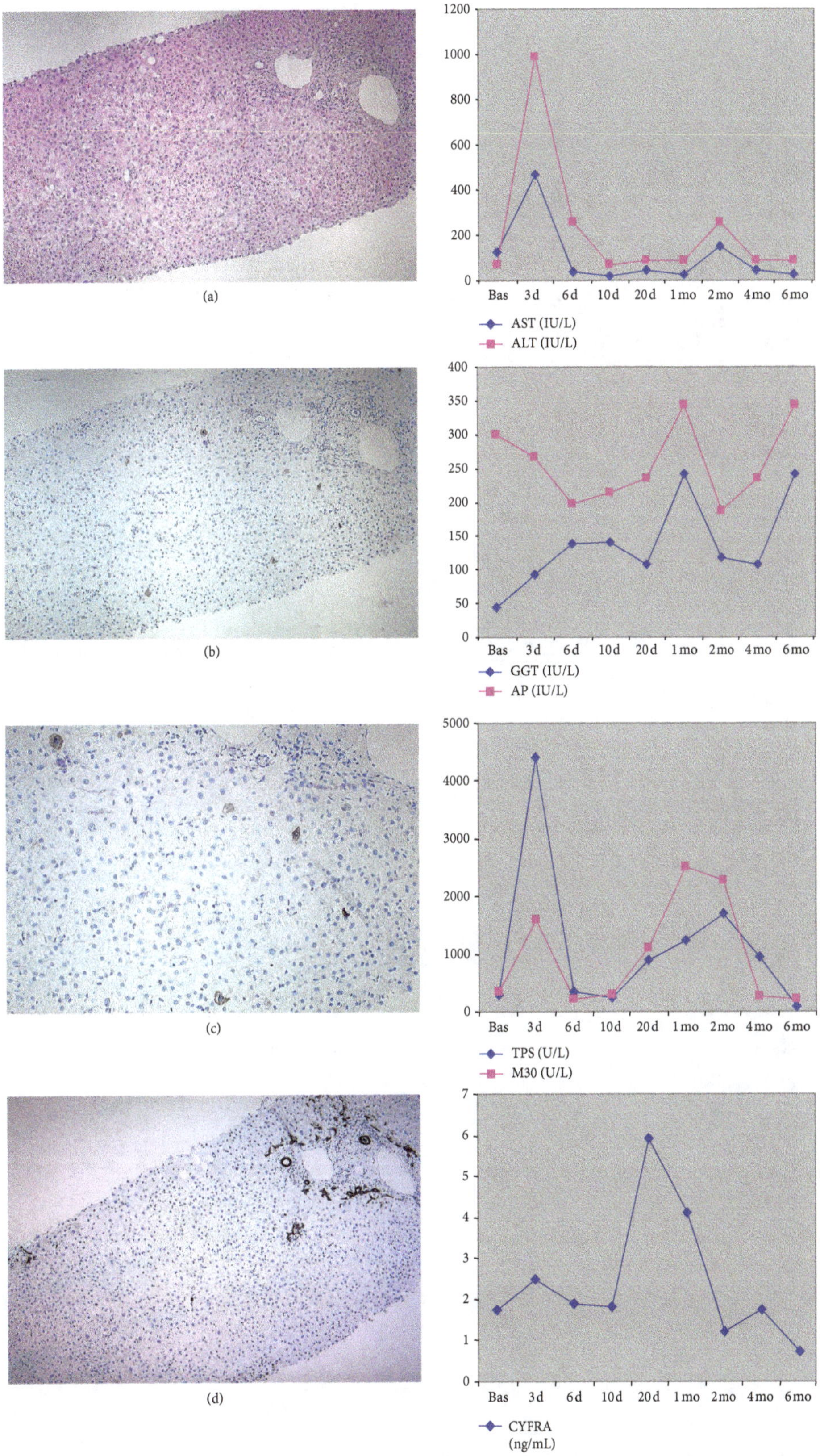

FIGURE 4: Individual data from Patient 10, who had HCV recurrence after liver transplantation. Liver biopsy (left panels) was performed 3 months after transplantation. (a) Hematoxylin-eosin staining revealed typical signs of HCV recurrence. (b and detail in c) Immunostaining for the M30 neoepitope revealed positivity in apoptotic hepatocytes throughout the liver lobule. (d) Immunostaining for K19 revealed only the normal positivity in bile ducts. Time-course changes in standard biochemical markers (AST, ALT, GGT, and alkaline phosphatase (AP)) and serum keratins (TPS, M30, and CYFRA 21-1) are presented in the right panels. d, day; mo, month.

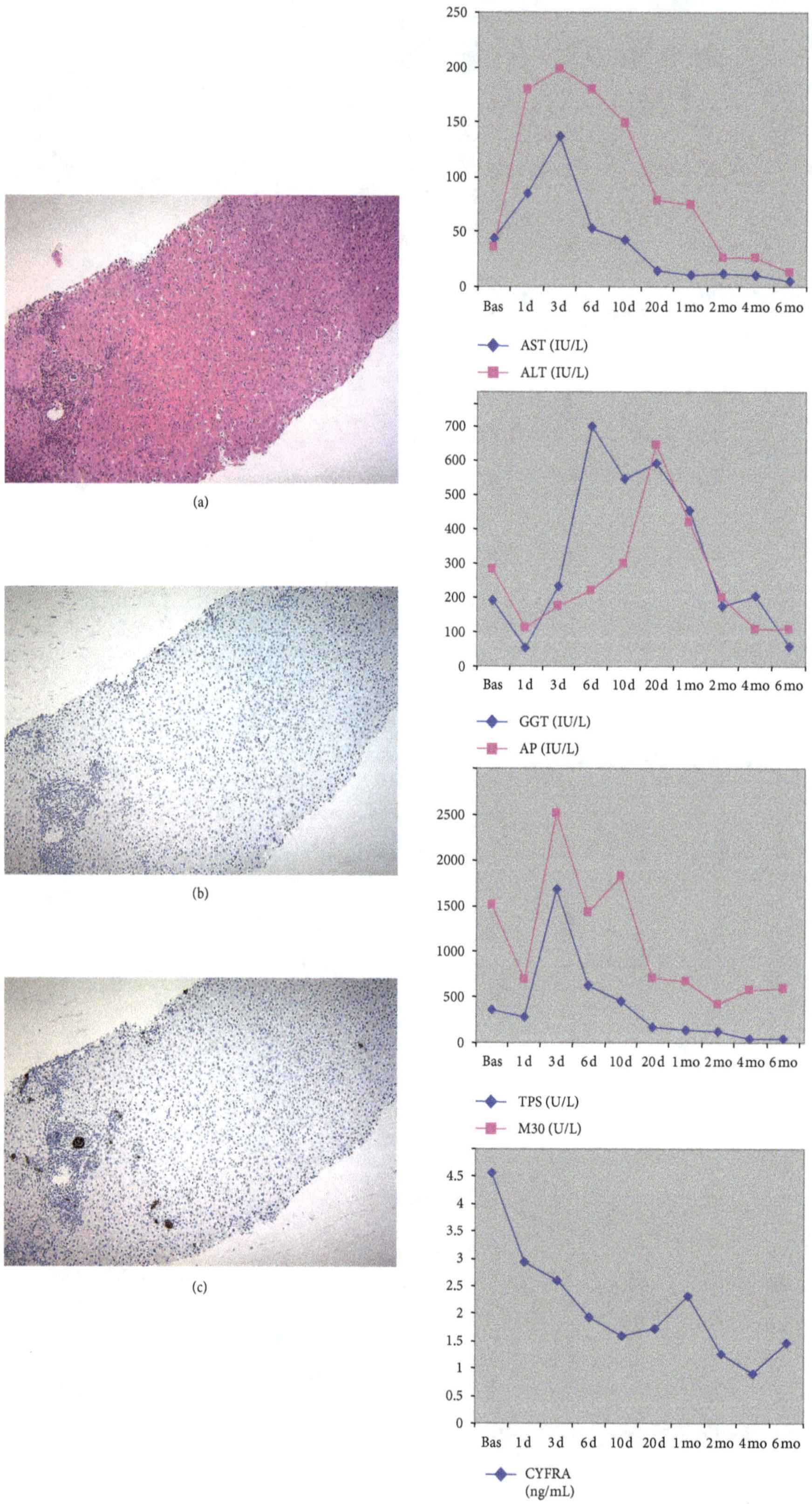

FIGURE 5: Individual data from Patient 4, who had acute cellular rejection after liver transplantation. Liver biopsy (left panels) was performed on day 33 after transplantation. (a) Hematoxylin-eosin stain revealed typical signs of rejection. (b) Immunostaining for the M30 neoepitope was negative. (c) Immunostaining for K19 revealed the normal positivity in the bile ducts and in a few scattered hepatocytes. Time-course changes in standard biochemical markers (AST, ALT, GGT, and alkaline phosphatase (AP)) and serum keratins (TPS, M30, and CYFRA 21-1) are presented in the right panels. d, day; mo, month.

the diagnostic value of serum keratins in this particular setting. Although data from individual case observations should be interpreted with caution, our preliminary results may serve as a basis for further studies of the diagnostic utility of serum keratins for the detection and diagnosis of complications after liver transplantation. It should be noted that keratins are expressed in most simple epithelial cells and are, therefore, not liver-specific [3, 6]. However, the high concentration of keratins in hepatocytes and the time-course changes in their serum concentrations relative to specific events after transplantation strongly indicate that serum keratins measured in our patients originated primarily in the liver.

Measuring the serum levels of keratin fragments may improve our understanding of liver diseases [3, 6]. From a mechanistic standpoint, serum keratins offer a means of measuring necrosis and apoptosis, both of which are important features of liver disease. In this regard, the development of antiapoptotic drugs to prevent early liver transplant-associated liver injury will be of great interest. From a diagnostic standpoint, serum keratin fragments are promising markers of liver disease. For this purpose, key hepatocyte proteins such as keratins may be more robust indicators than standard markers such as enzyme activity, which can be influenced by factors such as drugs in the absence of true liver damage [54]. Assays to determine the concentration of keratin fragments are commercially available, and concentrations may be easily determined with clinically used standard platforms [25]. Here, we have delineated the normal evolution of K18 and K19 fragments after liver transplantation. No conclusions can be drawn from single case reports but may generate discussion to evaluate this biomarker in cases of liver injury, specifically posttransplant complications including rejection. Further studies are warranted to evaluate the utility of keratin fragments as markers of disease in liver transplant patients.

Acknowledgments

This study was supported by funds (PS 08/69) from the Consellería de Sanidade (Xunta de Galicia, Spain).

References

[1] P. Van Eyken and V. J. Desmet, "Cytokeratins and the liver," *Liver*, vol. 13, pp. 113–122, 1993.

[2] M. B. Omary, N.-O. Ku, and D. M. Toivola, "Keratins: guardians of the liver," *Hepatology*, vol. 35, no. 2, pp. 251–257, 2002.

[3] M. B. Omary, N.-O. Ku, P. Strnad, and S. Hanada, "Toward unraveling the complexity of simple epithelial keratins in human disease," *Journal of Clinical Investigation*, vol. 119, no. 7, pp. 1794–1805, 2009.

[4] K. Zatloukal, C. Stumptner, A. Fuchsbichler et al., "The keratin cytoskeleton in liver diseases," *The Journal of Pathology*, vol. 204, no. 4, pp. 367–376, 2004.

[5] N.-O. Ku, P. Strnad, B.-H. Zhong, G.-Z. Tao, and M. B. Omary, "Keratins let liver live: mutations predispose to liver disease and crosslinking generates mallory-denk bodies," *Hepatology*, vol. 46, no. 5, pp. 1639–1649, 2007.

[6] P. Strnad, C. Stumptner, K. Zatloukal, and H. Denk, "Intermediate filament cytoskeleton of the liver in health and disease," *Histochemistry and Cell Biology*, vol. 129, no. 6, pp. 735–749, 2008.

[7] V. Barak, H. Goike, K. W. Panaretakis, and R. Einarsson, "Clinical utility of cytokeratins as tumor markers," *Clinical Biochemistry*, vol. 37, no. 7, pp. 529–540, 2004.

[8] J. M. G. Bonfrer, E. M. Groeneveld, C. M. Korse, A. van Dalen, L. C. J. M. Oomen, and D. Ivanyi, "Monoclonal antibody M3 used in tissue polypeptide– specific antigen assay for the quantification of tissue polypeptide antigen recognizes keratin 18," *Tumor Biology*, vol. 15, no. 4, pp. 210–222, 1994.

[9] S. Linder, "Cytokeratin markers come of age," *Tumor Biology*, vol. 28, no. 4, pp. 189–195, 2007.

[10] H. Bodenmüller, B. Ofenloch-Hähnle, E. B. Lane, A. Dessauer, V. Böttger, and F. Donié, "Lung cancer-associated keratin 19 fragments: development and biochemical characterisation of the new serum assay enzymun-test CYFRA 21-1," *The International Journal of Biological Markers*, vol. 9, no. 2, pp. 75–81, 1994.

[11] R. Einarsson and L. Rydlander, "Tissue polypeptide specific antigen (TPS) detects a specific epitope structure on human cytokeratin," *Anticancer Res*, vol. 17, pp. 3121–3124, 1997.

[12] M. A. Sheard, B. Vojtesek, M. Simickova, and D. Valik, "Release of cytokeratin-18 and -19 fragments (TPS and CYFRA 21-1) into the extracellular space during apoptosis," *Journal of Cellular Biochemistry*, vol. 85, no. 4, pp. 670–677, 2002.

[13] M. P. G. Leers, W. Klgen, V. Bjrklund et al., "Immunocytochemical detection and mapping of a cytokeratin 18 neo-epitope exposed during early apoptosis," *The Journal of Pathology*, vol. 187, no. 5, pp. 567–572, 1999.

[14] B. Schutte, M. Henfling, W. Kölgen et al., "Keratin 8/18 breakdown and reorganization during apoptosis," *Experimental Cell Research*, vol. 297, no. 1, pp. 11–26, 2004.

[15] T. Ueno, M. Toi, and S. Linder, "Detection of epithelial cell death in the body by cytokeratin 18 measurement," *Biomedicine & Pharmacotherapy*, vol. 59, pp. S359–S362, 2005.

[16] G. Kramer, H. Erdal, H. J. M. M. Mertens et al., "Differentiation between cell death modes using measurements of different soluble forms of extracellular cytokeratin 18," *Cancer Research*, vol. 64, no. 5, pp. 1751–1756, 2004.

[17] D. G. Tiniakos and G. V. Papatheodoridis, "Serum markers of hepatocyte apoptosis: current terminology and predictability in clinical practice," *Hepatology*, vol. 51, no. 2, pp. 717-718, 2010.

[18] D. Moraglio, M. Pagano, D. Galeazzi, A. Arnelli, and L. Bertero, "Tissue polypeptide specific antigen (TPS) in liver disease," *Clinica Chimica Acta*, vol. 224, no. 2, pp. 209–214, 1994.

[19] A. Gonzalez-Quintela, N. Mallo, C. Mella et al., "Serum levels of cytokeratin-18 (tissue polypeptide-specific antigen) in liver diseases," *Liver International*, vol. 26, no. 10, pp. 1217–1224, 2006.

[20] A. Gonzalez-Quintela, C. Mella, L. F. Perez, I. Abdulkader, A. M. Caparrini, and S. Lojo, "Increased serum tissue polypeptide specific antigen (TPS) in alcoholics: a possible marker

of alcoholic hepatitis," *Alcoholism: Clinical and Experimental Research*, vol. 24, no. 8, pp. 1222–1226, 2000.

[21] A. Gonzalez-Quintela, C. Mella, I. Abdulkader et al., "Serum levels of tissue polypeptide specific antigen are correlated with hepatocyte cytokeratin expression in alcoholic liver disease," *Alcoholism: Clinical & Experimental Research*, vol. 28, no. 9, pp. 1413–1418, 2004.

[22] A. Gonzalez-Quintela, J. García, J. Campos et al., "Serum cytokeratins in alcoholic liver disease: contrasting levels of cytokeratin-18 and cytokeratin-19," *Alcohol*, vol. 38, no. 1, pp. 45–49, 2006.

[23] G. Tarantino, C. Mazzarella, M. Tarantino, M. N. D. Di Minno, and P. Conca, "Could high levels of tissue polypeptide specific antigen, a marker of apoptosis detected in nonalcoholic steatohepatitis, improve after weight loss?" *Disease Markers*, vol. 26, no. 2, pp. 55–63, 2009.

[24] G. Tarantino, P. Conca, A. Coppola, R. Vecchione, and G. Di Minno, "Serum concentrations of the tissue polypeptide specific antigen in patients suffering from non-alcoholic steatohepatitis," *European Journal of Clinical Investigation*, vol. 37, no. 1, pp. 48–53, 2007.

[25] A. Gonzalez-Quintela, S. Lojo, E. Otero, and L. F. Perez, "Keratin-18 as a marker of steatohepatitis," *Hepatology*, vol. 45, no. 2, p. 545, 2007.

[26] L. P. Bechmann, C. Jochum, P. Kocabayoglu et al., "Cytokeratin 18-based modification of the MELD score improves prediction of spontaneous survival after acute liver injury," *Journal of Hepatology*, vol. 53, no. 4, pp. 639–647, 2010.

[27] E. Yagmur, C. Trautwein, M. P. G. Leers, A. M. Gressner, and F. Tacke, "Elevated apoptosis-associated cytokeratin 18 fragments (CK18Asp386) in serum of patients with chronic liver diseases indicate hepatic and biliary inflammation," *Clinical Biochemistry*, vol. 40, no. 9-10, pp. 651–655, 2007.

[28] Y. Yilmaz, E. Dolar, E. Ulukaya et al., "Soluble forms of extracellular cytokeratin 18 may differentiate simple steatosis from nonalcoholic steatohepatitis," *World Journal of Gastroenterology*, vol. 13, no. 6, pp. 837–844, 2007.

[29] A. Wieckowska, N. N. Zein, L. M. Yerian, A. R. Lopez, A. J. McCullough, and A. E. Feldstein, "In vivo assessment of liver cell apoptosis as a novel biomarker of disease severity in nonalcoholic fatty liver disease," *Hepatology*, vol. 44, no. 1, pp. 27–33, 2006.

[30] C. Wei, Z. Caiyan, S. Chuan, and W. Yadong, "Cytokeratin 18, alanine aminotransferase, platelets and triglycerides predict the presence of nonalcoholic steatoheatitis," *PLoS One*, vol. 8, Article ID e82092, 2013.

[31] J. Bissonnette, J. Altamirano, C. Devue et al., "A prospective study of the utility of plasma biomarkers to diagnose alcoholic hepatitis," *Hepatology*, vol. 66, no. 2, pp. 555–563, 2017.

[32] B. L. Woolbright, B. W. Bridges, W. Dunn, J. C. Olson, S. A. Weinman, and H. Jaeschke, "Cell death and prognosis of mortality in alcoholic hepatitis patients using plasma keratin-18," *Gene Expression*, vol. 17, no. 4, pp. 301–312, 2017.

[33] H. Bantel, A. Lügering, J. Heidemann et al., "Detection of apoptotic caspase activation in sera from patients with chronic HCV infection is associated with fibrotic liver injury," *Hepatology*, vol. 40, no. 5, pp. 1078–1087, 2004.

[34] A. Gonzalez-Quintela, I. Abdulkader, E. Otero, M. A. Freire, and S. Tomé, "Relationship between serum concentrations of keratin-18 and apoptosis in chronic hepatitis C," *Clin Chem Lab Med*, vol. 48, pp. 897–899, 2010.

[35] A. Parfieniuk-Kowerda, T. W. Lapinski, M. Rogalska-Plonska et al., "Serum cytochrome c and m30-neoepitope of cytokeratin-18 in chronic hepatitis C," *Liver International*, vol. 34, no. 4, pp. 544–550, 2014.

[36] G. V. Papatheodoridis, E. Hadziyannis, E. Tsochatzis et al., "Serum apoptotic caspase activity as a marker of severity in HBeAg-negative chronic hepatitis B virus infection," *Gut*, vol. 57, no. 4, pp. 500–506, 2008.

[37] C. B. Bae, S. S. Kim, S. J. Ahn et al., "Caspase-cleaved fragments of cytokeratin-18 as a marker of inflammatory activity in chronic hepatitis B virus infection," *Journal of Clinical Virology*, vol. 58, no. 4, pp. 641–646, 2013.

[38] F. Eren, Y. Yilmaz, S. Kose et al., "Caspase-cleaved fragments of cytokeratin 18 in patients with chronic hepatitis B," *Clinica Chimica Acta*, vol. 411, no. 23-24, pp. 2029–2032, 2010.

[39] T. Luft, M. Conzelmann, A. Benner et al., "Serum cytokeratin-18 fragments as quantitative markers of epithelial apoptosis in liver and intestinal graft-versus-host disease," *Blood*, vol. 110, no. 13, pp. 4535–4542, 2007.

[40] S. Kanzler and P. R. Galle, "Apoptosis and the liver," *Seminars in Cancer Biology*, vol. 10, no. 3, pp. 173–184, 2000.

[41] H. Malhi, G. J. Gores, and J. J. Lemasters, "Apoptosis and necrosis in the liver: a tale of two deaths?" *Hepatology*, vol. 43, no. S1, pp. S31–S44, 2006.

[42] M. G. Neuman, "Apoptosis in diseases of the liver," *Critical Reviews in Clinical Laboratory Sciences*, vol. 38, no. 2, pp. 109–166, 2001.

[43] J. M. Schattenberg, P. R. Galle, and M. Schuchmann, "Apoptosis in liver disease," *Liver International*, vol. 26, no. 8, pp. 904–911, 2006.

[44] B. Li, B. Chen, G. Zhang, K. Wang, L. Zhou, and S. Hu, "Cell apoptosis and fas gene expression in liver and renal tissues after ischemia-reperfusion injury in liver transplantation," *Transplantation Proceedings*, vol. 42, no. 5, pp. 1550–1556, 2010.

[45] E. E. Montalvo-Jave, T. Escalante-Tattersfield, J. A. Ortega-Salgado, E. Piña, and D. A. Geller, "Factors in the pathophysiology of the liver ischemia-reperfusion injury," *Journal of Surgical Research*, vol. 147, no. 1, pp. 153–159, 2008.

[46] W. H. Xu, Q. F. Ye, and S. S. Xia, "Apoptosis and proliferation of intrahepatic bile duct after ischemia-reperfusion injury," *Hepatobiliary & Pancreatic Diseases International: HBPD INT*, vol. 3, no. 3, pp. 428–432, 2004.

[47] B. Eksteen and J. M. Neuberger, "Mechanisms of disease: the evolving understanding of liver allograft rejection," *Nature Clinical Practice Gastroenterology & Hepatology*, vol. 5, no. 4, pp. 209–219, 2008.

[48] S. Faubel and C. L. Edelstein, "Caspases as drug targets in ischemic organ injury," *Current Drug Targets - Immune, Endocrine & Metabolic Disorders*, vol. 5, no. 3, pp. 269–287, 2005.

[49] H. Farnik, C. M. Lange, W. P. Hofmann et al., "Nucleos(t)ide analogue treatment reduces apoptotic activity in patients with chronic hepatitis B," *Journal of Clinical Virology*, vol. 52, no. 3, pp. 204–209, 2011.

[50] P. Georgiev, F. Dahm, R. Graf, and P. Clavien, "Blocking the path to death: anti-apoptotic molecules in ischemia/reperfusion injury of the liver," *Current Pharmaceutical Design*, vol. 12, no. 23, pp. 2911–2921, 2006.

[51] S. Ulukaya, E. Ulukaya, I. Alper, A. Yilmaztepe-Oral, and M. Kilic, "Soluble cytokeratin 18 biomarkers may provide information on the type of cell death during early ischemia and reperfusion periods of liver transplantation," *Clinical Transplantation*, vol. 24, no. 6, pp. 848–854, 2010.

[52] T. Brenner, C. Rosenhagen, H. Brandt et al., "Cell death biomarkers as early predictors for hepatic dysfunction in patients after orthotopic liver transplantation," *Transplantation Journal*, vol. 94, no. 2, pp. 185–191, 2012.

[53] A. Gonzalez-Quintela, I. Abdulkader, J. Campos, L. Fernandez-Hernandez, and S. Lojo, "Serum levels of keratin-18 fragments [tissue polypeptide-specific antigen (TPS)] are correlated with hepatocyte apoptosis in alcoholic hepatitis," *Digestive Diseases and Sciences*, vol. 54, no. 3, pp. 648–653, 2009.

[54] A. Gonzalez-Quintela, S. Tomé, C. Fernandez-Merino, J. Rey, L. Meijide, and F. Gude, "Synergistic effect of alcohol consumption and body mass on serum concentrations of cytokeratin-18," *Alcoholism: Clinical and Experimental Research*, vol. 35, no. 12, pp. 2202–2208, 2011.

43

Chronic Hepatitis C with Cyanosis

Mahmood Alawainati,[1] Jawad Khamis,[2] Muneer Abdulla,[2] and Saeed Alsaeed[2]

[1]*Department of Family Medicine, Ministry of Health, Manama, Bahrain*
[2]*Department of Medicine, Salmaniya Medical Complex, Manama, Bahrain*

Correspondence should be addressed to Mahmood Alawainati; mja91@live.com

Academic Editor: Manuela Merli

Background. There are multiple aetiologies for dyspnea in patients with liver disease, including pneumonia, pulmonary embolism, hepatic hydrothorax, portopulmonary syndrome, and hepatopulmonary syndrome. The aim of this paper is to emphasize the importance of early diagnosis and management of hepatopulmonary syndrome. *Case Presentation.* We report a case of a 65-year-old male who was known to have chronic hepatitis C presented with one-year history of shortness of breath and cyanosis. The initial impression of pulmonary embolism was excluded by comprehensive diagnostic investigations. The correlation between the clinical picture and investigations raised the possibility of hepatopulmonary syndrome which was confirmed by contrast-enhanced transthoracic echocardiography. *Conclusions.* High suspicion is required to diagnose hepatopulmonary syndrome in patients with liver disease and hypoxemia. Screening for this complication is appropriate in liver transplant candidates, and diagnosed patients should be evaluated extensively for liver transplant.

1. Background

Shortness of breath is commonly encountered in patients with liver diseases [1]. Some studies showed that more than 50% of patients with hepatic diseases reported respiratory symptoms but only 30% of these patients present pulmonary diseases as the underlying cause of their symptoms [2, 3]. Of note, some diagnostic entities should be screened for and considered in any patient with liver disease presenting with shortness of breath. Hepatopulmonary syndrome (HPS) is a rare but devastating manifestation of acute or chronic liver disease with unspecific clinical manifestations. To date, the pathogenetic processes of this syndrome are still not fully clear but are thought to induce a formation of intrapulmonary vascular dilatation, and, less commonly, direct arteriovenous connections [4]. In this case report, we are presenting a case of a man with chronic hepatitis C who was diagnosed with HPS after correlating the clinical and radiological features. Multidisciplinary approach is the best methodology to detect, treat, and follow up patients with this complication.

2. Case Presentation

A 65-year-old male known to have chronic viral hepatitis C presented to accident and emergency department with 1-year history of shortness of breath and blue discoloration of his fingers.

His shortness of breath worsened with the time; it was exertional initially, but recently it was noticed even at rest. It was aggravated by walking and setting, but relieved by lying flat and oxygen therapy. It limited his activities of daily living, sexual intercourse, and self-care (modified medical research council MMRC grade = 4). In addition, he reported that his shortness of breath was associated with generalized fatigue, blue discoloration of his hands, feet, mouth, and nose, and bilateral hand tremor that occurred mainly during exercises. He also had intermittent generalized nonradiating, moderately severe pressure like headache but no sensory or motor symptoms were noticed. Furthermore, this shortness of breath was not associated with chest pain, cough, sputum production, palpitation, or loss of consciousness. There was no leg swelling, abdominal distension, abdominal

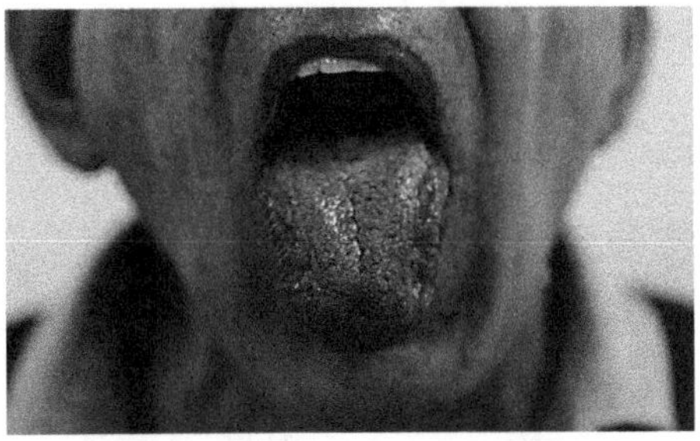

FIGURE 1: Central and peripheral cyanosis.

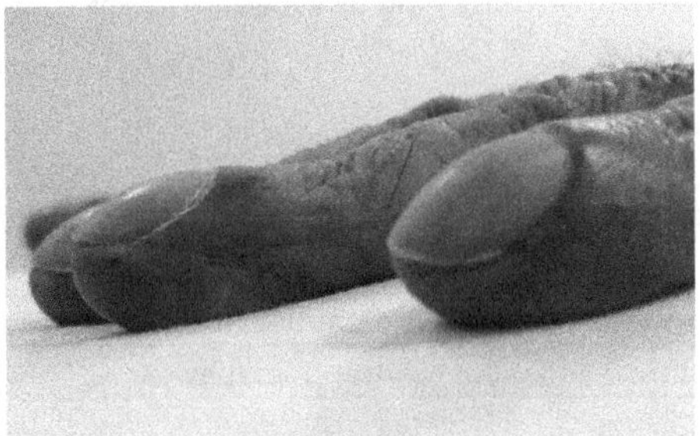

FIGURE 2: Digital clubbing.

pain, vomiting, jaundice, or change in bowel or urine habits.

Our patient was known to have chronic hepatitis C infection, which was not treated because of nonadherence issues. His social history revealed that he smoked cigarettes and consumed alcohol for more than forty years but quitted one year back. He also stopped using illicit drugs and shared needles after more than thirty years of consumption.

On physical examination he had peripheral and central cyanosis (Figure 1), grade 4 clubbing (Figure 2), muscle wasting, needle marks, palmar erythema, and bilateral resting tremor but no asterixis. The patient had scattered telangiectasia over his body. The abdominal, cardiovascular, respiratory, and neurological examinations were normal.

Initial laboratory investigations demonstrated a low platelet count 104×10^9 per L (reference range (RR) 150 -400×10^9/L), normal white and red cell counts, and normal haemoglobin level. In addition, his coagulation profile, renal function, and electrolytes were almost within normal limits. Liver function test revealed elevated total bilirubin 34 μmol/L (RR 5-21 μmol/L) and direct bilirubin 17 μmol/L (RR 0-5 μmol/L). Total protein 82 g/L including albumin (39 g/L), globulin 39 g/L (RR 15-30 g/L), G-Glutamyl transferase, and alkaline phosphatase was within normal ranges. Alanine transaminase level was 108 U/L (RR < 41 U/L) and his alpha fetoprotein was 13.3 μg/L (RR < 9 μg /L). Electrocardiogram was normal, but chest X-ray showed bibasal nodular opacities. Hepatitis profile revealed a positive anti-HCV Antibodies, HCV genotype 3, and HCV viral load of 251188.640 IU/mL.

At this point, pneumonia and hepatic hydrothorax were extremely less likely based on the mentioned clinical and basic laboratory investigations.

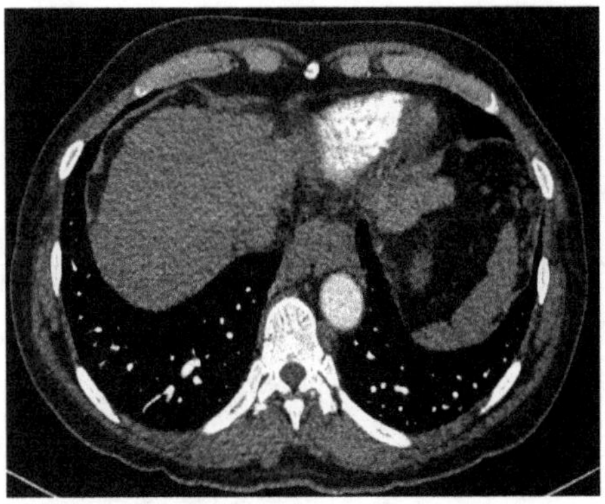

FIGURE 3: Chest CT scan showing the prominent pulmonary vasculatures and irregular borders of the liver.

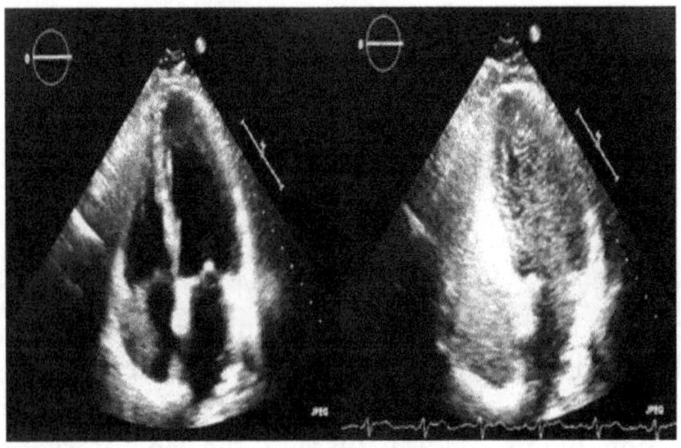

FIGURE 4: Contrast-enhanced transthoracic echocardiography showing contrasts' microbubbles in the left side of the heart.

Arterial blood gases (ABG) showed severe hypoxemia with improvement on lying down as follows: While setting, ABG readings were PH= 7.43, SO2= 57%, PO2=33.5 mmHg, PCO2= 31.9 mmHg, and HCO3=21 mmol/L. However, while lying down, his ABG results were PH= 7.438, SO2= 71.6%, PO2= 37.6 mmHg, PCO2= 29.3 mmHg, and HCO3= 21 mmol/L). A-a gradient increased in supine position from 76 mmHg to 78 mmHg. Abdominal Ultrasound showed liver surface nodularity and an incidental renal cyst. Gastroscopy confirmed the prescience of oesophageal varices hepatic gastropathy. As a result, his Child-Pugh score was 5 points (Class A) and MELD score (9 points)

His pulmonary function test showed normal forced expiratory volume to forced vital capacity ratio (FEV1/FVC) but reduced FEV1 and FVC. Chest computed tomography scan showed bibasal prominent pulmonary arterial dilatation and irregular borders of the liver, but no emphysematous or fibrotic changes. Contrast-enhanced transthoracic echocardiography was performed. Within 5 heart cycles from appearing in the right atrium, contrasts' microbubbles appeared in the left atrium and left ventricle (Figures 3 and 4).

Based on the history, physical examination, and laboratory investigations, our patient was diagnosed with hepatopulmonary syndrome (Table 1)

We treated him for his underling liver disease with Sofosbuvir and Daclatasvir, and for HPS he was managed symptomatically with long term oxygen therapy (LTOT).

TABLE 1: Differential diagnosis of hepatopulmonary syndrome.

	Parameter	HPS	PPH	HHTS	HH	Pneumonia
History	Liver disease	+	+	+/-	+	+/-
	Epistaxis	+/-	+/-	+	+/-	-
	Genetic predisposition	+/-	+/-	+ (AD)	-	-
Physical examination	Cyanosis	+	-	-	-	Usually -
	Telangiectasia	+/-	+/-	+	+/-	-
	Hypoxemia	Severe	Mild	+/-	Mild	+/-
	Other findings	Platypnea	Loud P2 ↑ JVD		Unilateral ↓ air entry	Dullness

HPS: hepatopulmonary syndrome, PPH: portopulmonary hypertension, HHS: hereditary Hemorrhagic Telangiectasia Syndrome, HH: Hepatic Hydrothorax, AD: autosomal dominant, JVD: jugular venous distension.

TABLE 2: Diagnostic criteria for HPS.

Liver disease	Acute or chronic, with or without portal hypertension
Impaired oxygenation	A-a oxygen gradient ≥15 mmHg or A-a oxygen gradient ≥ 20 mmHg in patients > 64 years old
Intrapulmonary vascular dilatation	Contrast-enhanced echocardiography

Subsequently, he was closely followed up in the outpatient department by hepatologists and pulmonologists every 3 months, advised to receive vaccination for hepatitis A and hepatitis B, and assessed for liver transplant. After the completion of his medical therapy, the laboratory results confirmed the resolution of hepatitis C infection.

3. Discussion

The prevalence of hepatopulmonary syndrome varies among the studies because it depends on the diagnostic criteria used (AaPO2 and PaO2 cut-offs), the population selected (cirrhotic vs noncirrhotic patients, acute vs chronic liver disease), and the confirmatory test selected. Most studies indicate that the prevalence lies between 10 and 25% in patients with chronic liver disease. However, this syndrome may be of a higher prevalence due to undiagnosed cases [4, 5].

The exact pathogenesis of HPS is not fully understood, but there are multiple proposed mechanisms, including translocation of bacteria from the gastrointestinal tract that leads to secretion of cytokines especially Tumour Necrosis Factor-a (TNF-a) from the accumulated macrophages in the lungs. Consequently, TNF-a induces Nitric Oxide synthase (NOS) to produce Nitric Oxide (NO) which is a known vasodilator of pulmonary capillaries. The other mechanism proposes that the damaged hepatocytes fail to clear vasodilators which leads to formation of new vessels. Additionally, inhibition of vasoconstrictors and release of vasodilators by the damaged hepatocytes may enhance this process [6].

In HPS, progressive vasodilatation of the capillaries occurs predominantly in the lung bases and results in more blood supply to these alveoli that have a normal ventilation. Thus, the partial pressure of oxygen in the alveoli is insufficient to achieve equilibration with blood moving near the centre of the affected capillaries causing a decrease in blood oxygenation. As a result, ventilation perfusion quotient (V/Q) will decrease and the end outcome will be the arterial hypoxemia.

Generally, the clinical manifestations of HPS are nonspecific and variable [7]. For example, shortness of breath, cyanosis, spider angioma, and palmar erythema can be caused by different respiratory, cardiac, or hepatic pathologies, possibly reflecting the difficulties in the diagnostic process. Therefore, screening for HPS is recommended in all hepatic transplant candidates [8].

To diagnose HPS, the triad of liver disease, impaired oxygenation, and the presence of intrapulmonary vascular dilatation must present (Table 2).

However, some studies showed that PaO2 value of <65 mm Hg in cirrhotic patients presenting with idiopathic cause of dyspnea will predict all patients with underlying HPS (PPV= 100%) [9]. Furthermore, HPS is classified based on PaO2 level into four categories as shown in Table 3.

The relationship between HPS and severity of hepatic dysfunction or portal hypertension is not yet clear. Conflicting conclusions exist in the studies regarding the correlation between HPS and the severity of liver disease. On the one hand, some studies reported that HPS is clearly correlated with the degree of liver disease, but on the other hand, some studies reported no correlation.

Laboratory investigations including full blood count, liver function test, renal function, and coagulation profile are essential for prioritizing the list of differential diagnoses. Though the X-ray of patients with HPS is typically normal, it is an extremely essential tool to determine the likelihood of pneumonia, hepatic hydrothorax, and pulmonary edema. In addition, ABG test is required to assess the level of oxygenation and to fulfill the diagnostic criteria of HPS; pulse oximeter is a rapid, almost always accessible and reasonable screening tool to detect hypoxemia in asymptomatic adults who are candidates for liver transplant. Chest CT scan may show suggestive findings of HPS such as prominent

Table 3: Severity of HPS.

Severity of HPS based on PaO2			
Mild	Moderate	Severe	Very severe
≥80 mmHg	≥60 mmHg and <80 mmHg	≥50 mmHg and <60 mmHg	<50 mmHg

pulmonary vasculatures, but it is also important to rule out other possible aetiologies such as pulmonary embolism. Overall, contrast (microbubble) echocardiography remains the most useful test to diagnose HPS. Macroaggregated albumin (MAA) is an alternative to contrast (microbubble) echocardiography with a lower sensitivity.

Although there are no established medical therapies for HPS, surprisingly, some publications reported spontaneous resolution of HPS [10]. Inferences of findings between the studies about effective experimental treatments are hindered by the relatively small number of participants and inconsistent results [11, 12]. Thus, in its recent guidelines, the European Association for the Study of the Liver concluded that there are insufficient data to recommend the placement of Transjugular Intrahepatic Portosystemic Shunt (TIPS) or other medical options. Currently, liver transplantation and oxygen therapy remain the only recommended interventions for HPS, but still, the management plan must be individualized.

Recent studies proposed the usage of Sorafenib, a kinase inhibitor indicated, in the treatment of HPS. In animal models, Sorafenib prevents angiogenesis in the lungs and reduces intrapulmonary shunting. However, a recent randomised controlled trial run by university of Pennsylvania which compared Sorafenib and placebo was terminated in phase 2 [13, 14].

The literature provides no consensus regarding the follow-up recommendations, best treatment approach in patients with very severe symptoms, and the therapeutic measures. Thus, future studies should tackle these aspects and identify the exact pathogenetic processes of this syndrome aiming to target the vasodilating and angiogenetic factors by therapeutic agents. It will be interesting to follow up the patient's condition after surgery to establish the influence of the surgery on the future relapses, thus providing more areas of interest for research. Moreover, the potential effect of smoking, alcohol, and illicit drug misuse on the pathogenesis of HPS remains unclear, and well-designed studies are needed to determine this possibility.

4. Conclusion

The lessons we learned from this case study are as follows: Firstly, a high index of suspicion for hepatopulmonary syndrome should be maintained, when evaluating patients with hepatic diseases. This will prevent further over-investigations (Quaternary prevention) and more ineffective treatment and will decrease the morbidity of this syndrome. Secondly, although liver transplant remains the only curative intervention, occasionally, the symptomatic treatment is the best approach especially in critically ill patients. Finally, the effect this syndrome on other organs and systems is still largely unknown, and the pre- and posttransplantation outcomes are yet to be studied.

Authors' Contributions

Mahmood Alawainati wrote the article, reviewed it, did the literature review, and provided the radiological images. Jawad Khamis, Muneer Abdulla, and Saeed Alsaeed reviewed the manuscript. All authors read and approved the final manuscript.

References

[1] S. A. Wahls, "Causes and evaluation of chronic dyspnea," *American Family Physician*, vol. 86, pp. 173–182, 2012.

[2] P. Y. Kwo, "Shortness of Breath in the Patient with Chronic Liver Disease," *Clinics in Liver Disease*, vol. 16, no. 2, pp. 321–329, 2012.

[3] B. Sureka, K. Bansal, Y. Patidar, S. Kumar, and A. Arora, "Thoracic perspective revisited in chronic liver disease," *Gastroenterology Report*, vol. 3, no. 3, pp. 194–200, 2015.

[4] A. E. Mansour, A. A. Elgamal, and M. Zaghlol, "Prevalence and predictors of hepatopulmonary syndrome in liver transplant candidates," *Egyptian Journal of Chest Diseases and Tuberculosis* vol. 63, no. 4, pp. 1071–1075, 2014.

[5] A. Al-Harbi, K. Abdullah, A. Al-Abdulkareem, A. Alghamdi, and H. Al-Jahdali, "Prevalence, severity, and prognostic effect of hepatopulmonary syndrome in liver transplant candidates," *Annals of Transplantation*, vol. 21, pp. 180–184, 2016.

[6] R. Rodríguez-Roisin, M. J. Krowka, P. Hervé, and M. B. Fallon, "ERS Task Force Pulmonary-Hepatic Vascular Disorders (PHD) Scientific Committee Pulmonary-Hepatic vascular Disorders (PHD)," *European Respiratory Journal*, vol. 24, pp. 861–880, 2004.

[7] S. Soulaidopoulos, E. Cholongitas, G. Giannakoulas, M. Vlachou, and I. Goulis, "Review article: Update on current and emergent data on hepatopulmonary syndrome," *World Journal of Gastroenterology*, vol. 24, no. 12, pp. 1285–1298, 2018.

[8] M. J. Krowka, M. B. Fallon, S. M. Kawut et al., "International liver transplant society practice guidelines: Diagnosis and management of hepatopulmonary syndrome and portopulmonary hypertension," *Transplantation*, vol. 100, no. 7, pp. 1440–1452, 2016.

[9] P. Schenk, V. Fuhrmann, C. Madl et al., "Hepatopulmonary syndrome: Prevalence and predictive value of various cut offs for arterial oxygenation and their clinical consequences," *Gut*, vol. 51, no. 6, pp. 853–859, 2002.

[10] S. M. Ghayumi, M. Rohani, S. Hasanzadeh, S. Sadeghi, A. Roozbehi, and S. Jokar, "Epstein-Barr virus hepatitis can cause transient hepatopulmonary syndrome," *Respiratory Medicine Case Reports*, vol. 24, pp. 50-51, 2018.

[11] M. C. Wallace, A. L. James, M. Marshall, and N. Kontorinis, "Resolution of severe hepato-pulmonary syndrome following transjugular portosystemic shunt procedure," *BMJ Case Reports*, 2012.

[12] J. Tsauo, N. Weng, H. Ma, M. Jiang, H. Zhao, and X. Li, "Role of Transjugular Intrahepatic Portosystemic Shunts in the Management of Hepatopulmonary Syndrome: A Systemic Literature Review," *Journal of Vascular and Interventional Radiology*, vol. 26, no. 9, pp. 1266–1271, 2015.

[13] W. Yang, J. Zhang, B. Hu et al., "The role of receptor tyrosine kinase activation in cholangiocytes and pulmonary vascular endothelium in experimental hepatopulmonary syndrome," *American Journal of Physiology-Gastrointestinal and Liver Physiology*, vol. 306, no. 1, pp. G72–G80, 2014.

[14] C.-C. Chang, C.-L. Chuang, F.-Y. Lee et al., "Sorafenib treatment improves hepatopulmonary: Syndrome in rats with biliary cirrhosis," *Clinical Science*, vol. 124, no. 7, pp. 457–466, 2013.

44

Marked Hyperbilirubinemia Associated with Primary Myelofibrosis Responsive to Ruxolitinib

Sunny Sandhu,[1] **Hunza Chaudhry**,[1] **Sharon Zhang**,[2] **and Devang Prajapati**[3]

[1]*Department of Internal Medicine, University of California, San Francisco- Fresno, Fresno, CA, USA*
[2]*Department of Pathology, Community Medical Centers, Fresno, CA, USA*
[3]*Department of Gastroenterology & Hepatology, University of California, San Francisco- Fresno, Fresno, CA, USA*

Correspondence should be addressed to Sunny Sandhu; ssandhu91@gmail.com

Academic Editor: Mauro Vigano

Primary myelofibrosis (PMF) is a chronic myeloproliferative disorder seen in older adults which can present both with hepatosplenomegaly as well as mild nonspecific liver enzyme abnormalities. Mild elevations in bilirubin can occasionally be seen due to both intravascular hemolysis as well as extramedullary hematopoiesis. Marked hyperbilirubinemia as a presenting sign of PMF progression, however, has not been reported. We present the case of a patient with a remote diagnosis of PMF, who presented with marked hyperbilirubinemia with a notable response to ruxolitinib.

1. Introduction

Primary myelofibrosis (PMF) is a chronic myeloproliferative disorder most commonly seen in older adults which can commonly lead to liver and spleen involvement due to extramedullary hematopoiesis (EMH). Mild hyperbilirubinemia can also be seen due to increased red blood cell turnover. We describe an unusual case of cholestatic liver injury with marked hyperbilirubinemia in a patient with a remote diagnosis of PMF, who had a notable response to ruxolitinib. There are no other similar reported cases in the literature to the best of our knowledge.

2. Case Presentation

A 64-year-old male with a 10-year history of asymptomatic JAK-2-positive PMF under observation presented with progressive pruritus and jaundice for 3 days. Labs revealed ALT 49 IU/L, AST 35 IU/L, ALP 378 IU/L, total bilirubin (TB) 17 mg/dL, and direct bilirubin 10 mg/dL. LDH was 173 U/L, and the haptoglobin level was normal. Complete blood count with differential showed WBC 4.4×10^3/uL (85% neutrophils, 8% lymphocytes, and 4% monocytes), hemoglobin 7.4 g/dL, and platelets 103×10^9/L. Lipid panel showed total cholesterol 229 mg/dL, triglyceride 171 mg/dL, HDL 5 mg/dL, and LDL 193 mg/dL. Anti-mitochondrial antibody was negative with titer <1 : 20. Workup for metabolic, viral, autoimmune, alcoholic, and drug-induced liver disease otherwise was unrevealing. The patient denied the use of any drugs, including herbal supplements. CT scan showed hepatomegaly without biliary ductal dilatation, along with marked splenomegaly with a spleen size of 27 cm. MRCP failed to demonstrate findings of an obstructive etiology. Therefore, EUS and ERCP were performed which were also unremarkable. Given worsening hyperbilirubinemia, a liver biopsy was subsequently pursued which was suggestive of a nonspecific cholestatic liver injury (Figures 1–3). TB continued to increase to 25 mg/dL, and a repeat ERCP was performed which was unremarkable. During the ERCP, a sphincterotomy was performed with biliary sweep which was unremarkable with cytology showing benign reactive epithelial cells. Liver biopsy was also repeated which showed similar findings as prior. Throughout his course, the patient also did not have any fevers, right upper quadrant pain, or leukocytosis to suggest underlying infection including acute cholangitis. Bone marrow biopsy performed showed hypercellular (90%)

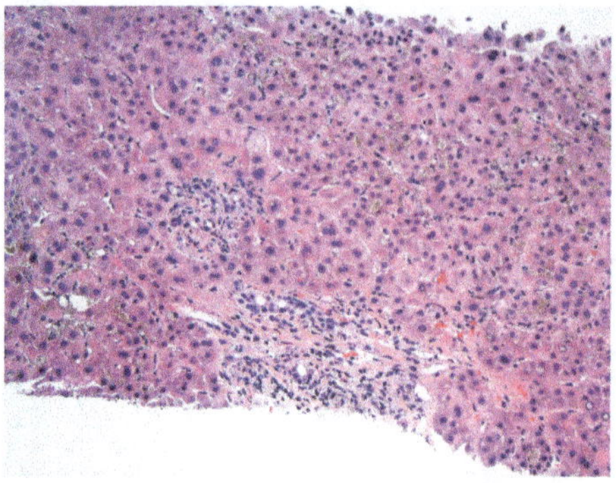

Figure 1: H&E stain (200×) showing marked canalicular cholestasis, portal and periportal fibrosis, bile duct injury, ductular reaction, and portal and lobular neutrophilic infiltrates, most suggestive of biliary obstruction.

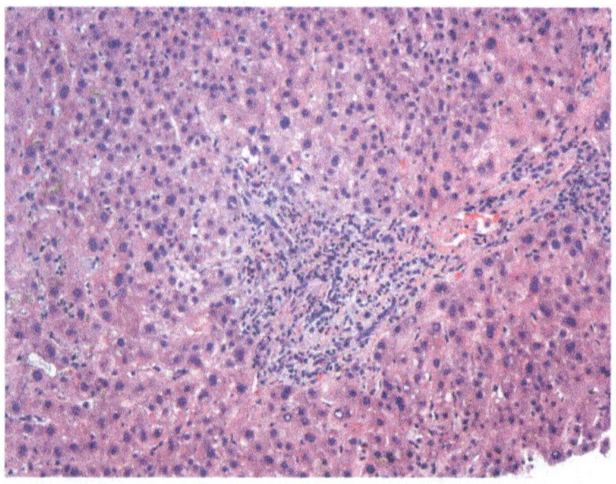

Figure 2: H&E stain (200×) showing marked canalicular cholestasis, portal and periportal fibrosis, bile duct injury, ductular reaction, and portal and lobular neutrophilic infiltrates, most suggestive of biliary obstruction.

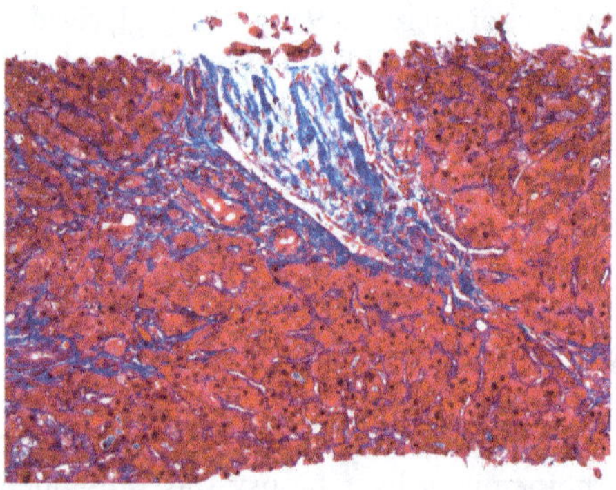

Figure 3: Trichrome stain (40×) showing portal and periportal fibrosis, as well as focal sinusoidal collagen deposition.

with 3+ reticulin fibrosis and no increased blasts, consistent with underlying primary myelofibrosis. TB continued to rise to 29 mg/dL, and given negative extensive workup otherwise, the decision was made to start empiric treatment for possible PMF-related disease. Dynamic International Prognostic Scoring System (DIPSS) score was 2, correlating with intermediate risk. Ruxolitinib was initiated with significant improvement of TB to 18 mg/dL. 3 weeks after initiation, ruxolitinib had to be temporarily held due to adverse effects of bone marrow suppression, and TB subsequently increased to 35 mg/dL over the next 5 weeks. Ruxolitinib was then resumed at a lower dose with improvement again of TB to 17 mg/dL (Figure 4). The patient's course was unfortunately complicated by renal failure secondary to biopsy-confirmed bile-acid nephropathy, ascites, functional decline, and eventually was transitioned to hospice.

3. Discussion

Primary myelofibrosis (PMF) is a chronic myeloproliferative disorder with an incidence of about 1.5 per 100,000 per year, and predominantly occurs in middle-aged and older adults [1]. The pathophysiology of the disease involves the release of growth factors by megakaryocytes, with subsequent fibroblast hyperactivity and bone marrow fibrosis which lead to the characteristic systemic findings [2].

Liver involvement is common in primary myelofibrosis, with hepatomegaly reported in 40%–70% of patients, and nonspecific liver enzyme elevations are also commonly seen [3]. Mild elevations in serum bilirubin can be related to the ineffective erythropoiesis which occurs due to bone marrow fibrosis. This, in turn, can lead to intravascular hemolysis with a resultant mild indirect hyperbilirubinemia, elevated LDH, and low haptoglobin [4]. Our patient, in contrast, had a much more profound direct hyperbilirubinemia in addition to normal LDH and haptoglobin levels, which made an underlying hemolytic process unlikely.

In addition, extramedullary hematopoiesis (EMH) is a well-known phenomenon that occurs in PMF. EMH, a process in which hematopoietic tissue and blood cells develop outside of the blood marrow, develops as a compensatory response to the bone marrow fibrosis seen in PMF, and the liver and spleen are well-known sites of EMH [5]. Given its predilection for liver involvement, EMH has been suggested to be a rare etiology of obstructive jaundice. Progression of liver involvement can also lead to portal hypertension and associated complications such as ascites [6]. Although the ascites were not fully investigated further as the patient was transitioned to hospice care, we suspect that this may have been the etiology. However, when associated with biliary obstruction, EMH has typically been shown to have specific histologic findings on liver biopsy, in which hematopoietic precursors including megakaryocytes are diagnostic for EMH [6, 7]. As mentioned previously, both biopsies in our patient were nonspecific which can potentially indicate an inadequate sensitivity for liver biopsy findings. Given the temporal relationship between myelofibrosis treatment and TB improvement, we speculate EMH was likely the underlying etiology of his cholestatic liver injury.

In regards to lab abnormalities, PMF has also been associated with mild liver enzyme elevations, with ALP elevation being the most common abnormality. In the literature, cases with EMH-related ALP elevation have been associated with worse outcomes. Hyperbilirubinemia, however, is extremely uncommon in PMF, and the majority of patients have normal bilirubin levels [8]. Marked

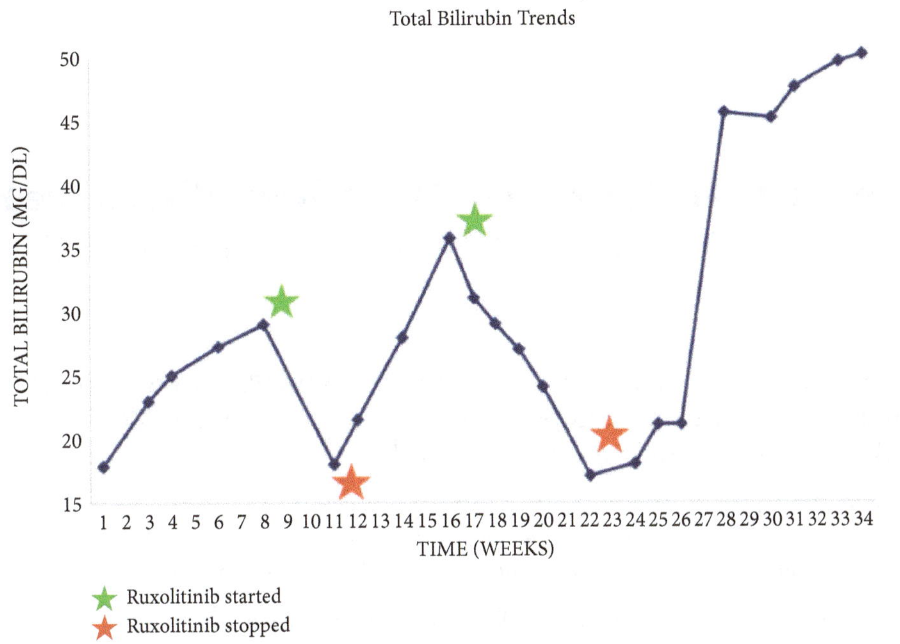

FIGURE 4: Total bilirubin trends with relation to initiation and discontinuation of ruxolitinib.

hyperbilirubinemia as a presenting sign of PMF progression has not been reported to date in the literature. We, therefore, suggest that even in patients with previously known and well-controlled PMF, a progression of disease should remain in the differential in cases of worsening hyperbilirubinemia.

Our case demonstrates that patients with PMF who present with hyperbilirubinemia can undergo extensive invasive workup before a diagnosis is made. Liver biopsy, although reported in the literature to be consistent with extramedullary hematopoiesis in such cases, can occasionally fail to show this as demonstrated in the 2 biopsies performed on our patient. In such cases, nonspecific findings of cholestatic liver injury can be suggestive of PMF-related liver injury. Furthermore, although ALP has been shown to be a prognostic marker, our case demonstrates that marked bilirubin elevations can also be associated with serious morbidity and even lead to complications including bile-acid nephropathy. When caring for patients with PMF that develop hyperbilirubinemia with unremarkable workup otherwise, we suggest a low threshold for empiric treatment of PMF, and as in our case, ruxolitinib can be extremely effective.

Authors' Contributions

S. Sandhu and H. Chaudhry reviewed the literature and drafted the manuscript. S. Zhang provided the pathology images. S. Sandhu, H. Chaudhry, and D. Prajapati revised the article for important intellectual content and were involved in the final approval of the version to be published. S. Sandhu is the article guarantor.

References

[1] R. A. Mesa, M. N. Silverstein, S. J. Jacobsen, P. C. Wollan, and A. Tefferi, "Population-based incidence and survival figures in essential thrombocythemia and agnogenic myeloid metaplasia: an Olmsted County Study, 1976-1995," *American Journal of Hematology*, vol. 61, no. 1, pp. 10–15, 1999.

[2] A. Tefferi, "Primary myelofibrosis: 2021 update on diagnosis, risk-stratification and management," *American Journal of Hematology*, vol. 96, no. 1, pp. 145–162, 2021.

[3] J. Murakami and Y. Shimizu, "Hepatic manifestations in hematological disorders," *International Journal of Hepatology*, vol. 2013, pp. 1–13, 2013.

[4] Z. L. Liu and H. D. Zhang, "Abnormally short erythrocyte LifeSpan in three patients with primary myelofibrosis despite successful control of splenomegaly," *The American Journal of the Medical Sciences*, vol. 361, no. 2, pp. 274–277, 2021.

[5] D. Cenariu, S. Iluta, A. A. Zimta et al., "Extramedullary hematopoiesis of the liver and spleen," *Journal of Clinical Medicine*, vol. 10, no. 24, p. 5831, 2021.

[6] M. S. Sherman, W. R. Samore, and D. S. Pratt, "Myelofibrosis and portal hypertension: the case for primary variceal screening," *ACG Case Reports Journal*, vol. 7, no. 2, Article ID e00333, 2020.

[7] S. Kamran, A. Al-Obaidi, Y. Al-Khazraji, J. Alderson, and P. S. Reddy, "Obstructive jaundice secondary to extramedullary hematopoiesis," *Cureus*, vol. 13, no. 9, Article ID e17927, 2021.

[8] D. Barraco, M. Mudireddy, S. Shah et al., "Liver function test abnormalities and their clinical relevance in primary myelofibrosis," *Blood Cancer Journal*, vol. 7, no. 4, p. e557, 2017.

45

Management of Acute Wilsonian Hepatitis with Severe Hemolysis: A Successful Combination of Chelation and MARS Dialysis

Jeremy Hassoun ,[1] Nathalie Hammer,[2] Giulia Magini ,[1] Belen Ponte ,[2] Marie Ongaro ,[1] Anne-Laure Rougemont ,[3] Nicolas Goossens ,[1] Jean-Louis Frossard ,[1] and Laurent Spahr [1]

[1]*Gastroenterology and Hepatology, University Hospitals of Geneva and Faculty of Medicine, Geneva, Switzerland*
[2]*Nephrology, University Hospitals of Geneva and Faculty of Medicine, Geneva, Switzerland*
[3]*Clinical Pathology, University Hospitals of Geneva and Faculty of Medicine, Geneva, Switzerland*

Correspondence should be addressed to Laurent Spahr; laurent.spahr@hcuge.ch

Academic Editor: Haruki Komatsu

Wilson's disease is a rare hereditary disorder of copper metabolism leading to progressive accumulation of copper in several organs including the brain and the liver. Acute liver failure is a relatively rare hepatic manifestation of WD which may require urgent liver transplantation if medical treatment fails. We report here the case of a young woman who presented with classic acute Wilsonian hepatitis complicated by liver and renal failure and a severe hemolysis related to massive nonceruloplasmin bound copper accumulation requiring repeated blood transfusions. The early initiation of a combined treatment including conventional chelation therapy and repeated MARS dialysis sessions allowed a rapid control of hemolysis, a progressive decrease of free copper overload, and clinical recompensation without liver transplantation.

1. Introduction

Acute liver failure is a rare hepatic manifestation of WD [1], which may require urgent liver transplantation (LT) if medical treatment fails [2]. We report here the case of a young woman presenting with classic acute wilsonian hepatitis (AWH) with liver and renal failure and severe hemolysis related to massive nonceruloplasmin bound copper accumulation requiring repeated blood transfusions. The early initiation of a combined treatment including chelation therapy [3] and repeated MARS dialysis sessions allowed a rapid control of hemolysis, a progressive decrease of free copper overload, and a survival without urgent LT.

2. Case Presentation

A 26-year-old female was admitted to our hospital following a 3-week history of anorexia, fatigue, and dark urines. She denied taking alcohol, recreative drugs, or any medications and had no family history of liver disease. On examination, except for jaundice, the patient had no signs of chronic liver disease, was alert, oriented, and afebrile. Blood pressure was 112/65 mmHg, and pulse rate was 88 beats per minute. At admission, blood tests showed mild AST elevation (3 times the upper limit of normal, ULN), normal ALT, low alkaline phosphatase (43 IU/L [N: >46], high gamma-glutamyl-transferase (GGT) at 190 IU/L [N: <38], and elevated total bilirubin (128 μmol/L [N: <2] with a conjugated form of 52 μumol/L [N: 0.5–9.5]. Albumin level was 26 gr/l [N: 28–35]. Coagulation parameters were altered, with an elevated international normalized ratio (INR) of 2.34 and factor V 44% [N: >70]. Cell blood count demonstrated normal leucocytes and platelets, but low hemoglobin value of 67 gr/l [N: 120–160] with a high reticulocyte count of 293 G/L [N: 20–120)]. In the absence of overt bleeding, anemia was predominantly related to hemolysis with undetectable serum haptoglobin, high lactate dehydrogenase (LDH) [4], and negative Coomb's test. Further testing excluded hepatitis A,

B, C, and E, as well as autoimmune hepatitis, based on normal total IgG level and absence of antismooth muscle antibodies. The ceruloplasmin level was 0.22 gr/l [N: 0.2–0.6]. No biliary tract disease or vascular alterations were detected on abdominal echography. Acute hepatitis due to WD was considered as the most likely diagnosis. Histological features observed at liver biopsy obtained by the transjugular route were consistent with the diagnosis, showing cirrhosis associated with chronic inflammatory changes, mild (10%) macrovesicular steatosis, and few ballooned hepatocytes. Increased hepatocyte copper-associated protein deposition was observed in periportal areas using Victoria blue stain (Figure 1). A quantification of 8071 μg/gr in liver tissue [N: 10–35] was consistent with a massive accumulation of copper [1, 3]. Additional studies included a major increase in serum and urinary copper values of 2205 μg/l [N: 70–175] and 4130 μg/24 h [N: 15–60], respectively. A slit-lamp examination was inconclusive regarding Kayser–Fleischer's ring. Brain magnetic resonance imaging (MRI) was not performed at that time. Thus, according to the Leipzig score [3, 5], a diagnosis of AWH with cirrhosis and liver insufficiency was made, and a combined treatment of oral D-penicillamine (1200 mg/d) and zinc gluconate (90 mg/day) was promptly initiated on day 1 after admission. However, the following days were associated with a rapid clinical deterioration and majoration of hemolytic anemia with low hemoglobin levels in the range of 60 to 70 gr/l, necessitating repeated blood transfusions (Figure 2). At this stage, with a MELD score of 31, the patient did not reach Clichy criteria for urgent LT [6, 7] (no hepatic encephalopathy and a factor V level of 35%). Nevertheless, a WD prognostic index [8] of 11 indicated a poor prognosis with medical treatment alone. Therefore, considering the role of massive copper overload in the severe hemolysis coexistent with acute liver and renal failure (serum creatinine 177 μmol/l [N: 44–80]), we decided to combine conventional chelation therapy with a mechanical method to rapidly remove excess serum copper. In spite of a very limited experience in the literature, a multidisciplinary team including hepatologists, nephrologists, and intensive-care specialists decided to use the Molecular Adsorbent Recirculating System (MARS) (MARS-Flux, Gambro, Lund, Sweden) as an albumin-based dialysis able to remove free exchangeable copper molecules in addition to other albumin-bound toxins associated with liver failure [9]. This technique has been preferred to therapeutic plasma exchange (TPE), reported to bring benefits as a bridge for liver transplantation in anecdotal reports [10, 11], because the use of fresh frozen plasma replacement would have influenced coagulopathy as a criterion to decide urgent listing [7].

MARS is a hemodialysis system coupled to a closed circuit containing an albumin-rich dialysate with a carbon filter and an anion exchanger. The device aims to mimic the liver detoxification mechanisms at the hepatocyte membrane level. The plasma albumin loaded with toxins will, at the level of the MARS filter, transfer the albumin-bound toxins *via* a membrane permeable to toxins but not to proteins (cut-off 30 kDa) [12], therefore minimizing the depletion in hormones, proteins, and platelets. From a technical point of view, MARS therapy is coupled with hemodiafiltration using the MARS Prismaflex system which includes both one filter in contact with blood (MARS-FLUX) and one in contact with albumin. The MARS set also includes one adsorber column filled with carbon charcoal (diaMARS AC250) eliminating nonpolar compounds (i.e., fatty acids) and another column filled with ion-exchanger resin (diaMARS IE250) to eliminate anionic molecules including bilirubin and copper. The MARS system was administered to our patient using a 13F dialysis catheter in the femoral vein according to the manufacturer's recommendations adapted to our institution's guidelines. A total of 9 MARS dialysis sessions (each session lasting 6–8 hours) were administered starting from day 6 to day 17, with an excellent clinical tolerance, no bleeding complications, and only a marginal decrease in platelet count. Figure 3 depicts the MARS device and the dark-brown-colored adsorber cartridge filled with copper. The patient rapidly recovered from hemolysis, as no further blood transfusions were necessary after day 7 (see Figure 2). The evolution of WD prognostic index during the hospitalization is depicted in Figure 4. On day 21, the MELD score was 14, hemoglobin level was 87 gr/l, LDH had decreased from 2004 U/L to 327 U/L [N: 87–210], and the patient's general condition was good. She left the hospital on a combined treatment of penicillamine 1200 mg/d and zinc gluconate 90 mg/d and received also dietary counseling. At the outpatient visit 3 weeks later, hemoglobin was 133 gr/l, and the urinary copper excretion value was reduced at 1080 μg/24 h compared to baseline measure (−74%). Determination of serum copper level was not repeated thereafter. The brain MRI scan did not show T2 hyperintensity in basal ganglia.

3. Discussion

This is a typical clinical presentation of AWH with background chronic liver disease, presenting as an acute-on-chronic liver failure [13]. Wilson's disease is a rare autosomal recessive disorder of copper metabolism resulting in a progressive accumulation of copper in several organs including the liver and the brain [3]. Clinical presentation includes neurological symptoms, paucisymptomatic chronic liver disease, or acute liver injury [13] which accounts for approximately 10% of acute liver failure cases referred for urgent LT [14]. Laboratory values of AWH may show typical alterations including a low alkaline phosphatase and modest elevations of transaminases levels, while serum ceruloplasmin, the concentration of which is expected to be low, may be normal under the influence of inflammation. A Coombs-negative hemolytic anemia is suggestive of the diagnosis of acute WD [15]. High values of non-ceruloplasmin-bound copper and 24-hour cupruria are typical of AWH, but similar alterations may also be observed in acute hepatitis of other etiologies due to passive release of copper from hepatocytes. Thus, when interpretation is difficult, a liver biopsy with quantification of hepatic copper, as in our case, helps to make a final diagnosis.

Liver failure due to AWH is a clinical challenge. Once the diagnosis is established, it is crucial to determine early if

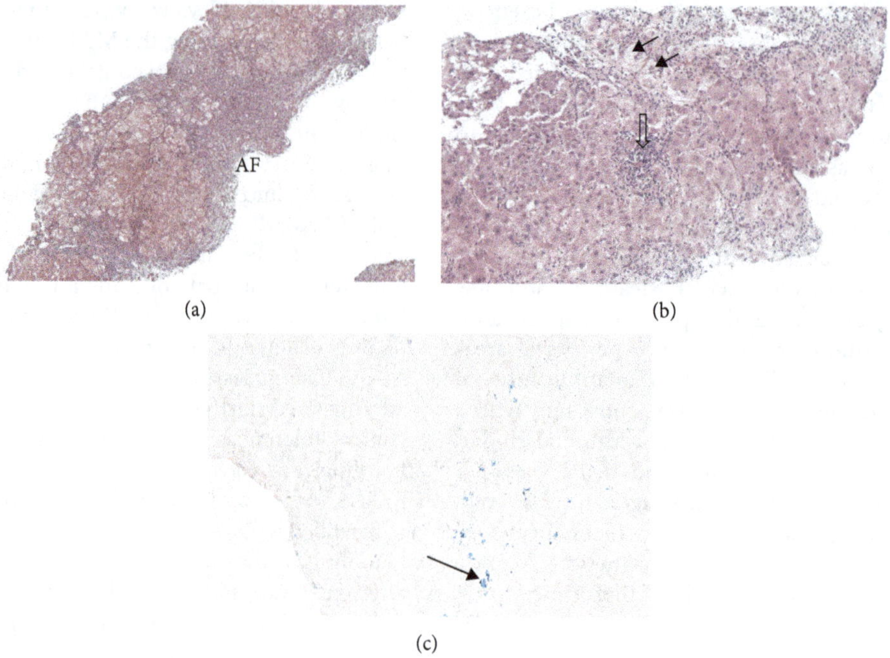

FIGURE 1: Liver biopsy specimen. (a) Annular fibrosis (AF) surrounding hepatocyte nodules (Masson trichrome staining, original magnification × 50). (b) Chronic hepatitis with lobular activity (open arrow), ballooned hepatocytes (black arrows), and mild steatosis (H&E staining, original magnification × 50). (c) Black arrows indicate Victoria blue staining deposits in periportal areas.

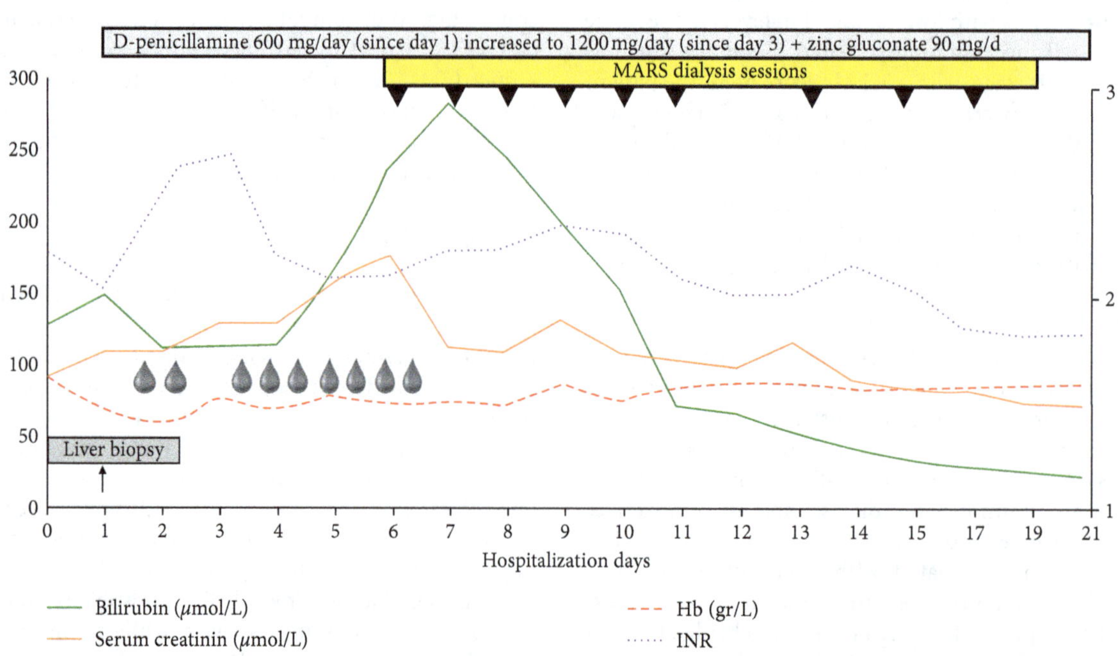

FIGURE 2: Graphical illustration of the patient's course during hospitalization. Each cartoon drop indicates a blood transfusion. The violet line indicates INR, and the red dotted line corresponds to hemoglobin level. The orange line and the green solid line illustrate serum creatinine and total bilirubin values, respectively. Black triangles correspond to the individual MARS dialysis session.

pharmacological chelation therapy will be efficient enough to remove excess copper and progressively improve liver function [16] or if urgent liver transplantation is required [3]. On the one hand, according to a value of 11 in the New Wilson Prognostic Index published by Dhawan et al. [8], there was a high risk of death without transplantation. On the other hand, Clichy's criteria used in our institution for the management of fulminant hepatic failure were not met and, thus, the patient was not immediately listed for urgent LT. In spite of a rapid initiation of both the copper-chelating agent (penicillamine) and an intestinal absorption copper blocker (zinc gluconate), biological tests continued to deteriorate with renal and hematological complications. It was considered that massive copper overload was primarily

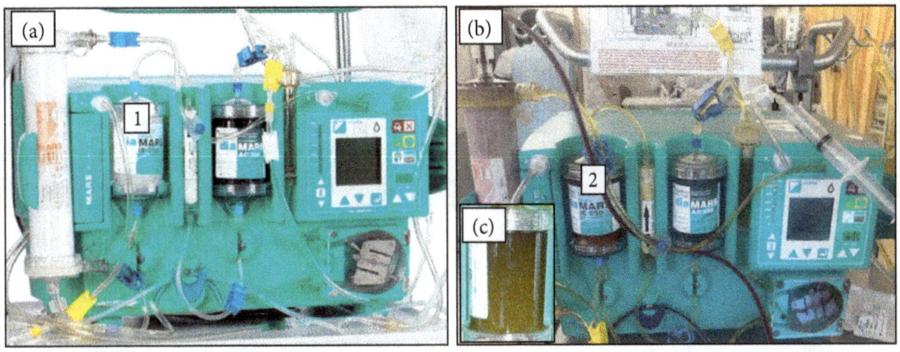

FIGURE 3: Illustration of the MARS device prior to use (a) and at the end of the initial session (b). The initially colorless diaMARS IE250 adsorber cartridge (1) became dark brown at the end of the procedure due to massive copper deposits (2). (c) A cartridge from a historical case of alcoholic cirrhosis and hepatorenal syndrome under MARS therapy showing, instead, a yellowish brown color due to bilirubin pigments.

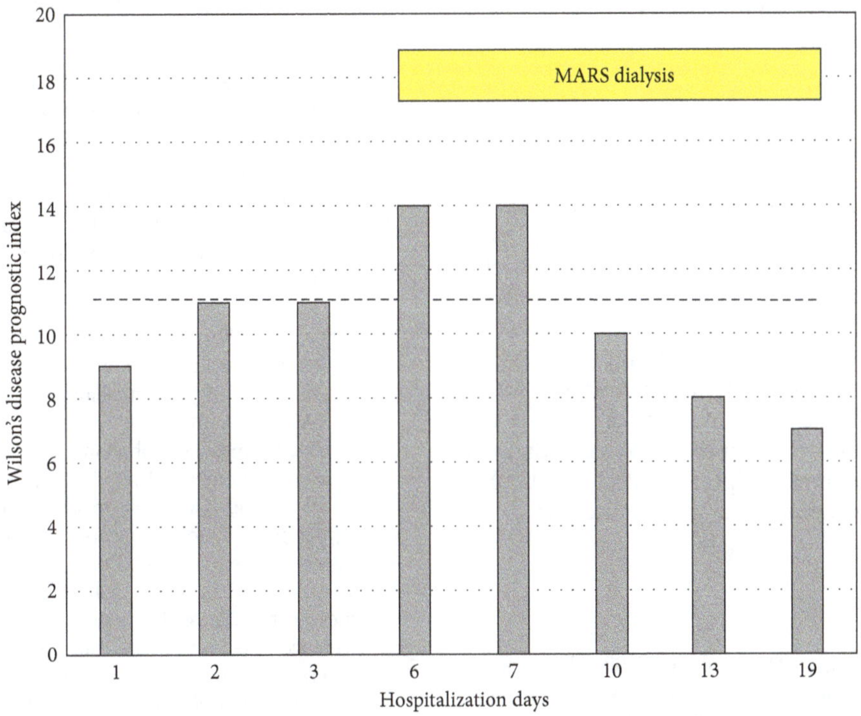

FIGURE 4: Evolution of Wilson's disease prognostic index during hospitalization. A score ≥ 11 (dashed line) is associated with a high probability of death without LT according to [8].

responsible for both the development of acute tubular injury with renal failure and the severe intravascular hemolysis [17] requiring repeated blood transfusions.

The extracorporeal detoxification methods that are available to rapidly remove excess copper in acute WD include TPE and MARS dialysis. According to recent American guidelines on apheresis, TPE is the first-line therapy as a bridge to liver transplantation in WD, although the recommendation level is low [18]. TPE removes both ceruloplasmin and albumin-bound copper, improves coagulation parameters due to concomitant plasma administration, is available in most healthcare settings, but uses citrate which is not recommended in acute liver failure. The MARS system combines a separate albumin circuit and two columns including a large ion-exchanger resin cartridge that can be used until saturation and uses unfractionated heparin during the procedure. These technical characteristics make this particular extracorporeal detoxification device a suitable option in this clinical situation [19–21]. In addition, conventional dialysis combined with MARS clears water-soluble substances such as creatinine, urea, and ammonium that participate in hepatic encephalopathy and hepatorenal syndrome [22].

In our patient, repeated MARS dialysis combined with conventional medical treatment allowed a rapid control of hemolysis, as blood transfusions were no longer necessary after the second MARS session. This improvement was associated with a progressive decrease in LDH level as a marker of hemolysis [4].

The survival benefit of MARS in acute-on-chronic liver failure is not proven [23]. Based on few case series [5, 20, 24] and clinical practice guidelines on WD from India [25], MARS dialysis could stabilize the patient's condition and may serve as a bridge to LT. Our observation demonstrates that MARS sessions administered to target massive copper-overload-associated hemolysis reduced the need for repeated blood transfusions and have contributed to the patient's survival without urgent LT.

Abbreviations

Hb: Hemoglobin
INR: International Normalized Ratio
WD: Wilson's disease
AWH: Acute Wilsonian hepatitis
MARS: Molecular adsorbents recirculating system
TPE: Therapeutic plasma exchange
MELD: Model for end-stage liver disease
LT: Liver transplantation.

Authors' Contributions

JH collected data, performed critical analysis, and wrote the manuscript. NH collected data, performed critical analysis, and participated in redaction of this paper. GM collected data and critically reviewed the manuscript. BP collected data, performed + critical analysis of data, and reviewed the manuscript. MO collected data and critically reviewed the manuscript. ALR collected data and performed critical analysis. NG collected data, performed critical analysis, and participated in redaction of this paper. JLF collected data and critically reviewed the manuscript. LS collected data, performed critical analysis, and wrote the manuscript.

References

[1] P. Steindl, P. Ferenci, H. Dienes et al., "Wilson's disease in patients presenting with liver disease: a diagnostic challenge," *Gastroenterology*, vol. 113, no. 1, pp. 212–218, 1997.

[2] P. Knoflach, "Diagnosis and current therapy of Wilson's disease," *Alimentary Pharmacology & Therapeutics*, vol. 19, no. 2, pp. 157–165, 2004.

[3] P. Ferenci, A. Czlonkowska, W. Stremmel et al., "EASL clinical practice guidelines: Wilson's disease," *Journal of Hepatology*, vol. 56, no. 3, pp. 671–685, 2012.

[4] W. Barcellini and B. Fattizzo, "Clinical applications of hemolytic markers in the differential diagnosis and management of hemolytic anemia," *Disease Markers*, vol. 2015, Article ID 635670, 7 pages, 2015.

[5] E. A. Roberts, "Update on the diagnosis and management of Wilson disease," *Current Gastroenterology Reports*, vol. 20, no. 12, p. 56, 2018.

[6] A. Pauwels, N. Mostefa-Kara, C. Florent, and V. G. Lévy, "Emergency liver transplantation for acute liver failure," *Journal of Hepatology*, vol. 17, no. 1, pp. 124–127, 1993.

[7] J. Wendon, J. Cordoba, A. Dhawan et al., "EASL Clinical Practical Guidelines on the management of acute (fulminant) liver failure," *Journal of Hepatology*, vol. 66, no. 5, pp. 1047–1081, 2017.

[8] A. Dhawan, R. M. Taylor, P. Cheeseman, P. De Silva, L. Katsiyiannakis, and G. Mieli-Vergani, "Wilson's disease in children: 37-year experience and revised King's score for liver transplantation," *Liver Transplantation*, vol. 11, no. 4, pp. 441–448, 2005.

[9] S. Sen and R. Jalan, "The role of the Molecular Adsorbents Recirculating System (MARS) in the management of liver failure," *Perfusion*, vol. 19, no. 1, pp. S43–S48, 2004.

[10] T. Hilal and R. S. Morehead, "Fulminant Wilson's disease managed with plasmapheresis as a bridge to liver transplant," *Case Reports in Medicine*, vol. 2014, Article ID 672985, 4 pages, 2014.

[11] H. P. Pham, J. Schwartz, L. Cooling et al., "Report of the ASFA apheresis registry study on Wilson's disease," *Journal of Clinical Apheresis*, vol. 31, no. 1, pp. 11–15, 2016.

[12] K. Wong, V. Stadlbauer, P. Krisper, and R. E. Stauber, "Effect of extracorporeal liver support by molecular adsorbents recirculating system and Prometheus on redox state of albumin in acute-on-chronic liver failure," *Therapeutic Apheresis and Dialysis*, vol. 13, no. 5, pp. 431–436, 2009.

[13] P. Ferenci, K. Caca, G. Loudianos et al., "Diagnosis and phenotypic classification of Wilson disease1," *Liver International*, vol. 23, no. 3, pp. 139–142, 2003.

[14] M. L. Schilsky, I. H. Scheinberg, and I. Sternlieb, "Liver transplantation for Wilson's disease: indications and outcome," *Hepatology*, vol. 19, no. 3, pp. 583–587, 1994.

[15] J. Roche-Sicot and J. P. Benhamou, "Acute intravascular hemolysis and acute liver failure associated as a first manifestation of Wilson's disease," *Annals of Internal Medicine*, vol. 86, no. 3, pp. 301–303, 1977.

[16] F. Durand, J. Bernuau, E. Giostra et al., "Wilson's disease with severe hepatic insufficiency: beneficial effects of early administration of D-penicillamine," *Gut*, vol. 48, no. 6, pp. 849–852, 2001.

[17] K. F. Adams, G. Johnson Jr., K. E. Hornowski, and T. H. Lineberger, "The effect of copper on erythrocyte deformability. A possible mechanism of hemolysis in acute copper intoxication," *Biochimica et Biophysica Acta (BBA)-Biomembranes*, vol. 550, no. 2, pp. 279–287, 1979.

[18] A. Padmanabhan, L. Connelly-Smith, N. Aqui et al., "Guidelines on the use of therapeutic apheresis in clinical practice-evidence-based approach from the writing committee of the American society for apheresis: the eighth special issue," *Journal of Clinical Apheresis*, vol. 34, no. 3, pp. 171–354, 2019.

[19] T. Zantek, A. Ochs, E. Bisse, C. Strey, and W. Grotz, "Liver support-a task for nephrologists? Extracorporeal treatment of a patient with fulminant wilson crisis," *Blood Purification*, vol. 21, no. 3, pp. 232–236, 2003.

[20] A. Chiu, N. S. Tsoi, and S. T. Fan, "Use of the molecular adsorbents recirculating system as a treatment for acute decompensated wilson disease," *Liver Transplantation*, vol. 14, no. 10, pp. 1512–1516, 2008.

[21] N. Rustom, M. Bost, F. Cour-Andlauer et al., "Effect of molecular adsorbents recirculating system treatment in children with acute liver failure caused by Wilson disease," *Journal of Pediatric Gastroenterology & Nutrition*, vol. 58, no. 2, pp. 160–164, 2014.

[22] A. A. Kaplan and M. Epstein, "Extracorporeal blood purification in the management of patients with hepatic failure," *Seminars in Nephrology*, vol. 17, no. 6, pp. 576–582, 1997.

[23] R. Banares, L. Ibanez-Samaniego, J. M. Torner et al., "Meta-analysis of individual patient data of albumin dialysis in acute-

on-chronic liver failure: focus on treatment intensity," *Therapeutic Advances in Gastroenterology*, vol. 12, 2019.
[24] M. A. Camarata, M. Gottfried, J. A. Rule et al., "Outcomes of acute liver injury in adults due to Wilson's disease: is survival without transplant possible?" *Liver Transplantation*, vol. 26, no. 3, pp. 330–336, 2020.
[25] A. Nagral, M. S. Sarma, J. Matthai et al., "Wilson's disease: clinical practice guidelines of the Indian national association for study of the liver, the Indian society of pediatric gastroenterology, hepatology and nutrition, and the movement disorders society of India," *Journal of Clinical and Experimental Hepatology*, vol. 9, no. 1, pp. 74–98, 2019.

A Devastating Case of Hepatitis C-Induced Mixed Cryoglobulinemia

Sameeha Khalid,[1] Dhuha Alhankawi,[2] Kamalmeet Kaur,[1] Ali Ali,[1] Anna Kazaryan,[3] and Marina Roytman[2]

[1]*Department of Internal Medicine, University of California San Francisco-Fresno, Fresno, CA, USA*
[2]*Department of Gastroenterology & Hepatology, University of California San Francisco-Fresno, Fresno, CA, USA*
[3]*Department of Rheumatology, University of California San Francisco-Fresno, Fresno, CA, USA*

Correspondence should be addressed to Sameeha Khalid; sameeha.khalid@ucsf.edu

Academic Editor: Mauro Vigano

Hepatitis C-induced mixed cryoglobulinemia leading to rapidly progressive gangrene, necessitating amputations, is a rare presentation. We describe a case of a 55-year-old man with untreated chronic hepatitis C virus (HCV) presenting with arthralgia and palpable purpura, which rapidly progressed to life-threatening gangrene of all extremities requiring amputations in the setting of mixed cryoglobulinemia. Treatment for HCV was initiated which led to the arrest of gangrene progression and the patient's survival. Patients with HCV-induced cryoglobulinemia should be closely monitored and started on early therapy with direct-acting antiviral therapy to prevent progression of vasculitis to gangrene. Universal screening for HCV can aid in early diagnosis and treatment to prevent devastating consequences.

1. Introduction

Mixed cryoglobulinemia is a rare condition, with a prevalence of 1 : 100,000 in the United States. The most common cause is chronic hepatitis C virus (HCV); however, a number of other etiologies including other infections, autoimmune diseases, and lymphoproliferative disorders are known to precipitate mixed cryoglobulinemia [1]. Meltzer coined the clinical triad of mixed cryoglobulinemia as palpable purpura, arthralgia, and weakness in 1966; however, it is unlikely for patients to present with all three, and palpable purpura is the most common presentation [2].

Chronic HCV infection is known to be the underlying disorder in a majority (80–90%) of cases of mixed cryoglobulinemia; however, only 5–10% of HCV patients are estimated to have symptomatic disease [2, 3]. In many cases, the extrahepatic manifestations of HCV can occur in patients without features of overt liver disease. The role played by HCV in the development of this disease is thought to stem from chronic stimulation of the immune system causing B-cell hyperactivation and selective expansion of cryoglobulin-producing B-cell clones which express rheumatoid factor (RF) and proliferate in the liver, serum, and lymph nodes [4, 5]. Circulating cryoglobulins precipitate at low temperatures below 37 degrees Celsius and deposit in small and medium vessels, leading to complement activation and inflammation and subsequently causing systemic vasculitis and damage to various end organs [4]. It is the circulation of these large cryoproteins that leads to increased blood viscosity causing hypoperfusion and subsequently gangrenes [2].

There is a wide spectrum of manifestations associated with cryoglobulinemia which can range from mild (>50%) to moderate or severe (35%) and even life-threatening conditions (<15%) [6]. Life-threatening cryoglobulinemia vasculitis can be diagnosed if any of the following are present: renal involvement, gastrointestinal involvement, lung involvement, CNS involvement, heart involvement, widespread vasculitis (multiorgan involvement), hyperviscosity syndrome, or liver failure in HCV-related mixed

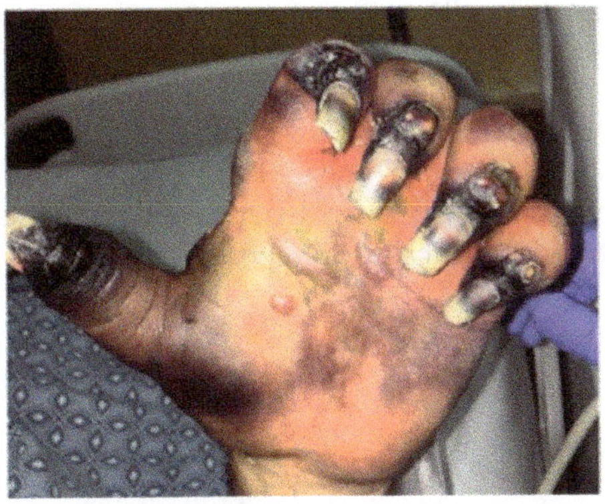

FIGURE 1: Patient's hand on initial presentation.

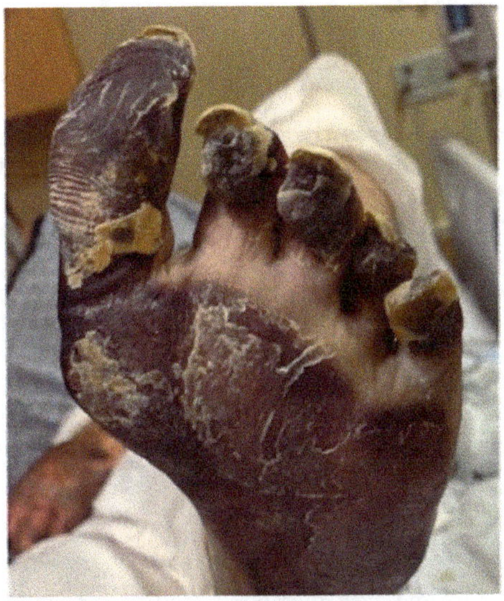

FIGURE 2: Patient's foot on initial presentation.

cryoglobulinemia [3]. Such life-threatening features carry a mortality rate between 20% and 80% and in almost two-thirds of cases may be the initial clinical manifestation of cryoglobulinemia [6]. HCV-induced mixed cryoglobulinemia leading to rapidly progressive gangrene of all four extremities, necessitating amputations, is a rare presentation of cryoglobulinemia that we present here.

2. Case Report

A 55-year-old man with treatment-naive HCV infection (genotype 1a) presented to the emergency room with bilateral hand pain and diffuse purpuric rash. He described associated arthralgias, purpuric lesions, weakness, and numbness. Physical examination showed palpable purpura and extensive gangrene affecting bilateral upper and lower extremities (Figures 1 and 2). Laboratory investigation revealed positive rheumatoid factor (>1,200 IU/mL), hypocomplementemia (C4 <8.0 mg/dL), HCV RNA 2,390,000 IU/mL, and positive cryoglobulins. Skin biopsy of the leg showed mixed, predominantly acute, infiltrate with scattered small to mid-sized vessels with features of fibrin thrombi with or without associated vasculitis. The patient

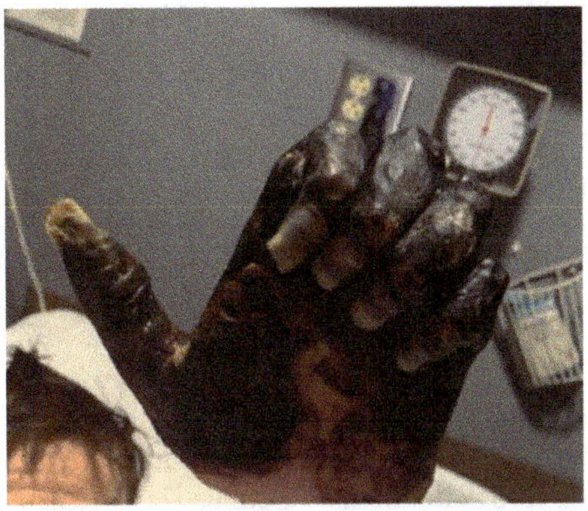

FIGURE 3: Progression of gangrene 10 days after initial presentation.

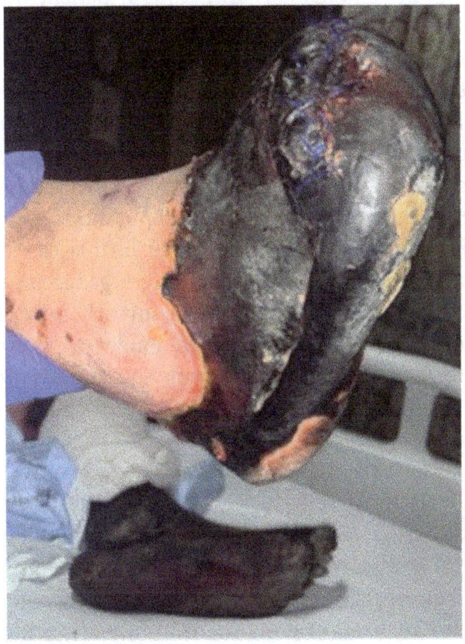

FIGURE 4: Bilateral gangrenous lower extremities 10 days after initial presentation.

was diagnosed with mixed cryoglobulinemia complicated by severe cutaneous vasculitis with ischemic limbs.

Plasmapheresis was initiated; however, gangrene continued to progressively worsen despite it (Figures 3 and 4). He was transitioned to immunosuppressive therapy with high-dose pulse steroids followed by prednisone 60 mg daily for four weeks in combination with rituximab without improvement. Given progressive gangrene despite multiple surgical debridements, inpatient treatment with sofosbuvir/velpatasvir was started for treatment of chronic HCV infection. After initiation of HCV treatment, the viral load went from 2,390,000 IU to <15 IU after four weeks and there was no further spread of gangrene. The necrotic limbs were unsalvageable, requiring serial limb amputations including bilateral above the knee amputations, right metacarpophalangeal disarticulation of fingers, right interphalangeal disarticulation of the thumb, and left wrist disarticulation. He was discharged to a skilled nursing facility. On follow-up with Hepatology, the patient achieved sustained virologic response week 12 (SVR-12) and has not had further recurrence of manifestations associated with mixed cryoglobulinemia.

3. Discussion

There is a wide spectrum of manifestations associated with cryoglobulinemia with severe and life-threatening presentations being relatively rare (<15% of cases) [6]. Most patients with such severe presentations do not survive. One case study by Manuel Ramos-Casals, MD, of 29 patient cases demonstrated a 66% mortality in patients presenting with severe, life-threatening cryoglobulinemia vasculitis [7]. It remains unclear why some patients manifest a severe form of cryoglobulinemia vasculitis, and information regarding clinical presentation and prognosis of these patients is limited. Our patient with HCV-related mixed cryoglobulinemia presented with severe cutaneous vasculitis progressing to gangrene of all extremities with the catastrophic result of unsalvageable limbs. Upon literature review, this is one of the most aggressive cases of mixed cryoglobulinemia vasculitis reported thus far that resulted in the patient's survival. There have been no other cases reported that have resulted in multiple limb amputations secondary to this extent of cryoglobulinemia. As such, this case serves to increase clinician awareness of the severe gangrene that may rapidly develop in mixed cryoglobulinemia. These cases require early recognition and aggressive treatment to prevent progression to the extent of limb amputation and even death.

The mainstays of treatment of HCV-induced mixed cryoglobulinemia include the eradication of HCV infection, deletion of underlying B-cell clonal expansions, and depletion of cryoproteins [1, 8]. Multiple studies agree that regardless of the severity of mixed cryoglobulinemia, an attempt to eradicate HCV should be pursued whenever possible and as soon as possible as suppression of viral replication may limit or halt the immunopathogenic process triggered by HCV [9, 10]. In the presence of life-threatening manifestations of mixed cryoglobulinemia, it is vital to begin rapid treatment with immunosuppressive therapy concomitantly with direct-acting antiviral (DAA) therapy. A prospective study showed that DAA therapy is highly effective and safe for patients with HCV-induced mixed cryoglobulinemia with an overall 100% clinical response rate for vasculitis [11].

This case notably highlights the necessity of universal screening for HCV and portrays the devastating effects that delayed screening and therefore delayed treatment may have. Universal screening is imperative for the early detection, treatment, and prevention of the intrahepatic and extrahepatic consequences of HCV, such as mixed cryoglobulinemia.

Disclosure

The abstract was presented earlier at the ACG Annual Scientific Meeting on October 23–28, 2020. The abstract was published in The American Journal of Gastroenterology: October 2020—Volume 115—Issue—p S1325.

Authors' Contributions

Sameeha Khalid, Kamalmeet Kaur, and Ali Ali were involved in direct patient care, conception of the work, drafting the work, and revising it. Dhuha Alhankawi, Anna Kazaryan, and Marina Roytman carried out direct patient care and revised the work critically for important intellectual content.

References

[1] G. Lauletta, S. Russi, V. Conteduca, and L. Sansonno, "Hepatitis C virus infection and mixed cryoglobulinemia," *Clinical and Developmental Immunology*, vol. 2012, Article ID 502156, 11 pages, 2012.

[2] E. D. Charles and L. B. Dustin, "Hepatitis C virus-induced cryoglobulinemia," *Kidney International*, vol. 76, no. 8, pp. 818–824, 2009.

[3] E. Rosenthal and P. Cacoub, "Extrahepatic manifestations in chronic hepatitis C virus carriers," *Lupus*, vol. 24, no. 4-5, pp. 469–482, 2015.

[4] D. Mebust, "Mixed cryoglobulinemia: an unusual presentation of hepatitis C," *The Permanente Journal*, vol. 17, no. 3, pp. e112–e113, 2013.

[5] F. Dammacco and D. Sansonno, "Therapy for hepatitis C virus-related cryoglobulinemic vasculitis," *New England Journal of Medicine*, vol. 369, no. 11, pp. 1035–1045, 2013.

[6] S. Retamozo, C. Díaz-Lagares, X. Bosch et al., "Life-threatening cryoglobulinemic patients with hepatitis C," *Medicine*, vol. 92, no. 5, pp. 273–284, 2013.

[7] M. Ramos-Casals, A. Robles, P. Brito-Zerón et al., "Life-threatening cryoglobulinemia: clinical and immunological characterization of 29 cases," *Seminars in Arthritis and Rheumatism*, vol. 36, no. 3, pp. 189–196, 2006.

[8] N. J. Schamberg and G. V. Lake-Bakaar, "Hepatitis C virus-related mixed cryoglobulinemia: pathogenesis, clinica manifestations, and new therapies," *Gastroenterology and Hepatology*, vol. 3, no. 9, pp. 695–703, 2007.

[9] M. E. Sise, A. K. Bloom, J. Wisocky et al., "Treatment of hepatitis C virus-associated mixed cryoglobulinemia with direct-acting antiviral agents," *Hepatology*, vol. 63, no. 2, pp. 408–417, 2016.

[10] M. Pietrogrande, S. De Vita, A. L. Zignego et al., "Recommendations for the management of mixed cryoglobulinemia syndrome in hepatitis C virus-infected patients," *Autoimmunity Reviews*, vol. 10, no. 8, pp. 444–454, 2011.

[11] L. Gragnani, M. Visentini, E. Fognani et al., "Prospective study of guideline-tailored therapy with direct-acting antivirals for hepatitis C virus-associated mixed cryoglobulinemia," *Hepatology*, vol. 64, no. 5, pp. 1473–1482, 2016.

47

Zinc Monotherapy as an Alternative Treatment Option for Decompensated Liver Disease due to Wilson Disease?

Hansa Haftu,[1] **Mohammed Mustefa,**[1] **and Teklu Gebrehiwot**[2]

[1]*Mekelle University, College of Health Science, Pediatric and Child Health Department, Tigray, Ethiopia*
[2]*Mekelle University, College of Health Science, Clinical Pharmacist, Tigray, Ethiopia*

Correspondence should be addressed to Hansa Haftu; hansahaftu21@gmail.com

Academic Editor: Melanie Deutsch

Background. Wilson disease is a rare metabolic disorder involving copper metabolism, and patients may present with a variable degree of hepatic, neurologic, and psychiatric manifestations. In the case of hepatic presentation, treatment is usually initiated with potentially toxic copper chelators (D-penicillamine or Trenton). Although zinc is of low toxicity and low cost for treatment of Wilson disease, it has been limited to the adjunctive as a single maintenance drug or for asymptomatic patients. The use of zinc monotherapy in patients suffering from a severe liver disease was not well studied. In our case report, we describe a pediatric patient who presented with liver failure and the use of zinc monotherapy in patients with severe hepatic manifestations. *Case presentation.* A 15-year-old male patient from Ethiopia presented with generalized body swelling (edema and ascites) with yellowish discoloration of his eyes and easy fatigability. He had hyperbilirubinemia, coagulopathy, hypoalbuminemia, and deranged liver enzymes. He had a Keyser–Fleischer ring visible with the naked eye, which was confirmed by slit-lamp examination. He had very low serum ceruloplasmin (<8 mg/L) and high 24-hour urine copper (150 mcg/dl). In accordance with the scoring system proposed by the 8th International Meeting on Wilson Disease and Menkes Disease, a diagnosis of Wilson disease was made. Zinc monotherapy with low copper diet was initiated for decompensated liver disease due to Wilson disease because of the inaccessibility of chelators (D-penicillamine or Trientine). After months of treatment with zinc, the patient experienced normalization of hepatic synthetic function and resolution of hypoalbuminemia and coagulopathy. The patient had also clinically stabilized (ascites, lower extremity swelling, edema, and jaundice were improved. Currently, the patient is on follow-up almost for the last four years in the gastrointestinal clinic. *Conclusion.* Our case shows that zinc has the potential for treatment in improving liver function. Though zinc has its own side effects, it is important and maybe an alternative treatment option in those with limited resources (not able to access chelators). This example hopefully will encourage future investigations and researches on zinc monotherapy for treating symptomatic decompensated hepatic Wilson disease.

1. Background

Wilson disease (WD) is a rare autosomal recessive genetic disorder of copper metabolism, which is a defective biliary excretion of copper, resulting in the accumulation of copper in the liver, brain, kidney, and cornea. The disease affects one in 100,000 individuals [1, 2]. Patients with WD have varying clinical presentations ranging from an asymptomatic state to acute life-threatening liver involvement (acute liver failure), which can cause high mortality reaching 95% without liver transplantation [1, 3, 4]. Other patients may present with chronic liver disease mimicking other etiologies and neuropsychiatric manifestations. Though acute liver failure (ALF) presentation is rare in pediatric age groups (only 3% of all ALF case series in children), it is dramatic and may result in suddenness [3]. Although Wilson disease is rarely diagnosed and reported in African children, it must be considered differential in any patient with liver disease. There are few reports regarding zinc monotherapy in patients with decompensated liver disease. Our case report documents the role of zinc monotherapy in clinical resolution and normalization of laboratory liver synthetic dysfunction in patients with the severe hepatic presentation of Wilson disease.

1.1. Case Presentation. A 15-year-old male child, from nonconsanguineous marriage, was referred to our hospital from a private clinic with a possible diagnosis of renal disease in December 2015. His main complaint was generalized body swelling of 3 months in duration. In the private clinic, he was given Lasix for the diagnosis of renal disease, but the symptoms got worse and he discontinued the medication. He had easy fatigability and shortness of breath at rest and loss of appetite associated with yellowish discoloration of the eye for two weeks. He was a grade seven student. He had no change in school performance, no difficulty in playing and writing, and no behavioral change or abnormal body movement. He had no history of vomiting, change in bowel habit, abdominal pain, drug, or herbal medication use, alcohol intake, previous history of jaundice or contact with a jaundiced person, and family history of similar illness. He also had no history of bleeding from any site. His developmental history was optimal. The physical examination showed that he was conscious and oriented to time, person, and place. He had icteric sclera, a well-formed Kayser–Fleischer ring visible with the naked eye (Figure 1), which was confirmed by slit-lamp examination, grossly distended abdomen with shifting dullness and fluid thrill, pitting pedal, and pretibial edema. Initial investigations showed deranged liver function (Table 1). His serum creatinine and blood urea nitrogen, serum electrolytes, lipid profile, and urine analysis were normal. A serologic test for the human immune deficiency virus (HIV), hepatitis B virus surface antigen (HBsAg), antinuclear antibody (ANA), and antibodies to the hepatitis C virus (HCV) were negative. Serum ceruloplasmin was very low, less than 8 mg/dl (normal 20–60 mg/dl), and the 24-hr urinary copper excretion was high (150 mcg/dl). Abdominal ultrasound showed that the liver size was normal, but it was coarse and nodular with ascites. For our patient, Wilson disease was diagnosed according to the scoring system proposed by the 8th International Meeting of Wilson Disease and Menkes Disease [4], with a total score of 4 (serum ceruloplasmin = 2, K-F ring = 2). The patient was admitted and started on diuretics, low protein and salt diet, bisacodyl metronidazole, multivitamins, and parental vitamin K. After Wilson disease was confirmed, the patient started on zinc acetate (neither penicillamine nor trientine was available, and even more, it was difficult to bring them from abroad) and was advised to avoid high copper-containing foods. The effectiveness of the treatment was assessed by clinical resolution of symptoms and serial determination of the liver enzymes, coagulation profile, serum albumin, and serum bilirubin (Table 1).

On follow-up, our patient started to improve clinically (the symptoms and signs disappeared), and the deranged laboratory findings also improved initially (Table 1). Finally, the patient was discharged with zinc acetate (25 mg PO TID) and low copper diet (the patient was given a written paper in the local language of what food to avoid). Our patient is still on follow-up in one of the pediatric clinics (GI-clinic) with normal laboratory findings and free of clinical symptoms. He also had an improvement in the Keyser–Fleischer ring both clinically (Figure 2) and on slit examination. On follow-up, the family (two younger siblings and his parents) were screened with serum ceruloplasmin, and his mother had a low level of ceruloplasmin, but she is asymptomatic.

2. Discussion and Conclusion

WD is rarely diagnosed and reported in African countries except in North African countries. In North African countries where consanguinity is common, autosomal recessive disease, including Wilson disease, is relatively common and reported. There are also reports from Senegal and Nigeria (two case reports). But the exact epidemiology of WD in Africa is not known because it is rare to diagnose and report. In those patients with signs and symptoms of liver disease which is not due to viral infections, WD must be considered and investigated because hepatic manifestations are common in children [4–7]. The diagnosis of WD relies on clinical manifestations like the pigmentation of the iris (Kayser–Fleischer rings, suggestive signs and symptoms of liver disease, and neuropsychiatric problems) with some laboratory pieces of evidence (low ceruloplasmin, elevated urine, and hepatic copper level) [5, 6]. However, the presence of Keyser–Fleischer rings and a low level of ceruloplasmin is sufficient to diagnose WD, especially in developing countries with limited resources [7]. Hepatic manifestation is more common in children with the symptoms ranging from an asymptomatic elevation of liver enzymes to a fulminant course [1, 8, 9]. So, in any patient with an unexplained liver disease, the disease must be investigated for possible WD and relatives of WD patients must also be screened for any asymptomatic WD with ceruloplasmin or urine copper, so that they will start early management [7].

Our patient had signs and symptoms of liver disease (jaundice, peripheral edema, and ascites) with elevated liver enzymes, hypoalbuminemia, hyperbilirubinemia, and coagulation abnormality. He had Kyser–Fleischer ring in both clinical (Figure 1) and slit-lamp examination. In addition to the K–F ring, our patient had laboratory evidence (high urinary copper and low ceruloplasmin) for WD. Laboratory tests, including alkaline phosphatase, bilirubin, and serum aminotransferases, were elevated. Medical therapy is effective, but WD is not yet curable, and it is progressive and fatal if not diagnosed and treated early [1, 10]. The American Association for the Study of Liver Diseases (AASLD) and the European Association for the Study of the Liver (EASL) recommend the use of a copper chelating agent, such as D-penicillamine or trientine, in the initial treatment of symptomatic patients. Zinc therapy can be initiated in those presymptomatic patients or for maintenance after chelators in symptomatic patients [10–13]. Till now, different guidelines, including the standard Nelson Textbook of Pediatrics, recommend that all symptomatic patients with Wilson disease receive a chelating agent [11, 13–15]. But chelators have many side effects with limited access, and most patients with neurologic WD symptoms may exacerbate as high as 50% and some may be intolerant [11, 15]. Although zinc is less effective than chelators in established Wilson disease treatment, data are limited and uncontrolled. While zinc treatment is effective in neurologic WD and in

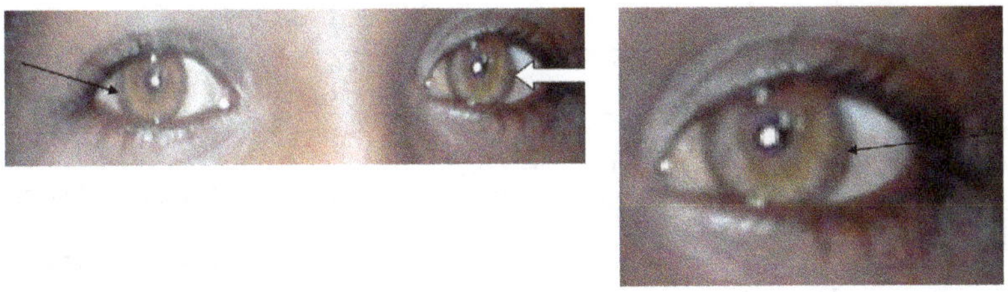

(a) (b)

FIGURE 1: (a, b) Both arrows (black and white arrows) show the Kayser-Fleischer ring before the treatment.

TABLE 1: Laboratory result at presentation and on follow-up.

Laboratory parameters	At presentation	Subsequent laboratory measurement on follow-up			
		2nd week	3rd week	5th week	7th week
WBC (4.0–10.5 × 10^3/L)	8.4				
Hemoglobin (12.5–16.1)	12				
Platelet (150–4500 × 10^3)	247				
AST (5–45 IU/L)	130	97	59	30	37
ALT (5–45 IU/L)	581	160	60	24	30
ALP (115 IU/L)	300				
Serum albumin (3.2–5.1 gm/L)	1.7	2.7	2.2	3.9	4
Total protein		9.3	8.4	8.5	8.7
PT (11–14 sec)	28.8	32.4	32	18.1	12
APTT (25–35 sec)	38.5	36.8	35	34.2	30
INR (0.8–1.2)	2.62	2.88	2.8	1.62	1.3
Total bilirubin (mg/dl)	5	5.3	3.2	0.8	1
Serum ceruloplasmin (20–60 mg/dl)	<8				
24 hr urine copper (mcg/dl)	150				
Slit lamp examination			Kayser-Fleischer rings		

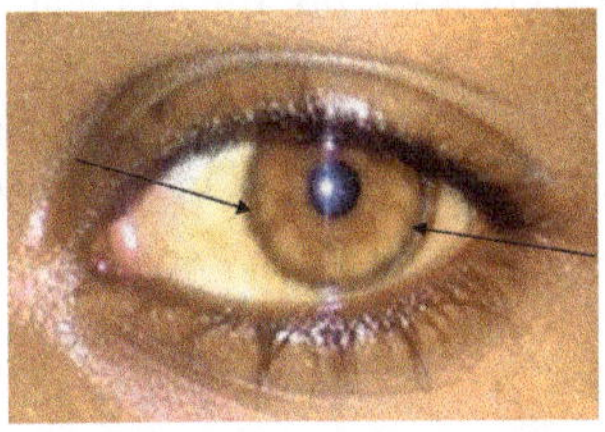

FIGURE 2: K-F ring on follow-up, which was after zinc treatment and has significantly decreased from the initial size of pigmentation.

asymptomatic patients, caution is needed in hepatic WD as there are reports of hepatic deterioration. This may be related to less efficient decoppering and any adverse effects of zinc with most common gastrointestinal irritations [14]. Thus, exclusive monotherapy with zinc in those with symptomatic WD is controversial [14, 15]. In cases of hepatic presentation, treatment is usually initiated with potentially toxic copper chelators (D-penicillamine or trientine). Although multiple studies have introduced zinc as less toxic, available in low cost for WD treatment, its use has been limited to adjunctive or single-agent maintenance options for asymptomatic patients [10]. From most observational studies, it has been found that zinc therapy is the best choice in presymptomatic patients as it is effective and has fewer adverse effects. Especially acutely ill hepatic patients might do better on D-penicillamine, as zinc acts too slowly in these patients [12]. The use of zinc monotherapy in patients suffering from decompensated liver disease has not been well documented with the controversial results, but there are few cases reported with successful treatment [10].

Milanino et al. used a 2-year course of zinc sulfate in the pediatric case and noted normalization of the liver function, negative copper balance, and reduction of inflammatory infiltration, necrosis, and fat deposition in the liver histology [16, 17]. Brewer et al. briefly commented on a patient presenting with hepatic failure who experienced marked improvement in hypoalbuminemia and resolution of ascites after 8 months of zinc acetate therapy after the initial 4 weeks of Trenton therapy. In the same study, the investigators reported on the histologic evaluation of consecutive liver biopsy examination in 7 patients undergoing zinc monotherapy. The pathologic review showed no progression of cirrhosis and in two cases showed a complete resolution of cirrhosis [18]. There was one case of a 58-year-old male patient reported in Virginia, admitted with acute liver failure caused by WD, who was initiated with zinc monotherapy while awaiting liver transplantation. Over a 1-year period with zinc monotherapy, the patient experienced normalization of hepatic synthetic function and resolution of hypoalbuminemia and coagulopathy. Clinical stabilization of variceal bleeding, ascites and lower-extremity edema was also observed. The patient was not a candidate for transplantation because of the improvement in symptoms and the stage of the disease which is assessed by the Child—Turcotte—Pugh score [10]. This was supported by a study done in Italy, which showed that zinc

Table 2: Summary of improved decompensated liver disease after zinc treatment.

No	Sex	Diagnosis	Country	Treatment	Publication details	Year of publication
1	M	Decompensated liver disease with CNS	Nigeria	Zinc	Christopher I., et al.; Wilson disease in a Nigerian child: a case report; BMJ	2012
2	F	Liver disease with CNS	Nigeria	Zinc	Longe A. C., Glew R. H., Omene J. A; Wilson's disease. Report of a case in a Nigerian; Arch neurol	1892
3	F	Decompensated liver disease	Virginia	Zinc	Vanessa D. L., Patrick G. N., and Carl L. B.; Resolution of decompensated cirrhosis from Wilson's disease with zinc monotherapy: a potential therapeutic option; Clinical Gastroenterology and Hepatology	2006
4	M	Decompensated liver disease	Italy	Zinc	Brewer G. J., et al.; Treatment of Wilson's disease with zinc: initial treatment studies; Clinical MED	1989
5	Twenty-two children with Wilson disease with different degree of liver disease treated and followed up for 10 years with zinc acetate, and they show liver function and symptom improvement with no complications.				J Lab Clin Med.; 145(3):139–43	2005
6	Zinc monotherapy is effective in 44 Wilson disease patients, with mild liver disease diagnosed in childhood:				Ranucci et al; Orphanet Journal of Rare Diseases, 9:41	2014

monotherapy is effective in controlling WD-related liver disease, both as first-line and as maintenance treatment in patients with milder liver disease diagnosed in childhood [18]. There was also a case report from Nigeria, an 8-year-old male patient, with decompensated liver disease with neurologic manifestations managed with zinc monotherapy because of the unavailability of copper chelator drugs, and the patient showed significant improvement in the clinical manifestations and laboratory abnormalities [6]. There are a few examples (Table 2) that summarize the improvement of decompensated liver on zinc treatment. In our current case report, there is documentation of clinical resolution and normalization of laboratory liver synthetic dysfunction with zinc treatment. There were no documented adverse effects on the time frame. So, zinc is less toxic, accessible, and inexpensive. This may give hope for countries with limited resources. And this example and other case reports hopefully will encourage future investigations on the monotherapeutic administration of zinc for symptomatic hepatic Wilson disease. This is especially important for developing countries which have no access to copper chelator drugs and liver transplantation options.

3. Strengths and Limitations

The strengths of this case report are that the patient fulfills the diagnostic criteria, there was no doubt about the diagnosis and the synthetic functions done, and the severity of liver dysfunction was also assessed. The patient is followed up until now in clinics, and the clinical and laboratory resolution of symptoms was assessed fully. Lack of diagnostic modality for liver biopsy and the genetic analysis might be considered as a limitation in this case report.

Abbreviations

WD: Wilson disease
ALF: Acute liver failure
K-F ring: Keyser-Fleischer ring
AST: Aspartate aminotransferase
ALT: Alanine aminotransferase
ALP: Alkaline phosphatase.

Authors' Contributions

HHL conceived and drafted the case report. MM and TGG reviewed the data. They were also involved in preparation and critical revision of the manuscript. All authors read and approved the final report.

Acknowledgments

The authors would like to thank pediatric residents, seniors, and other staffs in Ayder Comprehensive Specialized Hospital who contributed to the clinical management of the patient. The authors would also like to appreciate the patient and his mother for giving consent to publication of this case report and Dr. Mohamed and Mr. Teklu for their support in writing this case report.

References

[1] A. Ala, A. P. Walker, K. Ashkan, J. S. Dooley, and M. L. Schilsky, "Wilson's disease," *The Lancet*, vol. 369, no. 9559, pp. 397–408, 2007.

[2] D. Qin-Yun and W. Zhi-Ying, "Advance in the pathogenesis and treatment of Wilson disease," *Translational Neurodegeneration*, vol. 1, no. 1, p. 23, 2012.

[3] M. Patil, K. A. Sheth, A. C. Krishnamurthy, and H. Devarbhavi, "A review and current perspective on Wilson disease," *Journal of Clinical and Experimental Hepatology*, vol. 3, no. 4, pp. 321–336, 2013.

[4] K. S. More, K. Dee Park, C. Lalit et al., "Wilson's disease; a rare presentation, a case report," *Medpulse International Medical Journal*, vol. 1, no. 4, pp. 174–176, 2014.

[5] W. Ella, P. Orit, Peretz et al., "Late-onset fulminant Wilson's disease: a case report and review of the literature," *World Journal of Gastroenterology*, vol. 20, no. 46, pp. 17656–17660, 2014.

[6] C. I. Esezobor, N. Banjoko, A. Rotimi-Samuel, and F. E. Afolabi Lesi, "Wilson disease in a Nigerian child: a case report," *Journal of Medical Case Reports*, vol. 6, no. 1, 2012.

[7] M. L. Schilsky, "Diagnosis and treatment of Wilson's disease," *Pediatric Transplantation*, vol. 6, no. 1, pp. 15–19, 2002.

[8] J. D. Korman, I. Volenberg, J. Balko et al., "Screening for Wilson disease in acute liver failure: a comparison of currently available diagnostic test," *Hepatology*, vol. 48, no. 4, pp. 1167–1174, 2008.

[9] M. Aydinli, O. Harmanci, O. Ersoy et al., "Two unusual cases with Wilson's disease: hepatoma and fulminant hepatitis treated with plasma exchange," *Journal of the National Medical Association*, vol. 98, no. 12, pp. 1989–1991, 2006.

[10] D. L. Vanessa, G. N. Patrick, and L. B. Carl, "Resolution of decompensated cirrhosis from Wilson's disease with zinc monotherapy: a potential therapeutic option," *Clinical Gastroenterology, and Hepatology*, vol. 4, no. 8, pp. 1070-1071, 2006.

[11] G. M. Hill, G. J. Brewer, A. S. Prasad, C. R. Hydrick, and D. E. Hartmann, "Treatment of Wilson's disease with zinc; oral zinc therapy regimens," *Hepatology*, vol. 7, no. 3, pp. 522–528, 1987.

[12] M. Wiggelinkhuizen, M. E. C. Talinus, C. W. Bollen, and R. H. J. Houwen, "Systemic review: clinical efficacy of chelator agents and zinc in the initial treatment of Wilson disease," *Alimentary Pharmacology & Therapeutics*, vol. 29, no. 9, pp. 947–958, 2009.

[13] European Association for the Study of the Liver, "EASL clinical practice guidelines: Wilson's disease," *Journal of Hepatology*, vol. 56, no. 3, pp. 671–685, 2012.

[14] R. Santiago, F. Gottrand, D. Debray et al., "Zinc therapy for wilson disease in children in french pediatric centers," *Journal of Pediatric Gastroenterology and Nutrition*, vol. 61, no. 6, pp. 613–618, 2015.

[15] W. F. Balistreri and R. G. Carey, "Metabolic Diseases of the Liver," in *Nelson Textbook of Pediatrics*, pp. 1388–1393.e2, Elsevier, Amsterdam, Netherlands, 2018.

[16] R. Milanino, A. Deganello, M. Marrella et al., "Oral zinc as initial therapy in Wilson's disease: two years of continuous treatment in a 10-year-old child," *Acta Paediatrica*, vol. 81, no. 2, pp. 163–166, 1992.

[17] R. Milanino, M. Marrella, U. Moretti et al., "Oral zinc sulphate as primary therapeutic intervention in a child with Wilson disease," *European Journal of Pediatrics*, vol. 148, no. 7, pp. 654-655, 1989.

[18] G. J. Brewer, V. Yuzbasiyan-Gurkan, D. Y. Lee, and H. Appelman, "Treatment of Wilson's disease with zinc: initial treatment studies," *Journal of Clinical Medicine*, vol. 114, no. 6, pp. 633–638, 1989.

Lactulose to the Rescue: A Case of Toxic Hepatic Encephalopathy Caused by Portosystemic Shunting and Epistaxis in a Patient with Hereditary Hemorrhagic Telangiectasia

Ruchit N. Shah,[1,2] Michael Makar,[2] Nasir Akhtar,[3] and Erin Forster[3,4]

[1] *Geisinger Medical Center, Department of Internal Medicine, 100 N Academy Ave, Danville, PA 17822, USA*
[2] *Geisinger Commonwealth School of Medicine, 525 Pine Street, Scranton, PA 18510, USA*
[3] *Geisinger Medical Center, Department of Gastroenterology, 100 N Academy Ave, Danville, PA 17822, USA*
[4] *Medical University of South Carolina, 30 Courtenay Dr, Charleston, SC 29425, USA*

Correspondence should be addressed to Michael Makar; michaelmakar5@gmail.com

Academic Editor: Melanie Deutsch

Hereditary hemorrhagic telangiectasia (HHT) is an uncommon autosomal dominant disorder characterized by telangiectasias and arteriovenous malformations. Multiple organ systems are involved including the skin, lungs, gastrointestinal tract, and brain. Hepatic encephalopathy is an extremely rare complication of HHT and early diagnosis and treatment can be life-saving. We present a rare case of hepatic encephalopathy caused by HHT-induced portosystemic shunting treated with lactulose.

1. Introduction

Hereditary hemorrhagic telangiectasia (HHT) or Osler-Weber-Rendu syndrome is a rare autosomal dominant vascular disorder characterized by telangiectasias and arteriovenous malformations (AVMs). Multiple organ systems are involved including the skin, lungs, gastrointestinal tract and brain [1]. Common complications of HHT include bleeding disorders such as epistaxis, gastrointestinal bleeding, iron deficiency anemia, and neurologic sequelae including stroke and hemorrhage. Patients with liver involvement commonly present with symptoms of high-output cardiac failure, portal hypertension, and biliary disease [2]. Portosystemic shunting leading to encephalopathy is a rare complication likely secondary to portal hypertension and severe hepatocellular disease [3, 4]. This case highlights the importance of a multisystem approach to patients with HHT and reviews the treatment and management of hepatic complications.

2. Case Presentation

An 85-year-old male with a medical history pertinent for HHT and congestive heart failure presented with epistaxis, altered mental status, and melena. Physical exam revealed a lethargic male with generalized abdominal tenderness, asterixis, and telangiectasias on the lower lip and dorsal aspect of the hands. Ammonia level was 68 umol/L (ref: 11-35 umol/L), alkaline phosphatase 244 U/L (ref: 0-153 U/L), AST 25 and ALT 29 U/L (ref: 10-50 U/L), bilirubin 0.7mg/dL (ref: 0-1.2 mg/dL), INR 4.11 (ref: 0.87-1.17), and hemoglobin 6.8 g/dL (ref: 13.7-16.5 g/dL). Doppler abdominal ultrasound showed coarse liver parenchyma with multiple scattered hyperechoic lesions suggestive of hepatic AVMs (Figure 1). Computed tomography (CT) confirmed the presence of hepatic venous enhancements, consistent with AVMs (Figure 2). The patient was diagnosed with HHT-induced portosystemic encephalopathy secondary to AVMs and recurrent epistaxis. He was started on lactulose with complete resolution of his

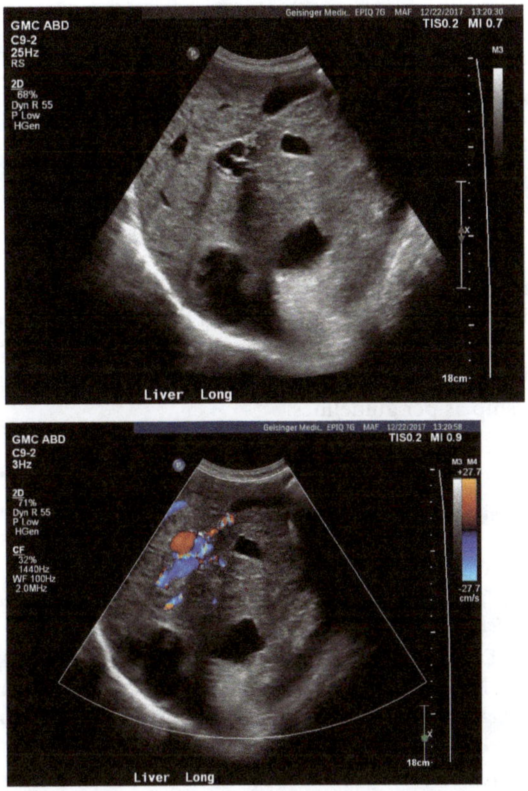

FIGURE 1: (a) Ultrasound gray scale image shows multiple anechoic structures in the liver with surrounding echogenicity. There is flow on color Doppler (b), consistent with hepatic arteriovenous malformations.

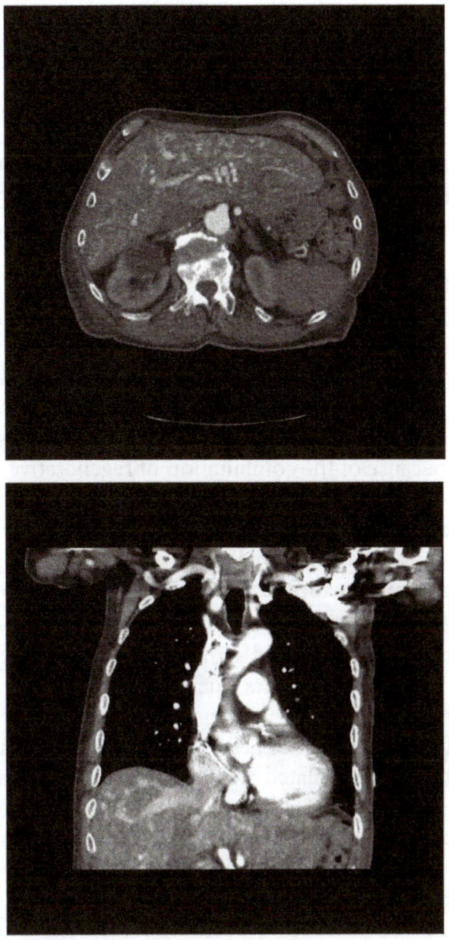

FIGURE 2: Computed Tomography in the axial (a) and coronal (b) arterial phase images showing an increased number of opacified hepatic arteries with early opacification of draining veins, consistent with multiple hepatic AVMs.

symptoms. Epistaxis was managed with nasal packing. He remained stable and was discharged.

3. Discussion

Hereditary hemorrhagic telangiectasia is a rare inherited autosomal dominant disease that may present with a variety of clinical manifestations. Multiple organ systems are involved including the skin, lungs, gastrointestinal tract and brain [1]. HHT-induced portosystemic encephalopathy (PSE) secondary to AVMs is a rare life-threatening complication.

Clinicians must maintain a high index of suspicion for hepatic encephalopathy in patients with HHT presenting with altered mental status and epistaxis. Symptoms from liver involvement are often misdiagnosed and early identification and treatment in these patients is life-saving. The Curacao criteria are used to diagnose HHT which include three of the following features: recurrent and spontaneous epistaxis, mucocutaneous telangiectasias, visceral involvement, and family history or first-degree relative with HHT [5]. Portosystemic encephalopathy is an extremely rare manifestation of HHT. Buscarini and colleagues studied the clinical manifestations in HHT patients with liver AVMs and reported only two out of one-hundred and fifty-four patients had developed portosystemic encephalopathy [6]. There are three types of portosystemic encephalopathy differentiated based on cause: Type A is associated with acute liver failure, Type B is a consequence of portosystemic shunts with no existing liver disease, and Type C is found in patients with cirrhosis and chronic liver disease [7]. Portosystemic encephalopathy secondary to HHT must be differentiated from other possible causes of encephalopathy related to concomitant conditions such as liver disease due to hepatitis or cirrhosis that may confound the diagnosis. Diagnosis with positive antibody titers for hepatitis B and C and using CT imaging to identify liver disease can be helpful in the initial workup. Further, clinicians must take into consideration the complete clinical picture and precipitating factors such as infections, gastrointestinal bleeding, and electrolyte disorders must be adequately identified and treated. The most common clinical symptoms from HHT are due to bleeding such as epistaxis or gastrointestinal hemorrhage from telangiectasias. Our patient presented with epistaxis and altered mental status and was diagnosed with portosystemic encephalopathy secondary to hepatic AVMs from HHT.

The majority of patients with liver AVMs are asymptomatic, as symptoms secondary to liver AVMs occur in only

5-8% of patients with liver AVMs [8, 9]. Symptomatic patients with hepatic involvement usually present with high-output cardiac failure, biliary ischemia, and portal hypertension [10]. Hepatic vascular malformations are widespread and various patterns of abnormal vascular communications can occur [11]. The three types of vascular shunts in patients with HHT are arteriosystemic shunts between a hepatic artery and a hepatic vein, arterioportal shunts between a hepatic artery and the portal venous system, and portosystemic venous shunts that form between a portal vein and a hepatic vein [12]. Shunts are common complications of hepatic AVMs and may lead to encephalopathy. "Pseudocirrhosis" is described as a morphologic sign in patients with hepatic manifestations of HHT because of the changes that mimic liver cirrhosis following chronic liver diseases. Patients may be misdiagnosed with cirrhosis because of the combination of regenerative nodules and fibrosis but the preservation of normal hepatocellular architecture has led to the term "pseudocirrhosis" [13, 14]. Many clinicians are involved in the care of these patients and being familiar with the various clinical manifestations is imperative for patient care.

Angiography is the gold standard for diagnosing AVMs but less invasive modalities such as Doppler ultrasound, magnetic resonance imaging, and CT imaging may also be used. Diagnosis on CT can be identified through diffuse liver telangiectasias and dilated hepatic arteries [13]. The three types of shunts in HHT are not easily distinguished and conventional imaging cannot easily identify portosystemic shunts. Recently, three-dimensional sonography has been used as a noninvasive method for examining the hepatic vasculature and visualizing portovenous shunts [15]. There are no standard medical therapies for patients with HHT and treatment is patient specific and varies with clinical manifestations. The mainstay of treatment for encephalopathy is medical management with osmotic laxatives. Prior studies have shown successful treatment with lactulose in patients with hepatic encephalopathy [6]. Candelli and colleagues studied the influence of hepatic AVMs on the liver first-pass effect on drugs in HHT patients and found a statistically significant reduced metabolism rate in HHT when compared to controls [16]. Shunt reduction via surgical ligation or transarterial embolization has also been performed in these patients [17]. In patients who are unresponsive to medications, liver transplantation is the only definitive treatment [18]. Systemic treatment options such as Bevacizumab have shown improvement in patients with hepatic complications [19, 20]. This case is an unusual presentation of hepatic encephalopathy caused by HHT-induced portosystemic shunting treated successfully with lactulose.

4. Conclusion

In patients with hereditary hemorrhagic telangiectasia and liver involvement, hepatic encephalopathy is a rare and life-threatening presentation. This case highlights the importance of a multisystem approach to patients with HHT and considers the management and treatment of hepatic complications. While HHT and its complications are underdiagnosed, there is an increasing understanding of this disease and its various presentations. This case report presents a patient with hepatic encephalopathy caused by portosystemic shunting in a patient with hereditary hemorrhagic telangiectasia.

Disclosure

This study was conducted at Geisinger Medical Center, Department of Gastroenterology at 100 N Academy Ave, Danville, PA 17822, USA. A version of this case was presented at the American College of Gastroenterology in Philadelphia, PA, October 5–10, 2018. All authors worked in all 4 aspects of authorship as per guidelines.

References

[1] A. E. Guttmacher, D. A. Marchuk, and R. I. White Jr., "Hereditary hemorrhagic telangiectasia," *The New England Journal of Medicine*, vol. 333, no. 14, pp. 918–924, 1995.

[2] J. W. Donaldson, T. M. McKeever, I. P. Hall, R. B. Hubbard, and A. W. Fogarty, "Complications and mortality in hereditary hemorrhagic telangiectasia: a population-based study," *Neurology*, vol. 84, no. 18, pp. 1886–1893, 2015.

[3] G. Román, M. Fisher, D. P. Perl, and C. M. Poser, "Neurological manifestations of hereditary hemorrhagic telangiectasia (rendu-osler-weber disease): report of 2 cases and review of the literature," *Annals of Neurology*, vol. 4, no. 2, pp. 130–144, 1978.

[4] G. M. Pepper, S. M. Brenner, C. Rodriguez, S. Sprayregen, and B. Burack, "Portosystemic encephalopathy. Resulting from liver involvement in hereditary hemorrhagic telangiectasia," *New York State journal of medicine*, vol. 81, no. 2, pp. 209–212, 1981.

[5] A. Kritharis, H. Al-Samkari, and D. J. Kuter, "Hereditary hemorrhagic telangiectasia: diagnosis and management from the hematologist's perspective," *Haematologica*, vol. 103, no. 9, pp. 1433–1443, 2018.

[6] E. Buscarini, G. Leandro, D. Conte et al., "Natural history and outcome of hepatic vascular malformations in a large cohort of patients with hereditary hemorrhagic teleangiectasia," *Digestive Diseases and Sciences*, vol. 56, no. 7, pp. 2166–2178, 2011.

[7] K. Weissenborn, "Hepatic encephalopathy: definition, clinical grading and diagnostic principles," *Drugs*, 2019.

[8] E. Buscarini, C. Danesino, C. Olivieri et al., "Doppler ultrasonographic grading of hepatic vascular malformations in hereditary hemorrhagic telangiectasia - results of extensive screening," *Ultraschall in der Medizin - European Journal of Ultrasound*, vol. 25, no. 05, pp. 348–355, 2004.

[9] A. A. S. Ianora, M. Memeo, C. Sabbà, A. Cirulli, A. Rotondo, and G. Angelelli, "Hereditary hemorrhagic telangiectasia: multi-detector row helical CT assessment of hepatic involvement," *Radiology*, vol. 230, no. 1, pp. 250–259, 2004.

[10] S. Khalid and G. Garcia-Tsao, "Hepatic vascular malformations in hereditary hemorrhagic telangiectasia," *Seminars in Liver Disease*, vol. 28, no. 03, pp. 247–258, 2008.

[11] C. Sabbà and M. Pompili, "Review article: the hepatic manifestations of hereditary haemorrhagic telangiectasia," *Alimentary Pharmacology & Therapeutics*, vol. 28, no. 5, pp. 523–533, 2008.

[12] T. E. McCann, L. M. Scoutt, and G. Gunabushanam, "Hepatic involvement of hereditary hemorrhagic telangiectasia: evaluation with ultrasound," *Ultrasound Quarterly*, vol. 30, no. 3, pp. 221–224, 2014.

[13] G. Garcia-Tsao, "Liver involvement in hereditary hemorrhagic telangiectasia (HHT)," *Journal of Hepatology*, vol. 46, no. 3, pp. 499–507, 2007.

[14] T. Cooney, E. C. Sweeney, R. Coll, and M. Greally, "Pseudocirrhosis, in hereditary haemorrhagic telangiectasia," *Journal of Clinical Pathology*, vol. 30, no. 12, pp. 1134–1141, 1977.

[15] M. Matsuo, M. Kanematsu, H. Kato, H. Kondo, K. Sugisaki, and H. Hoshi, "Osler-Weber-Rendu disease: visualizing portovenous shunting with three-dimensional sonography," *American Journal of Roentgenology*, vol. 176, no. 4, pp. 919-920, 2001.

[16] M. Candelli, M. Pompili, P. Suppressa et al., "Liver involvement in hereditary hemorrhagic telangiectasia: can breath test unmask impaired hepatic first-pass effect?" *Internal and Emergency Medicine*, vol. 7, no. 4, pp. 323–329, 2012.

[17] G. Garcia-Tsao, J. R. Korzenik, L. Young et al., "Liver disease in patients with hereditary hemorrhagic telangiectasia," *The New England Journal of Medicine*, vol. 343, no. 13, pp. 931–936, 2000.

[18] O. Boillot, F. Bianco, J. Viale et al., "Liver transplantation resolves the hyperdynamic circulation in hereditary hemorrhagic telangiectasia with hepatic involvement," *Gastroenterology*, vol. 116, no. 1, pp. 187–192, 1999.

[19] S. Dupuis-Girod, I. Ginon, J.-C. Saurin et al., "Bevacizumab in patients with hereditary hemorrhagic telangiectasia and severe hepatic vascular malformations and high cardiac output," *Journal of the American Medical Association*, vol. 307, no. 9, pp. 948–955, 2012.

[20] P. Bose, J. L. Holter, and G. B. Selby, "Bevacizumab in hereditary hemorrhagic telangiectasia," *The New England Journal of Medicine*, vol. 360, no. 20, pp. 2143-2144, 2009.

Permissions

All chapters in this book were first published by Hindawi Publishing Corporation; hereby published with permission under the Creative Commons Attribution License or equivalent. Every chapter published in this book has been scrutinized by our experts. Their significance has been extensively debated. The topics covered herein carry significant findings which will fuel the growth of the discipline. They may even be implemented as practical applications or may be referred to as a beginning point for another development.

The contributors of this book come from diverse backgrounds, making this book a truly international effort. This book will bring forth new frontiers with its revolutionizing research information and detailed analysis of the nascent developments around the world.

We would like to thank all the contributing authors for lending their expertise to make the book truly unique. They have played a crucial role in the development of this book. Without their invaluable contributions this book wouldn't have been possible. They have made vital efforts to compile up to date information on the varied aspects of this subject to make this book a valuable addition to the collection of many professionals and students.

This book was conceptualized with the vision of imparting up-to-date information and advanced data in this field. To ensure the same, a matchless editorial board was set up. Every individual on the board went through rigorous rounds of assessment to prove their worth. After which they invested a large part of their time researching and compiling the most relevant data for our readers.

The editorial board has been involved in producing this book since its inception. They have spent rigorous hours researching and exploring the diverse topics which have resulted in the successful publishing of this book. They have passed on their knowledge of decades through this book. To expedite this challenging task, the publisher supported the team at every step. A small team of assistant editors was also appointed to further simplify the editing procedure and attain best results for the readers.

Apart from the editorial board, the designing team has also invested a significant amount of their time in understanding the subject and creating the most relevant covers. They scrutinized every image to scout for the most suitable representation of the subject and create an appropriate cover for the book.

The publishing team has been an ardent support to the editorial, designing and production team. Their endless efforts to recruit the best for this project, has resulted in the accomplishment of this book. They are a veteran in the field of academics and their pool of knowledge is as vast as their experience in printing. Their expertise and guidance has proved useful at every step. Their uncompromising quality standards have made this book an exceptional effort. Their encouragement from time to time has been an inspiration for everyone.

The publisher and the editorial board hope that this book will prove to be a valuable piece of knowledge for researchers, students, practitioners and scholars across the globe.

List of Contributors

Victoria Green
Department of Internal Medicine, University of California, San Francisco, Fresno, CA, USA

Marina Roytman
Department of Gastroenterology & Hepatology, University of California San Francisco-Fresno, Fresno, CA, USA

Yoshiaki Sasaki and Hiroki Kajino
Department of Pediatrics, Abashiri-Kosei General Hospital, Abashiri, Hokkaido, Japan

Admir Kurtcehajic
Medical Faculty, University of Tuzla, Tuzla 75000, Bosnia and Herzegovina
Department of Internal Medicine, Medical Center "Plava Poliklinika", Plava Medical Group, Tuzla 75000, Bosnia and Herzegovina

Amar Habibovic
Department of Gastroenterology and Hepatology, University Clinical Center Tuzla, Tuzla 75000, Bosnia and Herzegovina

Ervin Alibegovic
Department of Gastroenterology and Hepatology, University Clinical Center Tuzla, Tuzla 75000, Bosnia and Herzegovina
Medical Faculty, University of Tuzla, Tuzla 75000, Bosnia and Herzegovina

Boris Ilic and Ahmed Hujdurovic
Department of Internal Medicine, Medical Center "Plava Poliklinika", Plava Medical Group, Tuzla 75000, Bosnia and Herzegovina

Edinka Smajic
Department of Radiology, Medical Center "Plava Poliklinika", Plava Medical Group, Tuzla 75000, Bosnia and Herzegovina

Darja Perkunic
Department of Biochemistry, Medical Center "Plava Poliklinika", Plava Medical Group, Tuzla 75000, Bosnia and Herzegovina

Prachi Rana and Shida Haghighat
Department of Internal Medicine, Los Angeles County Hospital/University of Southern California, USA

Hyosun Han
Department of Gastroenterology and Liver Diseases, Los Angeles County Hospital/University of Southern California, USA

Raphael P. Luber
Department of Gastroenterology, The Alfred Hospital, 55 Commercial Road, Melbourne, Victoria, Australia
Department of Gastroenterology and Liver Transplantation, The Austin Hospital, 145 Studley Road, Heidelberg, Melbourne, Victoria, Australia
Central Clinical School, Monash University, The Alfred Hospital, 99 Commercial Road, Melbourne, Victoria, Australia

Steve Lontos
Department of Gastroenterology and Liver Transplantation, The Austin Hospital, 145 Studley Road, Heidelberg, Melbourne, Victoria, Australia

William Kemp, Stuart K. Roberts and Ammar Majeed
Department of Gastroenterology, The Alfred Hospital, 55 Commercial Road, Melbourne, Victoria, Australia
Central Clinical School, Monash University, The Alfred Hospital, 99 Commercial Road, Melbourne, Victoria, Australia

Clarissa Rentsch
Department of Gastroenterology, The Alfred Hospital, 55 Commercial Road, Melbourne, Victoria, Australia
Central Clinical School, Monash University, The Alfred Hospital, 99 Commercial Road, Melbourne, Victoria, Australia
Department of Pharmacy, The Alfred Hospital, 55 Commercial Road, Melbourne, Victoria, Australia

Hans G. Schneider
Clinical Biochemistry Unit, The Alfred Hospital, 55 Commercial Road, Melbourne, Victoria, Australia
Department of Epidemiology and Preventive Medicine, Monash University, Melbourne, Australia

Jeffrey D. Pope
Clinical Biochemistry Unit, The Alfred Hospital, 55 Commercial Road, Melbourne, Victoria, Australia
Department of Forensic Medicine, Monash University, Melbourne, Australia

Ar Kar Aung
Department of Epidemiology and Preventive Medicine, Monash University, Melbourne, Australia
Department of General Medicine, The Alfred Hospital, 55 Commercial Road, Melbourne, Victoria, Australia

Eduardo A. Rodriguez, Raquel Teixeira Yokoda, David E. Payton, Rish Pai and Thomas J. Byrne
Mayo Clinic Arizona, 5777 E Mayo Blvd, Phoenix, AZ 85054, USA

Deanna K. Bauerlein
Veterans Affairs New Jersey Healthcare System, USA

Hashem N. Akbar
Tufts University Medical Center, USA

Erik C. von Rosenvinge and Preeti R. John
Veterans Affairs Maryland Healthcare System, University of Maryland School of Medicine, USA

Nora D. Loughry
Emory University School of Medicine, USA

Jordan Roussel
Department of Internal Medicine, Louisiana State University Health Sciences Center, Shreveport, LA, USA

Sudha Pandit, Paul Jordan, Moheb Boktor and Hrishikesh Samant
Department of Gastroenterology and Hepatology, Louisiana State University Health Sciences Center, Shreveport, LA, USA

Kurt Knowles and Nester Dela Cruz
Department of Pathology, Louisiana State University Health Sciences Center, Shreveport, LA, USA

Iman Abutineh
Department of Internal Medicine, University of Tennessee Health Science Center, Memphis, TN, USA

Kyle Kreitman and Jiten P. Kothadia
Methodist University Hospital, James D. Eason Transplant Institute, University of Tennessee Health Science Center, Memphis, TN, USA

Bilal Ali and Benedict J. Maliakkal
Methodist University Hospital, James D. Eason Transplant Institute, University of Tennessee Health Science Center, Memphis, TN, USA

Richa Jain and Ian Clark
Department of Pathology, Memphis Pathology Group, University of Tennessee Health Science Center, Methodist University Hospital, Memphis, TN, USA

Satheesh P. Nair
MUH James D. Eason Transplant Institute, University of Tennessee Health Sciences Center, 1265 Union Avenue, 4 Shorb Tower, Memphis, TN 38104, USA
Methodist University Hospital, James D. Eason Transplant Institute, University of Tennessee Health Science Center, Memphis, TN, USA

Ahmed I. Edhi and Seifeldin Hakim
Division of Gastroenterology & Hepatology, Department of Medicine, William Beaumont Hospital, 3535 W Thirteen Mile Rd, Royal Oak, MI 48073, USA

Christienne Shams
Department of Medicine, William Beaumont Hospital, Oakland University William Beaumont School of Medicine, 3535 W Thirteen Mile Rd, Royal Oak, MI 48073, USA

Damanpreet Bedi
Transplant Surgery, Department of Surgery, William Beaumont School of Medicine, 3601 W Thirteen Mile Rd, Royal Oak, MI 48073, USA

Mitual Amin
Department of Pathology, William Beaumont Hospital, Oakland University William Beaumont School of Medicine, 3601 W Thirteen Mile Rd, Royal Oak, MI 48073, USA

Mitchell S. Cappell
Division of Gastroenterology & Hepatology, Department of Medicine, William Beaumont Hospital, 3535 W Thirteen Mile Rd, Royal Oak, MI 48073, USA
Division of Gastroenterology & Hepatology, Department of Medicine, Oakland University William Beaumont School of Medicine, 3535 W Thirteen Mile Rd, Royal Oak, MI 48073, USA

Chen-Yu Wang and Bor-Jen Lee
Department of Critical Care Medicine, Taichung Veterans General Hospital, Taichung, Taiwan

Sz-Iuan Shiu
Division of Gastroenterology and Hepatology, Department of Internal Medicine, Taichung Veterans General Hospital, Taichung, Taiwan
Department of Critical Care Medicine, Taichung Veterans General Hospital, Taichung, Taiwan

Su Ann Yong
China Medical University, Taichung, Taiwan

Kuo-Lung Lai and Chih-Wei Tseng
Division of Allergy, Immunology and Rheumatology, Department of Internal Medicine, Taichung Veterans General Hospital, Taichung, Taiwan

Yi-Hsing Chen
Division of Allergy, Immunology and Rheumatology, Department of Internal Medicine, Taichung Veterans General Hospital, Taichung, Taiwan
Faculty of Medicine, National Yang-Ming University, Taipei, Taiwan

Chloe H. Williams, Kelli Hickle, Katherine Bakke and Adel Bozorgzadeh
UMass Memorial Medical Center, Department of Surgery, Worcester, MA 01655, USA

Sarah Jamshed
UMass Memorial Medical Center, Department of Pathology, Worcester, MA 01655, USA

Nazia Khan
Michigan State University, Department of Internal Medicine, East Lansing, MI, USA

Atinuke Aluko, Ikponmwosa Enofe and Jacob Burch
Michigan State University, Department of Internal Medicine, East Lansing, MI, USA
Sparrow hospital, Lansing, MI, USA

Julie Yam
Michigan State University, Gastroenterology Fellowship, East Lansing, MI, USA

Mohammad K. Choudhry and John Trillo
Department of Gastroenterology, NYCHH-Coney Island Hospital, Brooklyn, NY, USA

Bei Xiong and Antony Anandaraj
Department of Medicine, NYCHHC-Coney Island Hospital, Brooklyn, NY, USA

Hakima Abid, Mouna Figuigui, Sidi Adil Ibrahimi and Mohamed El Abkari
Department of Hepato-Gastroenterology, University Hospital Hassan II-Fez, Laboratory of Human Pathology, Biomedicine and Environment, Fes, Morocco
Faculty of Medicine and Pharmacy of Fez, Sidi Mohamed Ben Abdellah University Fez-Morocco, Fes, Morocco

Mohamed Mzyiene, Soufiane Ennaciri, Ouima Justin Ziba and Mohamed Jamal El Fassi
Faculty of Medicine and Pharmacy of Fez, Sidi Mohamed Ben Abdellah University Fez-Morocco, Fes, Morocco
Urology Department-University Hospital Hassan II-Fez, Fes, Morocco

Layla Tahiri Elousrouti and Laila Chbani
Faculty of Medicine and Pharmacy of Fez, Sidi Mohamed Ben Abdellah University Fez-Morocco, Fes, Morocco
Pathological Anatomy Department, University Hospital Hassan II of Fez, Fes, Morocco

Thaninee Prasoppokakorn and Sombat Treeprasertsuk
Division of Gastroenterology, Department of Medicine, Faculty of Medicine, Chulalongkorn University, Bangkok, Thailand

Kessarin Thanapirom
Division of Gastroenterology, Department of Medicine, Faculty of Medicine, Chulalongkorn University, Bangkok, Thailand
Center of Excellence in Liver Diseases, King Chulalongkorn Memorial Hospital, Thai Red Cross Society, Bangkok, Thailand
Liver Fibrosis and Cirrhosis Research Unit, Chulalongkorn University, Bangkok, Thailand

Naoki Ishimaru, Kazuya Niwa and Yoshifumi Kobayashi
Department of Surgery, Suwa Central Hospital, 4300 Tamagawa, Chino, Nagano 3918503, Japan

Hirohisa Fujikawa
Department of Medical Education Studies, International Research Center for Medical Education, Graduate School of Medicine,)e University of Tokyo, 7-3-1 Hongo, Bunkyo-ku, Tokyo 1130033, Japan
Department of Internal Medicine, Suwa Central Hospital, 4300 Tamagawa, Chino, Nagano 3918503, Japan

Maria Kosmidou, Eleftherios Klouras, Iro Rapti, Sebastien Filippas-Ntekouan and Haralampos Milionis
First Division of Internal Medicine, Faculty of Medicine, University of Ioannina, Ioannina, Greece

Patrick Lee and Seth Politano
Keck School of Medicine, University of Southern California, Los Angeles, CA 90033, USA
Department of Medicine, University of Southern California, Los Angeles, CA 90033, USA

Brandon K. K. Fields
Keck School of Medicine, University of Southern California, Los Angeles, CA 90033, USA
Scripps Mercy Hospital San Diego, San Diego, CA 92103, USA

Tom Liang
Keck School of Medicine, University of Southern California, Los Angeles, CA 90033, USA
Department of Pathology, University of Southern California, Los Angeles, CA 90033, USA

Michael P. Dubé
Keck School of Medicine, University of Southern California, Los Angeles, CA 90033, USA
Department of Infectious Diseases, University of Southern California, Los Angeles, CA 90033, USA

Victoria Costa, Zhen Zhao, Sabrina E. Racine-Brzostek and He S. Yang
Department of Pathology and Laboratory Medicine, New York Presbyterian Hospital, Weill Cornell Medicine, New York, NY, USA

Gadi Lalazar
Department of Gastroenterology and Hepatology, New York Presbyterian Hospital, Weill Cornell Medicine, New York, NY, USA

Brittany Miles, Rupak Kulkarni, Jeffrey Fair and Michael Kueht
Department of Surgery, Division of Transplant Surgery, UTMB Galveston=University of Texas Medical Branch, Galveston, TX, USA

Muhammad Mujtaba and Shehzad Merwat
Department of Internal Medicine, Division of Transplant Medicine, UTMB Galveston=University of Texas Medical Branch, Galveston, TX, USA

Pratishtha Singh, Kayle Warren and Victor Collier
Department of Internal Medicine, Grand Strand Medical Center, Myrtle Beach, SC, USA

Lucas Ramer, Nicolas Goossens, Jean-Louis Frossard and Laurent Spahr
Gastroenterology and Hepatology, University Hospitals of Geneva and Faculty of Medicine, Geneva, Switzerland

Matthieu Tihy and Laura Rubbia-Brandt
Clinical Pathology, University Hospitals of Geneva and Faculty of Medicine, Geneva, Switzerland

Jonathan David Hendrie and Mary Crouse Blumer
Prisma Health-Upstate, University of South Carolina School of Medicine-Greenville, Department of Medicine, 701 Grove Rd., Greenville, SC 29605, USA

Hubert Henry Fenton
Prisma Health-Upstate, Department of Pathology, 701 Grove Rd., Greenville, SC 29605, USA

Gary Anthony Abrams
Prisma Health-Upstate, University of South Carolina School of Medicine-Greenville Department of Medicine, Division of Gastroenterology & Liver Center, 890 W. Faris Rd., Suite 100, Greenville, SC 29605, USA

Francisco A. Durazo
Division of Transplant Surgery, Department of Surgery, Medical College of Wisconsin, Milwaukee, WI, USA
Division of Gastroenterology and Hepatology, Department of Medicine, Medical College of Wisconsin, Milwaukee, WI, USA

Kelly Kristbaum and Motaz Selim
Division of Transplant Surgery, Department of Surgery, Medical College of Wisconsin, Milwaukee, WI, USA

Kia Saeian
Division of Gastroenterology and Hepatology, Department of Medicine, Medical College of Wisconsin, Milwaukee, WI, USA

James Miller
Department of Pathology and Laboratory Medicine, Medical College of Wisconsin, Milwaukee, WI, USA

Johnny C. Hong
Division of Transplantation, Pennsylvania State University, College of Medicine Penn State Health Milton S. Hershey Medical Center Hershey, Pennsylvania, USA

Katsutoshi Ishihara
Department of Radiology, Yuai Memorial Hospital, 707 Higashiushigaya, Koga, Ibaraki, Japan

Brandon Swed, Omar Gandarilla and Gagandeep Brar
Division of Hematology and Medical Oncology, Department of Medicine, Weill Cornell Medicine/New-York Presbyterian, New York, New York, USA

Kenrry Chiu and Rhonda Yantiss
Department of Pathology and Laboratory Medicine, Weill Cornell Medicine/New-York Presbyterian, New York, New York, USA

Karim H. Halazun and Benjamin Samstein
Division of Liver Transplantation and Hepatobiliary Surgery, Department of Surgery, Weill Cornell Medicine/New-York Presbyterian, New York, New York, USA

Jennifer Yoon
Department of Internal Medicine, University of California, Fresno, CA, USA

Steve Hu and Adnan Ameer
Department of Gastroenterology and Hepatology, University of California, Fresno, CA, USA

Daniel Phillips
Department of Pathology, Community Regional Medical Center, Fresno, CA, USA

Amir Fathi
Department of Surgery, University of California, Fresno, CA, USA

Ilenia Mascherona
Ospedale La Carità, Medicina Interna, Locarno, Switzerland

Caterina Maggioli
AUSL di Bologna, Ospedale di Budrio, Bologna, Italy

Maira Biggiogero
Clinica Luganese Moncucco, Unità di Ricerca Clinica, Lugano, Switzerland

Oreste Mora and Lucia Marelli
Clinica Luganese Moncucco, Oncologia Medica, Lugano, Switzerland

Youssef Ghosn, Mohammed Hussein Kamareddine and Ahmad Baghdadi
Faculty of Medicine and Medical Sciences, University of Balamand, Achrafieh, Beirut, Lebanon

Ali Abdallah, Amine Geahchan, Abbas Chamseddine and Raja Ashou
Department of Diagnostic Radiology, Saint George Hospital University Medical Center, University of Balamand, Achrafieh, Beirut, Lebanon

Ziad El-Rassi
Department of General Surgery, Saint George Hospital University Medical Center, University of Balamand, Achrafieh, Beirut, Lebanon

Swapnali Sabhapandit
Department of Ophthalmology, AIG Hospitals, Hyderabad, India

Mithun Sharma, Anand Kulkarni, Soumya TR and Padaki Nagaraja Rao
Department of Hepatology and Liver Transplantation, Asian Institute of Gastroenterology, Hyderabad, India

Anuradha Sekaran
Department of Pathology, Asian Institute of Gastroenterology, Hyderabad, India

Balachandran Menon
Department of Liver Transplantation, Asian Institute of Gastroenterology, Hyderabad, India

Duvurr Nageshwar Reddy
Department of Gastroenterology, Asian Institute of Gastroenterology, Hyderabad, India

Ali R. Ahmadi and Marcel van den Berge
Department of Internal Medicine, Erasmus MC, Rotterdam, Netherlands
Department of Internal Medicine, Admiraal de Ruyter Ziekenhuis, Goes, Netherlands

Maria Chicco
Department of General Surgery, Wexham Park Hospital, Frimley Health NHS Trust, Frimley, UK

Riana Wurzburger
Department of Internal Medicine, University of New Mexico Hospital, UNM School of Medicine MSC08 47201, University of New Mexico, Albuquerque, NM 87131, USA

Lin Cheng
Department of Pathology, Rush University Medical Center, Chicago, IL, USA

Yajuan Liu and Wenjing Wang
Department of Pathology, University of Washington, Seattle, WA, USA

J. L. Merritt
Department of Pathology, University of Washington, Seattle, WA, USA
Department of Pediatrics, University of Washington, Seattle, WA, USA

Matthew Yeh
Department of Pathology, University of Washington, Seattle, WA, USA
Department of Medicine, University of Washington, Seattle, WA, USA

Tasuku Hara, Tomoya Ohara, Masashi Taniguchi, Toshiaki Sakai, Kohei Oka, Naoto Iwai, Toshifumi Tsuji, Takashi Okuda, Toshiyuki Komaki, Junichi Sakagami and Keizo Kagawa
Department of Gastroenterology and Hepatology, Fukuchiyama City Hospital, Atsunaka-chou 231, Fukuchiyama, Kyoto 620-8505, Japan

Sanaa Al-Nattah, Kusum Lata Sharma and William N. Rose
Department of Pathology and Laboratory Medicine, University of Wisconsin Hospital, 600 Highland Ave, Madison, WI 53792, USA

Matthew Caldis and Erin Spengler
Department of Medicine, University of Wisconsin Hospital, 600 Highland Ave, Madison, WI 53792, USA

Dimitrios Farmakiotis, Kendra Vieira and Joseph M. Garland
Division of Infectious Diseases, Department of Internal Medicine, Brown Alpert Medical School, Providence, RI, USA

Zoe Weiss
Department of Internal Medicine, Brown Alpert Medical School, Providence, RI, USA
Division of Infectious Diseases, Brigham and Women's Hospital and Massachusetts General Hospital, Harvard Medical School, Boston, MA, USA

Amy L. Brotherton
Department of Pharmacy, The Miriam Hospital, Providence, RI, USA

Paul Morrissey
Department of Surgery (Transplantation), Brown Alpert Medical School, Providence, RI, USA

Reginald Gohh
Division of Nephrology (Transplantation), Department of Internal Medicine, Brown Alpert Medical School, Providence, RI, USA

Lynn E. Taylor
Division of Infectious Diseases, Department of Internal Medicine, Brown Alpert Medical School, Providence, RI, USA
CODAC Behavioral Health, Providence, RI, USA

Edgar Blecker and Maryam Ehtsham
Department of Internal Medicine, Methodist Dallas Medical Center, Dallas, TX 75203, USA

Yathip M. Chokpapone
The University of Texas at Dallas, Dallas, 800 W Campbell Rd., Richardson, TX 75080, USA

Anne R. Murray
Clinical Research Institute, Methodist Health System, 1411 N. Beckley Ave, Pavilion III, Suite 168, Dallas, TX 75203, USA

Ashwini P. Mehta, Vichin C. Puri, Alejandro Mejia and Parvez Mantry
The Liver Institute, Methodist Dallas Medical Center, 1411 N. Beckley Ave, Pavilion III, Suite 268, Dallas, TX 75203, USA

Mohanad Soliman, Olalekan Akanbi, Ihab Almagdub, Kishore Karri, Pradeep Yarra and Saad Emhmed Ali
Department of Medicine, Division of Hospital Medicine, University of Kentucky, Lexington, KY, USA

Hanine El Haddad
Department of Medicine, Division of Infectious Diseases, University of Kentucky, Lexington, KY, USA

Cristina Macía, Jose Loureiro, Isabel Campos-Varela and Arturo Gonzalez-Quintela
Department of Internal Medicine and Hepatology, Complejo Hospitalario Universitario de Santiago, Santiago, Spain

Ihab Abdulkader
Department of Pathology, Complejo Hospitalario Universitario de Santiago, Santiago, Spain

Evaristo Varo
Liver Transplant Unit, Complejo Hospitalario Universitario de Santiago, Santiago, Spain

Esteban Otero and Santiago Tomé
Department of Internal Medicine and Hepatology, Complejo Hospitalario Universitario de Santiago, Santiago, Spain
Liver Transplant Unit, Complejo Hospitalario Universitario de Santiago, Santiago, Spain

Mahmood Alawainati
Department of Family Medicine, Ministry of Health, Manama, Bahrain

Jawad Khamis, Muneer Abdulla and Saeed Alsaeed
Department of Medicine, Salmaniya Medical Complex, Manama, Bahrain

Sunny Sandhu and Hunza Chaudhry
Department of Internal Medicine, University of California, San Francisco- Fresno, Fresno, CA, USA

Sharon Zhang
Department of Pathology, Community Medical Centers, Fresno, CA, USA

Devang Prajapati
Department of Gastroenterology & Hepatology, University of California, San Francisco- Fresno, Fresno, CA, USA

Jeremy Hassoun, Giulia Magini and Marie Ongaro
Gastroenterology and Hepatology, University Hospitals of Geneva and Faculty of Medicine, Geneva, Switzerland

Nathalie Hammer and Belen Ponte
Nephrology, University Hospitals of Geneva and Faculty of Medicine, Geneva, Switzerland

Anne-Laure Rougemont
Clinical Pathology, University Hospitals of Geneva and Faculty of Medicine, Geneva, Switzerland

Sameeha Khalid, Kamalmeet Kaur and Ali Ali
Department of Internal Medicine, University of California San Francisco-Fresno, Fresno, CA, USA

Dhuha Alhankawi
Department of Gastroenterology & Hepatology, University of California San Francisco-Fresno, Fresno, CA, USA

Anna Kazaryan
Department of Rheumatology, University of California San Francisco-Fresno, Fresno, CA, USA

Hansa Haftu and Mohammed Mustefa
Mekelle University, College of Health Science, Pediatric and Child Health Department, Tigray, Ethiopia

Teklu Gebrehiwot
Mekelle University, College of Health Science, Clinical Pharmacist, Tigray, Ethiopia

Ruchit N. Shah
Geisinger Medical Center, Department of Internal Medicine, 100 N Academy Ave, Danville, PA 17822, USA
Geisinger Commonwealth School of Medicine, 525 Pine Street, Scranton, PA 18510, USA

Michael Makar
Geisinger Commonwealth School of Medicine, 525 Pine Street, Scranton, PA 18510, USA

Nasir Akhtar
Geisinger Medical Center, Department of Gastroenterology, 100 N Academy Ave, Danville, PA 17822, USA

Erin Forster
Geisinger Medical Center, Department of Gastroenterology, 100 N Academy Ave, Danville, PA 17822, USA
Medical University of South Carolina, 30 Courtenay Dr, Charleston, SC 29425, USA

Index

www.ingramcontent.com/pod-product-compliance
Lightning Source LLC
LaVergne TN
LVHW082138200926
848484LV00008B/2074